# Bridging the Boundaries:
# Human Experience in the Natural and Built Environment and Implications for Research, Policy, and Practice

D1742239

# Advances in People-Environment Studies

**David Uzzell;** PhD, FBPsS, FRSA, Prof., University of Surrey, UK, Past-President of the International Association for People-Environment Studies (IAPS).
(Series Editor)

The book series *Advances in People-Environment Studies*, published in collaboration with the International Association for People-Environment Studies (IAPS; http:// www.iaps-association.org), is a timely initiative to provide researchers with up-to-date reviews and commentaries on the diverse areas of people-environment studies that are of current concern. The series focuses on significant and currently debated themes. The books are interdisciplinary, drawing on expert authors from the social, environmental, and design disciplines, especially those who are working at the interface between the design (e.g., architects, landscape planners, urban designers, urban planners) and the social sciences (e.g., environmental psychologists, sociologists, geographers). Each volume reports on the latest research and applications of research in the field. The series is meant to provide a bridge, not only between disciplines but also between cultures. The authors and contributors come from many different countries and are undertaking research and practicing in culturally diverse environments. Books in the series are therefore a precious source for those who want to know what is going on in a specific field elsewhere and to find ideas and inspiration for their own work.

Advances in People-Environment Studies Vol. 5

# Bridging the Boundaries
## Human Experience in the Natural and Built Environment and Implications for Research, Policy, and Practice

Edward Edgerton
Ombretta Romice
Kevin Thwaites
(Editors)

HOGREFE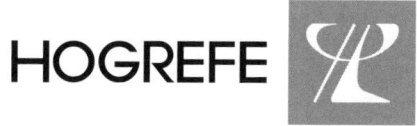

**Library of Congress Cataloging in Publication**

is available via the Library of Congress Marc Database under the
Library of Congress Control Number: 2014934798

**Library and Archives Canada Cataloguing in Publication**

Bridging the boundaries : human experience in the natural and built environment and implications for research, policy, and practice / Edward Edgerton, Ombretta Romice, Kevin Thwaites (editors).

(Advances in people-environment studies ; vol. 5)
"This book, volume five in the IAPS series Advances in People-Environment Studies, delivers selected peer reviewed papers developed by contributors to the 22nd IAPS International conference held at the University of Strathclyde, Glasgow, Scotland from 24–29th June 2012."–Preface.
Includes bibliographical references and index.
ISBN 978-0-88937-466-9 (pbk.).–ISBN 978-1-61676-466-1 (pdf).–ISBN 978-1-61334-466-8 (epub)

1. Human ecology–Congresses. 2. Architecture and society–Congresses. 3. Sustainability–Congresses. 4. Environmental health–Congresses.
I. Edgerton, Eddie, author, editor II. Romice, Ombretta Rossella Linda, editor III. Thwaites, Kevin, editor IV. International Association for People-Environment Studies. Conference (22nd : 2012 : Strathclyde University) V. Series: Advances in people-environment studies ; v. 5

GF3.B75 2014          304.2          C2014-901629-8

Cover illustration: Wilfried Moser (1914–1997). En ville. 1984. © Wilfried Moser Foundation

© 2014 by Hogrefe Publishing
www.hogrefe.com

PUBLISHING OFFICES
USA:          Hogrefe Publishing Corporation, 38 Chauncy Street, Suite 1002, Boston, MA 02111
              Phone (866) 823-4726, Fax (617) 354-6875; E-mail customerservice@hogrefe-publishing.com
EUROPE:    Hogrefe Publishing, Merkelstr. 3, 37085 Göttingen, Germany
              Phone +49 551 99950-0, Fax +49 551 99950-425; E-mail publishing@hogrefe.com

SALES & DISTRIBUTION
USA:          Hogrefe Publishing, Customer Services Department, 30 Amberwood Parkway, Ashland,
              OH 44805, Phone (800) 228-3749, Fax (419) 281-6883; E-mail customerservice@hogrefe.com
UK:            Hogrefe Publishing c/o Marston Book Services Ltd, 160 Eastern Ave., Milton Park, Abingdon,
              OX14 4SB, UK, Phone +44 1235 465577, Fax +44 1235 465556; E-mail direct.orders@marston.co.uk
EUROPE:    Hogrefe Publishing, Merkelstr. 3, 37085 Göttingen, Germany
              Phone +49 551 99950-0, Fax +49 551 99950-425; E-mail publishing@hogrefe.com

OTHER OFFICES
CANADA: Hogrefe Publishing, 660 Eglinton Ave. East, Suite 119-514, Toronto, Ontario, M4G 2K2
SWITZERLAND: Hogrefe Publishing, Länggass-Strasse 76, CH-3000 Bern 9

Hogrefe Publishing
Incorporated and registered in the Commonwealth of Massachusetts, USA, and in Göttingen, Lower Saxony, Germany

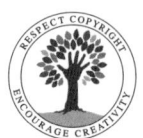

Printed and bound in Germany
ISBN: 978-0-88937-466-9

# Table of Contents

# Preface

This book, volume five in the IAPS series Advances in People-Environment Studies, delivers selected peer reviewed papers developed by contributors to the 22nd IAPS International conference held at the University of Strathclyde, Glasgow, Scotland from 24–29th June 2012. In the history of IAPS conferences, the 22nd conference was unique in that it was a collaborative event jointly organized by the University of Strathclyde (Dr. Ombretta Romice), the University of the West of Scotland (Dr. Edward Edgerton), and the University of Sheffield (Dr. Kevin Thwaites). This collaboration reflects and expresses an interdisciplinary framework of psychology, urban design, and landscape architecture as a foundation for knowledge exchange between research, policy, and practice within the overall theme of human experience in the natural and built environment. The intention behind the conference was to establish a broad agenda for increasing cross-disciplinary exchange and collaboration across the natural and social sciences, and between research and practice communities engaged with development, management, and design, as an essential response to the nature of growing, global socio-environmental challenges.

Contributors to the conference addressed a wide range of themes within the main areas of *geography and context, planning design and evaluation*, and *implementation and management*, reflecting developed and developing world contexts to optimize societal and environmental impact. Collectively this underpinned the delivery of a highly successful and well-attended scientific programme of exceptional breadth and quality including 21 symposia, 59 posters, and over 350 oral presentations and case studies within 48 paper sessions. Over 400 delegates attended the conference representing more than 50 countries worldwide. The richness, diversity, and quality of work delivered and discussed at the conference serves to demonstrate a global consensus of interest in the importance of developing greater understanding of the nature of human experience in the natural and built environments and the application of that understanding.

At the opening of the conference, Karen Anderson, Chair of A+DS asked questions of the delegates in terms of how their work related to the specific challenges of place making in Scotland. It was highlighted that first and foremost, place and placemaking is a political process involving people making decisions and that people should not have to adjust their lives to a set of man-made environmental contexts that do not consider their needs. This seemed to exemplify a central tenet of the IAPS community, the recognition that human-environment interactions are often mutually defining and that this should be reflected in approaches to research, policy-making, and practice.

A socially oriented emphasis on placemaking was also reflected in the contributions of the distinguished keynote speakers, Professors Ian Bentley, Nabeel Hamdi, and Gary Evans. Ian Bentley crossed scientific and design traditions to address the idea that we should apply ecological thinking to the design of human settlements in an attempt to better understand how to make human habitats that have benign ecological impacts. Nabeel

Hamdi focused on the changing nature of practice in the context of some of the big issues impacting people in the informal settlements of cities in the southern hemisphere, while Gary Evans reviewed some of the negative impacts of childhood poverty and their relationship to psycho-social, environmental, and physical risk factors.

Since its establishment in 1981 IAPS has developed into a worldwide international network, facilitating exchange, and communication of ideas between researchers and practitioners in the area of human-environment interactions. It can trace origins back further to the first debates in architectural psychology embodied in the 1st Architectural Psychology conference in Dalandhui, Scotland, 1969. It seems fitting then, that just after its 30th birthday, a chance to reflect on IAPS achievements and the theoretical and practical value of its work, should take place once more in Scotland, and especially at a time when the devolved government in Scotland is particularly supportive of innovation and change relating to socio-environmental improvement.

In 2005, the organizers of the 22nd IAPS Conference were involved in organizing a UK Environmental Psychology symposium (EPUK), which drew together over 100 delegates from around the world to focus on progress made in bridging the gap between research, practice, and policy making in the environment-behavior field. A book followed the discussion (Edgerton, Romice, & Spencer, 2007), which highlighted, after extensive dialogue with some of the major exponents in the field, that environmental psychology has, since its establishment, made considerable steps forward in making its research theoretically strong and influential as well as accessible and informative. There is significant evidence to support this achievement, such as the growth of major international journals, of professional associations, increasingly frequent and well-attended international events with organized, and accessible dissemination activities.

The conclusions offered many examples of insightful work being published in different formats, for different audiences, to develop new or reinforce existing theoretical constructs, to shape education, and to inform practice and policy making. Indeed, many examples were offered on how education, practice, and policy were opening up to the principles and investigations in environment-behavior studies (EBS). The publication concluded by stressing the potential benefits in bringing together EBS and urban design, the latter as a complex discipline lacking clear theoretical principles, and a defined and agreed object of investigation (Cuthbert, 2007).

Edward Edgerton
Ombretta Romice
Kevin Thwaites

# Introduction

# Bridging the Boundaries

Edward Edgerton,[1] Ombretta Romice,[2] and Kevin Thwaites[3]

[1]School of Social Sciences, Psychology Division, University of West Scotland, Paisky,
Scotland, UK
[2]Urban Design Studies Unit, Department of Architecture, University of Strathclyde,
Glasgow, Scotland, UK
[3]Department of Landscape, University of Sheffield, UK

The UN publishes yearly updates on urban growth and we have now surpassed the prophetic tipping point whereby urban dwellers outnumber rural dwellers. The urban population of developing countries will make up more than 80% of the urban population on the planet by the year 2030. The urban population in Africa and Asia is expected to double between 2000 and 2030, with some 1.7 billion new urbanites in the next 20 years expected to be poor. Much of this urbanization will occur, according to the UN, not in megacities, but in centers of around 500,000 people, in countries where planning systems are weak, or unequipped to guarantee locally, socio-environmentally sensitive development and lifestyles. In the developed part of the world, already between 80 and 90% urban at the turn of the Millennium, things are equally challenging, although the key problem here is about the regeneration of energy-intensive existing areas in relation to the urban model on which they are based and to surrounding areas. Decreasing densities, increased auto-dependency, and reliance on energy-rich lifestyles are claiming far beyond acceptable shares of ecological footprint, imposing unfair adjustments across the globe. This is logically not a compromise for much longer, and different practices for development which invest in environmental and social sustainability are now a necessity rather than a possibility (Frey & Yaneske, 2007).

Greater amounts of new, accessible knowledge and best practices are more than ever central to local, national, and international development and the margins of error we can afford are reducing: remediation is costly, from a human, environmental, and political point of view. Since development, at any scale, is considered to be a complex combination of human, economic, environmental, and psychological factors, the conference did not set out expecting to find solutions. Instead we were looking for approachable ways to look at problems and creative ways to address them, within a well described contextual setting. This has been one of the criteria of selection for the papers contained in this publication.

The seventeen papers that make up this volume have been organized into four themes reflecting the diversity of contributions to the conference, at the root of which is a central concern for human experience in a range of socio-environmental contexts at a range of scales. The papers include contributions of a theoretical and reflective nature, offering new ways of conceptualizing the way we think about human-environment interactions, providing alternative readings of environment from which to build innovative research responses in the future. There are also papers which have sought to overcome or review methodological challenges, developing new approaches in addition to focused research papers detailing findings from empirical work in a range of human-environment contexts. The papers reflect the diversity of disciplinary specializations that provide IAPS with its rich scientific foundations and collectively a set of foundations from which to build further on its unique cross-disciplinary potential thereby enabling it to continue to respond to present and future human-environment challenges at all scales and in all global contexts.

## Structure and Contents of the Volume

### Section 1: Environment, Health, and Well-Being

The first part of this volume reflects growing understanding about the varying ways in which the quality of an environment can impact on the health and well-being of populations in various contexts. *Hussain and Jorgensen*, for example, highlight the potential of recreational forests to provide urban inhabitants with benefits relating to health and well-being. Through analyses of participant responses to questionnaires and interviews about motivations for recreational forest use in Sengalor, Malaysia, the authors are able to identify seven factors active in motivations for forest use, enabling forest management practitioners to become better empowered to strengthen positive forest experiences. With a focus on the urban realm, *Weeks* reviews research into the relationship between urban form and encouragement of physical activity, particularly walking. This paper relates empirical evidence to policy implications for urban design which strengthen the case for mixed use, high density, walkable models of urbanism as infrastructures conducive to better levels of public health. Complimenting these contributions to the policy, planning and design frameworks of examples of natural and built environments, *Marquardt*, and *Ritchie and Edgerton* in different ways examine the implications of physical environments on vulnerable citizens, specifically those with dementia. The rising prevalence of dementia has been shown to hold particular implications for spatial organization in architectural and open space decision making. These papers together have the potential to inform overall spatial layout planning (*Marquardt*) and the provision and design of particular kinds of interior spaces for the benefit of dementia sufferers (*Ritchie and Edgerton*).

### Section 2: Environmental Perception, Behaviour, and Place-Identity

The second part gathers work on the relationship between places of a different nature, human choice and use, and the long term establishment of identity and attachment. The first paper provides an interesting new theoretical perspective, the identification of new types of spaces in our cities resulting from recent globalization and the consequent challenge of how to deal with them as a significant element in the already complex relationship between urban space and its users (*Castello*). The second paper presents with the findings of research on the relationship between childhood and adolescence, discussing how attitude, choice, and preference toward place can significantly be related to early familiar experience (*Nordström*). The three papers which conclude this part illustrate interesting new methodological approaches with design and space as focus. First, *De Saboya and colleagues* illustrate the strong impact that design decisions at different scales can have on the use of urban parks. *Vasilikou and Nikolopoulou*, then address how the use of walkways is influenced by variations in the microclimate of the public street network and finally, *Naoumova* discusses how the chromatic composition of street fronts plays a strong role in the perception of coherence and complexity in passers-by. The paper by *Naoumova* usefully engages with a discussion on the potential impact of its findings on planning, by discussing the relationship between the inclusion of new interventions as block-infill within existing contexts. Across their different focus, through an emphasis on both theory and practice, these papers alert readers to new challenges and possibilities in understanding and engaging with physical space.

## Section 3: Human Experience in Urban Sustainability

The broad theme of part three highlights the importance of human experience in dealing with large scale issues of urban sustainability. This is an important theme, needing advancements from several points of view: theoretical, policy, and implementation and development. The theoretical aspect is addressed by *Lucas*, who, while acknowledging the already established link between environment-behavior studies and social anthropology, urges the former to recognize broader important theoretical contributions in the latter related to areas of study more often linked to social and cultural studies but nevertheless fundamental in explaining environmental experiences. The next two papers discuss the fundamental role of human experience and expertise in dealing with environmental challenges of a different nature. *Wiesenfeld, Sánchez, & Giuliani* explain the benefits of user involvement in housing management and more importantly on policy, suggesting that local knowledge and skills can be usefully and successfully embedded in governance. *Kowaltowski and Colleagues* examine the problem from its roots, reflecting on the fundamental role that early education in human environmental experience can have on future practice, and offers several useful examples on how engaging curricula can be developed. Finally *Portella and Xavier* present a useful and practical tool for the assessment of the pre-development impact on perception that any infill development can have on street appearance, focusing on their experience of both practice and planning policy in Brazil.

## Section 4: Global Environment Challenges

The concluding part of the book addresses the  challenges linked to global or national phenomenon by addressing the relationships between scales of pertinence of these phenomena, the general attitude of the public toward them, and the possibility of establishing preventive forms of monitoring in order to reduce the impact of disasters on vulnerable groups. As such, the papers collected here present useful frameworks for policy making, illustrating the fine balance between local groups' perception and engagement with issues of global significance in relation to issues of pressing local relevance. This suggests that while the tendency might appear to be weighted toward a dismissal of broader, less immediately relevant problems, when appropriately related to more local issues, local groups could swing toward a conscious and positive assumption of responsibility and interest toward them (*Pedersen and Johansson*). Increasingly frequent large scale, temporary environmental problems, such as water shortage in Australia, are framed within another interesting debate, on the contemporary need for both broad (national) and very local, and individual measures. The role of the media is placed under scrutiny here; on the one side stressing its importance in highlighting and calling for individual responsibility and action, on the other the risk of it being hijacked for political discussion (*Chui*). This section also proposes an innovative approach to the evaluation of vulnerability of populations at risk of natural disasters. Focusing on a case in Tanzania, this paper proposes adaptive measures to reduce such vulnerability based on a multidimensional assessment of physical, social, individual and institutional characteristics, and a participatory approach to best implement findings (*John, Jean-Baptiste, & Kabisch*). Finally, a provocative paper by *Furtado, Alĉantara, & Bezerra* discusses how rapid development currently happening to Brazil in light of the 2014 World Cup ought to be thought of as a long term strategy to improve the infrastructure conditions of Recife and in particular of the water management system of coastal towns; an issue that strongly depends on even more global events.

# Environment, Health, and Well-Being

# Recreational Forests

## Use, Experience, and Motivation at Selected Sites in Selangor, Malaysia

Norhuzailin Hussain[1] and Anna Jorgensen[2]

[1]Department of Landscape Architecture, Faculty of Design and Architecture,
Universiti Putra Malaysia, Serdang, Malaysia
[2]Department of Landscape, The University of Sheffield, UK

### Abstract

Research suggests that recreational forests have the potential to provide many benefits to urbanites' health and well-being. Recreational forests were established in Peninsular Malaysia to preserve areas for recreation, ecotourism and to raise public awareness regarding forestry. Two study sites were selected namely: Ampang and Kanching Recreational Forests, both located in Selangor. This paper presents the results from the factor analysis of questionnaire data and semi-structured interviews dealing with the underlying factors influencing motivation for recreational forest use. Overall, seven factors explaining motivations for forest use, activities and experiences while in the forests were identified: forest amenities, restorative experience, intergenerational values, self-actualization, incivilities, natural threats in the forest and younger activity preference. Armed with this information forest managers can strengthen the opportunities to re-enforce positive forest experience and mitigate the impact of the detractors (incivilities and natural threats in the forest).

**Key words:** intergenerational values, motivation, recreational forest, restorative experience

## Introduction

Lack of exercise and sedentary life styles can result in many diseases such as obesity and coronary heart disease. Despite the knowledge that physical activity is known to combat obesity, at least 2.8 million people die around the world each year as a result of obesity-related diseases (World Health Organization, 2009). Michimi and Wimberly (2012) found that the occurrence of obesity decreased and the tendency for physical activity increased with a greater amount of both recreational opportunities and natural amenities.

Many current studies focus on the link between physical activity and green space use (e.g., Michimi & Wimberly, 2012; Toftager et al., 2011). Findings generally support the notion that people are more likely to use local green spaces for their health and well-being if these spaces are located close to their dwellings (Coombes, Jones, & Hillsdon, 2010; Nielsen & Hansen, 2007). Nielsen and Hansen (2007) also found that people who live less than 300 m from green spaces in Denmark used them regularly and were less likely to suffer from obesity and stress compared to those who live further away. This suggests that the provision of good access to green spaces in urban areas could help facilitate an increase in a local populations' physical activity. This previous empirical research has helped guide this research on Malaysia's obesity problem and the opportunities that convenient access to local green spaces and recreational forests can provide for the many urban dwellers.

Natural environments are rich in restorative qualities which offer restorative effects (Berman, Jonides, & Kaplan, 2008; Kaplan, 1995; Kaplan & Kaplan, 1989). Restorative environments are said to have four key characteristics, defined as: *being away, extent, fascination and compatibility* (Kaplan & Kaplan, 1989). For example, research by Garst, Williams, and Roggenbuck (2010), that focused on experience and meaning in relation to camping activities in the Mount Rogers National Recreation Area in Southwest Virginia, found that campers associated forests with "restoration," "family functioning," "experiencing nature," "special places," "self-identity," "social interaction" and "children's learning."

People's attitudes towards nature differ according to the stage they have reached in the life course (Lyons, 1983), and are related to their general beliefs: ". . . culture shapes our learning history, and thus, our attitudes" (Bell, Greene, Fisher, & Baum, 1996, p. 31). Thus beliefs about recreational forests could result in certain attitudes which in turn effect certain actions or behaviours (McFarlane & Boxall, 2003). Two factors are said to shape people's attitudes: their memories (O'Brien, 2006) and experiences (Proshansky, 1995). This paper will discuss the factors that motivate visitors to use Malaysian recreational forests and influence the activities they engage in whilst at the forests and the experiences they have in them.

## Background of Recreational Forests

There are 115 recreational forests in Peninsular Malaysia (State Department of Forestry, 2003) situated in various peri-urban and remote locations. Forestation is the dominant national landscape of Malaysia and still covers 50% of the land surface (Woon & Norini, 2002).

Two recreational forests were selected as case studies in this research – Ampang and Kanching Recreational Forests. Both recreational forests are located in the Selangor state, which is the most developed state in Malaysia (Abdullah & Nakagoshi, 2008). Ampang Recreational Forest is located in Ampang Jaya District; and is managed by the Ampang Jaya Municipal Council (Ludin, Abd Razak, Majid, & Rusli, n.d.). Kanching Recreational Forest is located in Rawang District and managed by the Selayang Municipal Council. These recreational forests were selected on the basis of their general similarities: Both having basic facilities such as parking areas, toilets, shelters and campsites, both opening to public in the 1980s, are similar in size (Ampang Recreational Forest, 637 ha. and Kanching Recreational Forest, 487 ha.), have water elements as attractions, namely rivers (both recreational forests) and waterfalls (Kanching Recreational Forest only), and are easy to access by private or public transport.

## Research Objective

The study as a whole examined a broad range of issues relating to recreational forest use, but this paper focuses on users' underlying motivations for visiting the recreational forests.

## Research Methods

Two approaches were used: A self-administered questionnaire and semi-structured interviews with selected results from both discussed in this paper. The questionnaire consisted of six sections (Section 1: Visits to the recreational forest, 2: Attitudes towards physical features, 3: Motivations for using the forests, 4: Feelings when in the forest, 5: Expectations towards the forest and 6: Demographic information). Sections 2–5 of the questionnaire consisted of attitudinal statements to which the research participants were invited to respond using a bipolar Likert scale (1 – strongly disagree, 2 – disagree, 3 – not sure, 4 – agree and 5 – strongly agree).

Overall, 413 recreational forest users were surveyed (Ampang $N = 208$, Kanching $N = 205$ respondents) and 40 interviews were conducted at the two sites. Both the surveys and interviews were conducted on weekdays and weekends in April and May 2010 in similar climatic conditions. The survey and interview samples were separate from each other.

Principal Components Analysis (PCA) with Varimax rotation was used to analyse the data from Sections 2 (Attitudes towards physical features), 3 (Motivations for using the forest) and 4 (Feelings when in the forest). The items in those sections were tested for reliability (Table 1). Seven factors explaining users' forest experiences and motives for forest use were extracted and labelled according to the constructs that the clusters of questionnaire items seemed to represent: forest amenities, restorative experience, intergenerational experience, self-actualisation, incivilities, natural threats in the forest, and younger activity

**Table 1.** Factor loadings after rotation, use for, motivation, and experience in the recreational forests

| Factors | Factor loading | Variance explained | Cumulative variance explained | Cronbach's $\alpha$ |
|---|---|---|---|---|
| **Factor 1: Forest amenities** | | 19.12 | 19.12 | 0.91 |
| Questionnaire items** | | | | |
| Where there are boards telling me about the forest | 0.745 | | | |
| That has basic facilities (e.g. toilet, shelter, prayer room) | 0.744 | | | |
| Where there are signs that lead me through the forest | 0.739 | | | |
| Where there are signs that lead me to the forest | 0.735 | | | |
| That is tidy in appearance | 0.693 | | | |
| That has available parking spaces | 0.673 | | | |
| That is free of rubbish | 0.652 | | | |
| That is fenced off and has secured environment | 0.638 | | | |
| That is easy to get into | 0.619 | | | |
| That clearly indicates that visitors are welcome | 0.600 | | | |
| Where there are streams, rivers or waterfall | 0.592 | | | |
| Where the paths are free from obstruction | 0.569 | | | |
| That has areas of open space | 0.543 | | | |
| That I can get to by car, bus or motorcycle | 0.496 | | | |
| **Factor 2: Restorative experience** | | 7.10 | 26.22 | 0.84 |
| To relax and forget my worries | 0.630 | | | |
| To view the scenery | 0.604 | | | |
| To go walking | 0.602 | | | |
| To experience the calm and comfort of a forest | 0.581 | | | |
| To experience the silence of the forest | 0.527 | | | |
| I feel alive: I can be in contact with the elements of nature | 0.517 | | | |
| To lift my spirits when I am depressed | 0.487 | | | |

(continued on next page)

**Table 1.** Continued.

| Factors | Factor loading | Variance explained | Cumulative variance explained | Cronbach's $\alpha$ |
|---|---|---|---|---|
| To watch birds and animals | 0.450 | | | |
| To get fresh air | 0.427 | | | |
| To enjoy the sights, smell and sounds of nature (e.g., insects, birds, water etc.) | 0.389 | | | |
| To be alone in the forest | 0.336 | | | |
| **Factor 3: Intergenerational experience** | | 6.81 | 33.03 | 0.81 |
| To teach my children about the outdoor environment | 0.751 | | | |
| So my children can play | 0.603 | | | |
| It links me to the future: I used to play, now my children do so as well | 0.583 | | | |
| To be with my family members | 0.558 | | | |
| To spend quality time with my family | 0.500 | | | |
| To go running/jogging/take exercise | 0.472 | | | |
| It brings back childhood memories of play | 0.395 | | | |
| **Factor 4: Self-actualisation** | | 3.94 | 36.97 | 0.73 |
| I feel equal to everyone else here | 0.652 | | | |
| I free from human influences | 0.635 | | | |
| I feel peaceful in the forest | 0.612 | | | |
| I feel joyful in the forest | 0.575 | | | |
| I feel safe in the forest | 0.572 | | | |
| I feel attached to nature, here there is order and a sequence of events (life cycle) | 0.548 | | | |
| To be myself, here no one expects anything from me | 0.422 | | | |

(continued on next page)

**Table 1.** Continued.

| Factors | Factor loading | Variance explained | Cumulative variance explained | Cronbach's $\alpha$ |
|---|---|---|---|---|
| **Factor 5: Incivilities** | | 3.52 | 40.49 | 0.71 |
| It is a place for vandalism | 0.599 | | | |
| It is a place people can hide | 0.588 | | | |
| It is a place for rubbish dumping | 0.561 | | | |
| I feel isolated in the forest | 0.552 | | | |
| I feel lonely in the forest | 0.546 | | | |
| It is a place for drug addicts | 0.545 | | | |
| It is boring in the forest | 0.461 | | | |
| I don't like being in the middle of dense vegetation | 0.341 | | | |
| **Factor 6: Natural threats in the forest** | | 3.00 | 43.49 | 0.79 |
| I am fear of seeing snake | 0.768 | | | |
| I fear having an accident in the forest | 0.768 | | | |
| I am afraid of getting bitten by insects | 0.767 | | | |
| The pathway is slippery, I might fall | 0.634 | | | |
| I might get lost | 0.489 | | | |
| **Factor 7: Younger activity preference** | | 2.70 | 46.19 | 0.73 |
| To take photographs | 0.653 | | | |
| To bathe/go swimming | 0.630 | | | |
| That has stalls that sell food and drinks | 0.534 | | | |
| To play (e.g., kicking a ball, jumping into the water, etc.) | 0.508 | | | |
| To have a picnic | 0.437 | | | |

**Originally coded on a 5-point Likert-type scale with: (1) = strongly disagree, (2) = disagree, (3) = not sure, (4) = agree, (5) = strongly agree. Total % variance explained = 46.19.

preference. These factors are discussed in more detail below, and compared with the findings from the rest of the questionnaire data and qualitative data, where relevant.

## Results and Discussion

The seven factors accounted for 46.2% of the total variance. Factor 1 "Forest amenities" consisted of 14 items and accounted for 19.1% of the variance (see Table 1). Forest amenities mainly included items relating to: access, parking, wayfinding, basic facilities (e.g., toilets, shelter, and prayer room), maintenance and security, indicating that basic forest infrastructure and maintenance are important incentives for recreational forest use. This factor also corroborated other research factors indicating that streams, rivers and waterfalls were very important attractors within the context of recreational forests in Malaysia.

Factor 2 "Restorative experience" consisted of 11 items accounting for 7.1% of the variance (Table 1). The loadings onto this factor indicate the importance of the restorative experience in the forest visit and link this with the physical qualities of the forest, including: the presence of birds and animals, the fresh air and the sensory engagement with nature. Some of the items are linked to the four characteristics proposed by Kaplan and Kaplan (1989): *being away, extent, fascination and compatibility.* For instance users came to recreational forests: to relax and forget their worries, be fascinated by watching birds and animals, view the scenery, as well as appreciating the silence, calm and comfort of the forest environment. The interview results highlighted variances in perceptions of the physical characteristics and ambiance between Kanching and Ampang forests. In the Kanching forest the spectacular waterfalls were the feature associated with a restorative experience whereas in the Ampang forest it was the peaceful ambiance due to limited development cited as the contributing factor in the restorative experience. Elderly users also associated fresh air early in the morning and engaging in activities such as: brisk walking, exercising and strolling, with health and well-being.

Factor 3 "Intergenerational values" consisted of seven items accounting for 6.8% of the variance (Table 1). This factor links a series of items relating to family interaction, and experience through the life course, suggesting that the recreational forests provided valued opportunities for users to spend time with their families. Contributing to a sense of emotional continuity and existential fulfilment connected to the ability to pass on aspects of the forest experience to one's children: the next generation. The recreational forests also offered opportunities for extended families to get together and share experiences. Data derived from other parts of the study confirmed that a popular family activity was running, jogging or exercising together as a family. The interviews revealed that, for some male forest users, forest visits provided an opportunity to pass on aspects of their childhood experience of visiting recreational forests with their parents to their own children.

Factor 4 "Self-actualisation" consisted of seven items accounting for 3.9% of the variance (Table 1). "Self-actualisation" reflects a sense of the forest as an alternative space in which normal pressures and constraints do not apply, allowing people both to be themselves and to feel more aware of the natural world going on around them. At Ampang

Forest this was articulated by some interviewees who explained how they connected with the natural world by understanding the forests' characteristics. Drawing parallels between the flow of the river and their own lives and seeing trees as living organisms or part of nature and giving hope. Ampang Forest in particular provides a tranquil environment for users to meditate by themselves.

Factor 5 "Incivilities" consisted of eight items accounting for 3.5% of the variance (Table 1). The "Incivilities" factor was a cluster of negative perceptions about the forest, centring on the idea that the forest is a lonely and isolating place in which one may be exposed to anti-social behaviour. Fears of crime and incivilities included fear of being mugged by snatch thieves and were mentioned mostly by women interviewees, some of whom felt unsafe being alone in the forest. The interview results showed that fear of crime and incivilities were related to forest characteristics such as thick bushes, which might conceal hostile individuals, for example, thieves.

Factor 6 "Natural threats in the forest" consisted of five items accounting for 3.0% of the variance (Table 1). This factor was a group of items that related anxiety to the physical characteristics of the forest such as steep slopes, dense vegetation or trees. Some respondents associated negative feelings with these characteristics, such as fear of having an accident and getting lost in the forest. Factors 5 and 6 may deter some users, especially women or older people from fully utilising the recreational forests. Interviewees in Ampang Forest mentioned environmental hazards including sharp pebbles in the water or vehicles entering the forest. Some interviewees in Kanching Forest felt wary of elements associated with the waterfalls such as the slippery pathway and steeply sloping waterfall areas, fearing that they would have an accident.

Factor 7 "Younger activity preference" consisted of five items accounting for 2.7% of the total variance (Table 1). Younger respondents, aged 19–25 years old, liked to engage in activities such as: taking photographs, bathing or swimming, and having a picnic. Recreational forests also functioned as a social medium to gather with friends and as a place to escape from their home or studies. The physical character of the forest also attracted younger people to use the recreational forest. The Kanching Recreational Forest has waterfalls that attracted this group to bathe/go swimming and have picnics. This age group was greater in numbers in Kanching Forest than at Ampang.

## Conclusion

The factor analysis revealed seven factors that influenced people to use the recreational forests and to engage in particular activities once they were there. Five factors of those mentioned above ("Forest amenities," "Restorative experience," "Intergenerational values," "Self-actualisation" and "Younger activity preference") motivated respondents to use the recreational forests and influenced the activities and experience they had. However, there were two factors – "Incivilities" and "Natural threats in the forest" that could deter users (especially women and older users) from full use of the recreational forests.

This study found that Malaysians come to recreational forests for a variety of complex reasons that have some similarities and differences with the motivations for forest use revealed by previous research. Malaysians are attracted to recreational forests for their restorative and stress-relieving qualities. These are closely linked to forest characteristics including: fresh air, forest ambiance, and their social function related to family activities mentioned in the "Intergenerational values" factor. Results show that users had mostly positive experiences when visiting the recreational forests, except for women and older users, who expressed some fears about their safety. Older users visited the recreational forest for health benefits such as fresh air, especially in the early morning. Men valued intergenerational experiences as a "rite of passage," passing on their experiences with their parents, when they were children, to the next generation. In contrast, women and older users expressed fear about crime and incivilities, and natural threats in the forest, more frequently than other user groups. These factors provide insights for policy makers and forest managers on how to strengthen opportunities to re-enforce positive forest experience and mitigate the potential impact of the detractors from the experience. Some factors in the work presented in this paper such as restorative experience and intergenerational values are likely to be relevant in other settings; but more research is needed to establish the role of the forest environment in these experiences. For example, do people derive the same benefits from other landscape types, for example, deserts, and how do cultural differences impact on this?

# References

Abdullah, S. A., & Nakagoshi, N. (2008). Changes in agricultural landscape pattern and its spatial relationship with forestland in the state of Selangor, peninsular Malaysia. *Landscape and Urban Planning, 87*, 147–155.

Bell, P. A., Greene, T. C., Fisher, J. D., & Baum, A. (1996). *Environmental psychology* (4th ed.). Fort Worth, TX: Harcourt Brace College.

Berman, M. G., Jonides, J., & Kaplan, S. (2008). The cognitive benefits of interacting with nature. *Psychological Science, 19*, 1207–1212.

Coombes, E., Jones, A. P., & Hillsdon, M. (2010). The relationship of physical activity and overweight to objectively measured green space accessibility and use. *Social Science and Medicine, 70*(6), 816–822.

Garst, B. A., Williams, D. R., & Roggenbuck, J. W. (2010). Exploring early twenty-first century developed forest camping experiences and meanings. *Leisure Sciences, 32*(1), 90–107.

Kaplan, S. (1995). The restorative benefits of nature: Toward an integrative framework. *Journal of Environmental Psychology, 15*, 169–182.

Kaplan, R., & Kaplan, S. (1989). *The experience of nature: A psychological perspective*. New York, NY: Cambridge University Press.

Ludin, A. N. M., Abd Razak, W. J. W., Majid, M. R., & Rusli, N. (n.d.). *A study on urban land use planning and its influence on drug related crime in high density areas of Ampang Jaya District of Kuala Lumpur, Malaysia*. Retrieved from http://uitm.academia.edu/NoradilaRusliRusliN/Papers/580761/A_STUDY_ON_URBAN_LAND_USE_PLANNING_AND_ITS_INFLUENCE_ON_

Lyons, E. (1983). Demographic correlates of landscape preference. *Environment and Behavior, 15*(4), 487–511.

McFarlane, B. L., & Boxall, P. C. (2003). The role of social psychological and social structural variables in environmental activism: An example of the forest sector. *Journal of Environmental Psychology, 23*(1), 79–87.

Michimi, A., & Wimberly, M. C. (2012). Natural environments, obesity, and physical activity in nonmetropolitan areas of the United States. *Journal of Rural Health, 28*(4), 398–407.

Nielsen, T. S., & Hansen, K. B. (2007). Do green areas affect health? Results from a Danish survey on the use of green areas and health indicators. *Health and Place, 13*(4), 839–850.

O'Brien, L. (2006). Social housing and green space: A case study in Inner London. *Forestry, 79*(5), 535–551.

Proshansky, H. M. (1995). Place identity: Physical world socialization of the self. In L. Groat (Ed.), *Giving places meaning* (pp. 87–113). London, UK: Academic Press.

State Department of Forestry. (2003). Recreational forests in Selangor. In *Annual Report*. Shah Alam, Malaysia: State Department of Forestry.

Toftager, M., Ekholm, O., Schipperijn, J., Stigsdotter, U., Bentsen, P., Grønbæk, M., & Kamper-Jørgensen, F. (2011). Distance to green space and physical activity: A Danish national representative survey. *Journal of Physical Activity and Health, 8*(6), 741–749.

Woon, W.-C., & Norini, H. (2002). Trends in Malaysian forest policy. *Policy Trend Report 2002*, pp. 12–28. Retrieved from http://enviroscope.iges.or.jp/modules/envirolib/upload/371/attach/02-Malaysia.pdf

World Health Organization. (2009). Global health risks: Mortality and burden of disease attributable to selected major risks. Geneva, Switzerland: Author.

# Objectively Healthy Cities

## Urban Design for the 21st Century

George Weeks

The Prince's Foundation for Building Community, London, UK

### Abstract

"Healthy City" initiatives are widespread, but what makes a healthy 21st century city? At present, the biggest cause of preventable death in the developed world is heart disease, whilst rates of depression and mental illness have increased steadily since the 1970s (Putnam, 2000). Much of this is attributable to a widespread lack of physical activity, essential for human health (Sallis, Frank, Saelens, & Kraft, 2004). Over the past decade, increasing amounts of research have been undertaken, investigating the relationship between the design of the built environment and human behaviour, particularly with respect to people's tendency to undertake sufficient physical activity. This paper reviews existing research on the relationship between physical activity, health and urban design. It examines how the form of the built environment – particularly walkability – can be objectively measured and positively correlated with physical activity and health, irrespective of expressed preferences for exercise. There are major policy implications for urban design and its potential to improve public health, social cohesion, and environmental quality that are reflected in recent UK studies, such as the Marmot Report (Geddes et al., 2011). This paper has particular relevance for urban policymakers, planners, and designers wishing to demonstrate an epidemiological basis for mixed-use, high density walkable urbanism, and the relationship between human behaviour and urban design.

**Key words:** health, urban design, utilitarian activity

## Introduction

The current paper reflects a review of previous research between design affordances the physical urban form provides for people's activity levels and health. The World Health Organization (WHO) defines health as follows: "Health is a state of complete physical, mental and social well-being and not merely the absence of disease or infirmity" (WHO, 1947, p. 1).

A healthy city could thus be described simply as one which is conducive to the achievement of such a state. However the UN's *Healthy Cities* programme (1986) is more specific in its definitions; not least that the act of being a healthy city is a *process*, not an *outcome*.

## Shifts in Policy Priorities: Urban Epidemiological Transition

The mention of an "unhealthy city" may suggest images of Dickensian squalor or over-crowded shantytowns. This is, however, a misleading image because the evolution of public health has undergone an epidemiologic transition over the course of human history (Frank, Engelke, & Schmid, 2003). Whilst the *Age of Pestilence and Famine* (Frumkin, Frank, & Jackson, 2004, p. 45) lasted for millennia, the *Age of Receding Pandemics* was characterised by the rise of immensely overcrowded industrial cities, where, in 1900, around a quarter of the population could expect to die from pneumonia or tuberculosis history (Frank et al., 2003, p. 40).

The post-industrial city has given rise to the *Age of Degenerative and Man-Made Diseases*, where cancer and cardiovascular diseases are the predominant causes of death. The image of the polluted Victorian mill town is thus merely a representation of the second stage in urban epidemiology; the first being pre-industrial plague and famine; the third being inactivity, heart disease, and obesity (see Figure 1; Frumkin et al., 2004).

Recent empirical research has integrated the previously separate yet overlapping approaches of built environment and health professionals into various integrated models. The task for public policymakers is to synthesise this research into actions that will address the challenge of an increasingly sedentary population (Bassett, Pucher, Buehler, Thompson, & Crouter, 2008). In order to pursue this objective research needs to be carried out on the correlations of urban design and the variations in affordances, alternative designs provide, that facilitate a more active lifestyle. This is a complex problem that requires an interdisciplinary or transdisciplinary approach, drawing on experiences of design and health professionals as well as laypeople.

## Initial Integrated Research

Correlations between physical inactivity and chronic health problems first emerged in the 1970s. Whilst research into the relationship between obesity and density was carried out in the 1990s (Solomon & Manson, 1997), health research tended to focus on the psychological and social variables of individuals undertaking recreational exercise (Sallis, Frank, Saelens, & Kraft, 2004). Concurrently, transport and urban planning research (e.g., Holtzclaw, 1994) examined the incidence of physical activity as a utilitarian activity

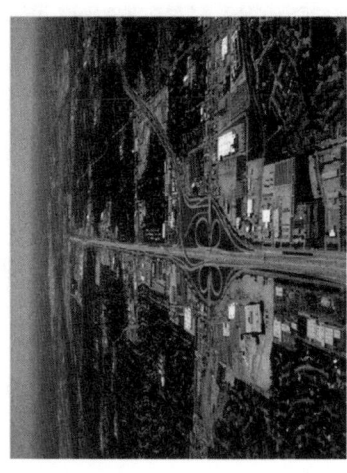

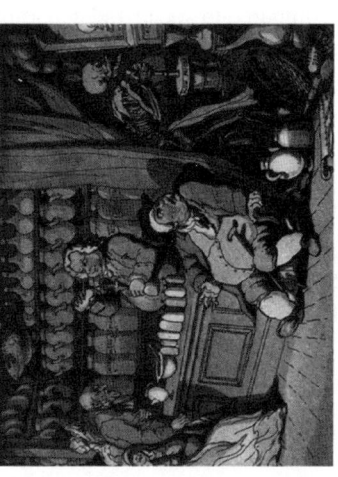

**Figure 1.** Urban epidemiological transition. (Source: left image: Ephemeral Scraps; middle image: Paul Townsend; right image: La Citta Vita)

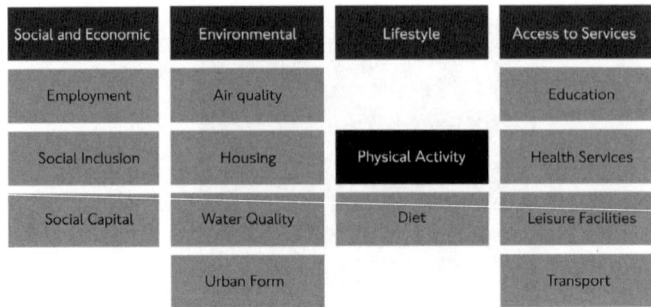

**Figure 2.** Urban factors that determine health and well-being. (Adapted from: Barton, Grant, & Guise, 2010)

affected by environmental variables at a community scale. It was not until the early 2000s that health researchers started to become interested in the environmental correlates of physical activity (Saelens, Sallis, Frank, & Chen, 2003).

An integrated approach between the health and built environment professions began to enter the mainstream with publications by Frank et al. (2003), Sallis et al. (2004), and Frumkin et al. (2004). This research field has since grown substantially and organisations such as The Glasgow Centre for Population Health (GCPH) and the WHO Collaborating Centre for Healthy Cities at the University of the West of England have come into being, specifically to promote healthy urban planning. Similar conclusions were reached at a national level in the USA, where the Transportation Research Board (2005, p. 2) concluded that "built environments designed to facilitate more active lifestyles and to reduce barriers to physical activity are desirable."

The urban characteristics that can affect human health can be categorised via the table shown in Figure 2 below: physical activity, like diet, operates at the scale of the individual (Barton, Grant, & Guise, 2010). Compared to social and economic determinants these life-style factors are perhaps more straightforward for a willing individual to alter themselves (Barton, 2009).

## Priorities for Public Health

Physical activity[1] or lack thereof, is associated with a large number of undesirable health outcomes (Bell, Ge, & Popkin, 2002). The leading causes of preventable death in the USA (and much of the western world) are heart disease and cancer (Frumkin et al., 2004).

---

[1]   In public health literature, an "active" adult is conventionally accepted as obtaining at least 30 minutes of moderate exercise per day, as recommended by the Chief Medical Officer (NHS Livewell); a sedentary person does not reach this threshold. This convention is followed throughout this study.

The total deaths in the USA attributable to inactivity are greater than those from road accidents and pollution combined, by a factor of four (Sallis et al., 2004). Physical inactivity is closely associated with coronary heart disease and is the leading cause of death in the UK. It kills around 100,000 people per year with the risk doubled for people who are sedentary versus active (British Heart Foundation).

The Royal Commission on Environmental Pollution's 26th report, entitled *The Urban Environment* (2007) ranked obesity, caused mainly by inactivity, as being responsible for around 34,000 premature deaths per year. Urban morphology is often eclectic with new developments incrementally adding to the shape and accessibility of the city. Although planners and architects do take cognisance of the need for movements of large volumes of people and transportation links, they more often than not do not take into account the academic and applied understanding of other disciplines such as health professionals. The affordances that built environments provide for healthy living and general well-being is perhaps a significant factor on ill health and mortality rates. Obesity is linked to increased mortality rates and incidences of cancer, coronary artery disease, hypertension, and type 2 diabetes (Solomon & Manson, 1997) resulting in obesity rates increasing steadily for decades (ibid). In the USA obesity is second only to smoking as the leading cause of preventable death (Allison, Fontaine, Manson, Stevens, & VanItallie, 1999). This has prompted studies into the factors that make a city "obesogenic" (Barton et al., 2010). Significantly, the problems associated with a sedentary lifestyle can be significantly reduced by relatively moderate increases in activity (Frank et al., 2003, p. 41). This problem is by no means restricted to the western world. Economic and social changes in China have caused an explosive growth in urbanisation and car ownership, with corresponding falls in levels of physical activity (Bell et al., 2002).

## Physical Activity and Health

Recommendations by the Chief Medical Officer and generally in public health literature, suggest that an "active" adult is conventionally accepted as one obtaining at least 30 min of *moderate* exercise per day whilst for children, the threshold is higher, at 60 min per day (Department of Health, 2011). Thirty minutes of moderate exercise for adults could encompass a wide range of activities from some as innocuous as walking or gardening, facilitated by the urban environment, to more sporting activities. The marginal increases in benefit are a lot more significant for a sedentary person starting to exercise than they are for an already active person taking *more exercise*. Human beings have evolved a physiology suited to a hunter-gatherer lifestyle which entails movement and high levels of energy expenditure (Katzmarzyk, 2010); it is unnatural to be sedentary.

Figure 3 illustrates a study on relative morbidly based upon data obtained form 13,000 Harvard University graduates in the 1960s. The relative risk of mortality falls with increasing levels of physical fitness, however the greatest fall is seen between the two lowest

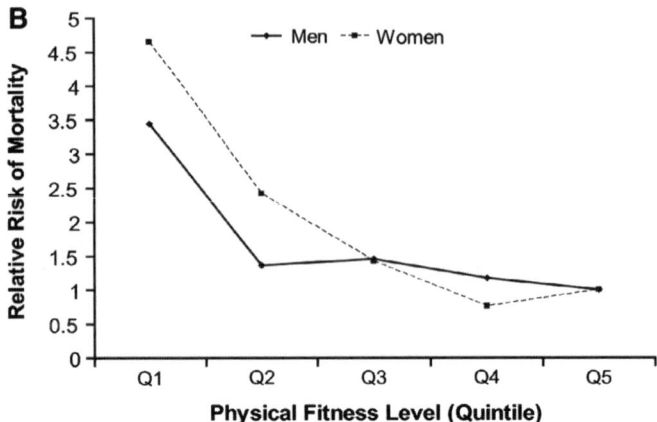

**Figure 3.** Exercise and health. (Source: Katzmarzyk, 2010, © 2010 by the American Diabetes Association)

quintiles. In other words, simply commencing a less sedentary lifestyle has a greater marginal significance for an adult's health than a subsequent devotion to athleticism (Katzmarzyk, 2010). More recently, a systematic review by Woodcock et al. (2011) has argued that that non-vigorous physical activity reduces all-cause mortality.

## Recreational vs. Utilitarian Activity

Physical activity can be categorised as recreational and/or utilitarian and embarked upon for different underlying reasons (Frank et al., 2003; Van Dyck, Deforche, Cardon, & DeBourdeaudhuij, 2009). As set out in Figure 4, recreational activity has its own utility and the decision to undertake recreational activity is subject to individual behavioural factors, for example enjoyment of playing a sport. Recreational activity requires time, effort, money, and willingness. Utilitarian activity is an indirect (i.e., derived) demand where some form of utility is obtained from the achieved result of completing a task. Whether a person is walking to a railway station, cycling to work, or walking down the high street on a Saturday morning, utilitarian exercise takes place as part of some other activity and is mediated much more by environmental factors (Frank et al., 2003).

    This distinction is not absolute; some considerations such as children's play can be affected by behaviour and circumstance with the built environment having a significant bearing on well-being (Gill, 2008). Nonetheless, it is important to highlight the differences between utilitarian and recreational exercise because the appropriate policy responses are very different in each case. Promotion of recreational activity must take place at a behaviour-based, individual scale. This entails a huge amount of targeted persuasion to

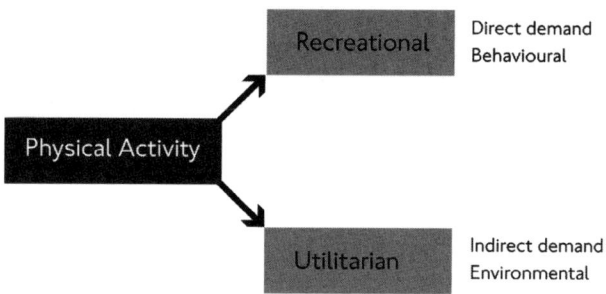

**Figure 4.** Recreational and utilitarian exercise. (Adapted from Van Dyck et al., 2009)

encourage people to take up and, just as importantly, maintain levels of exercise (Frank et al., 2003). Utilitarian exercise, on the other hand, is undertaken as a consequence of *circumstances*, for instance if it makes sense for people to walk to work, they will do so. This gives credence to the theory of creating walkable urbanism to increase levels of physical activity (Saelens, Sallis, Frank, & Chen, 2003).

## Relevance to Urban Planning: Planning for Walkability

Utilitarian exercise is linked to walkability (Barton et al., 2010) which is a straightforward concept in principle, but can be measured in various ways. It can be characterised by relatively high built densities, mixed land uses and high levels of connectivity (Frank et al., 2003). Walkability is reduced by lack of pavement provision, cul-de-sacs, single use land zoning and development at a scale intended for car drivers, not pedestrians (Holtzclaw, 1994). Research by Lopez (2004) uses density as a walkability metric and, whilst straightforward, does not take account of land use mix or street patterns. Alternatively, Saelens et al. (2004) amongst other studies (e.g., SMARTRAQ) utilise a measure based upon density, connectivity (i.e., street layouts), and mixed uses. Randall and Baetz (2001) examine pedestrian connectivity using a measure called the pedestrian route directness (PRD ratio), which equals route distance/geodetic[2] distance. A perfectly connected area will have a PRD ratio of 1 which tends to be lower in area with small blocks and multiple through routes. PRD can be used in conjunction with a pedshed threshold (often 400 m/5 min walk) to examine connectivity.

Walkability is not the only environmental factor affecting utilitarian physical activity; the accessibility and aesthetic attributes of the built environment are also relevant (Humpel, Owen, & Leslie, 2002). Nonetheless, walkability is popular because it is relatively straightforward to quantify objectively and accurately. Leyden (2003) found a strong

---

[2] geodetic = "as the crow flies"

statistical correlation ($p < .0001$) between residents' assessment of their neighbourhoods' walkability and researchers' own prior assessment of degrees of walkability. Thus indicating that neighbourhood type may be assessed objectively in a way that closely reflects subjective perception.

## Walkability

- Density
- Mix of use ⎫
- Connectivity ⎭ – Proximity

## Research Into Walkability and Walking

Frank, Schmid, Sallis, Chapman, and Saelens (2005) produced one of the first individual-based studies on the relationship between objectively measured physical activity and neighbourhood walkability. Having assessed areas of Atlanta, USA, with the metrics shown above, study participants were issued with pedometers to record how much they walked (357 sets of results used). After controlling for demographic and other factors, the study concluded that "An objectively measured walkability index was significantly related to objectively measured, moderate intensity physical activity in adults." In other words, all things being equal people walk more in walkable environments. The dramatic extent to which street connectivity affects accessibility is shown in Figure 5.

## Academic Consensus

Numerous studies have been carried out in this subject area, with remarkable consistency evident in the results. This was identified in an extensive literature review on the built environment and health behaviour by Hanlon, Walsh, and Whyte (2006) at the GCPH. A total of 65 studies were examined, from the USA, Canada, UK, Australia, and Japan. The consistency was striking: In every one of the 65 studies, residents of walkable neighbourhoods *always* tended to undertake more physical activity.

Walkability is a particularly significant determinant of physical activity because it encourages exercise irrespective of whether or not people have an expressed preference for it. Van Dyck et al. (2009) found that people with an expressed preference for passive (i.e., motorised) transport took significantly more steps per day when living in a walkable neighbourhood compared to a non-walkable neighbourhood. Walkable urban design can successfully encourage physical activity where behavioural initiatives have failed to change preferences.

The distinction between utilitarian and recreational activity must be emphasised. Saelens et al. (2003) found that neighbourhood walkability levels had a significant impact on

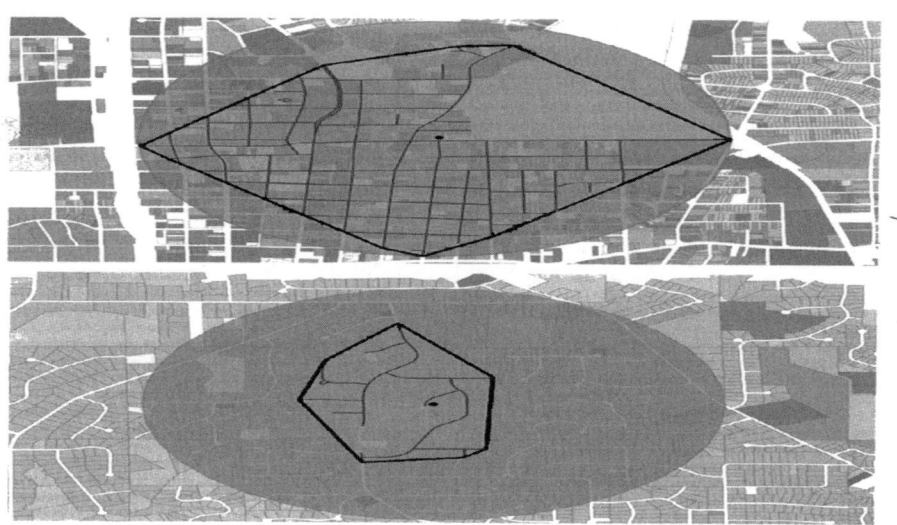

**Figure 5.** Connected streets and accessibility. (Source: Frank, Schmid, Sallis, Chapman, & Saelens, 2005)

utilitarian walking but no impact on recreational walking. This suggests that recreational activity is not significantly determined by environmental factors. If urban policymakers are looking to increase walking levels through design, the focus should be on utility walking.

## Implications for Planning and Policy

From these reviews, there is a clear and demonstrable link between the built environment, lifestyles, and health. Specifically;

1. Neighbourhood walkability, as defined by connectivity, density, and land use mix can be measured objectively (Leyden, 2003)
2. Walkability correlates with physical activity (Hanlon et al., 2006; Saelens et al., 2003)
3. Physical activity correlates with significantly lower levels of chronic and man-made illness and better physical, mental, and social health (Barton et al., 2010)
4. Walkable mixed use environments can contribute significantly to public health.

Governments and policymakers should focus unambiguously on ensuring that future cities are healthy cities (NICE, 2008). The strength of this argument is reflected in its recent emergence in UK public policy, such as the Health and Social Care Act (2012) which makes local authorities responsible for public health. This builds upon the publications of NICE PHG 8 (2008) Building Environments That Promote Physical Activity and The Urban Environment (Royal Commission on Environmental Pollution, 2007). Despite these encouraging movements, it appears that such measures are being adopted at a slower rate than is required to offset underlying trends in obesity and diabetes.

The implications extend beyond health, encompassing such considerations as inequality. The Marmott Review (Geddes, Allen, Allen, & Morrisey, 2011) specifically recommends investing in better walking and cycling routes as a means to reduce health inequalities. Walkable urbanism has its share of detractors (e.g., Cox, 2011; O'Toole, 2007), regarding walkable development as "elitist" and a limit to choice. As a counterpoint to this, it is prudent to illustrate that the provision of urban environments that differ radically from mainstream production is a manifestation of an increase in choice (Frumkin et al., 2004). The emergence of evidence favouring walkability as a way to improve public health is a further substantial contribution in support of well-connected streets, mixed uses, and relatively high building densities. There are other social and environmental implications, such as SMARTRAQ that showed un-walkable, single-use sprawl is especially inconvenient for families because most activities depends upon chauffeuring of children, with logistics further complicated by an average commute of 16 miles (Frank et al., 2005). Saunders, Green, Petticrew, Steinbach, and Roberts (2013) highlight the benefits of the reductions in pollution and carbon emissions arising from higher rates of active travel.

## Conclusion

To conclude, we have seen that the health effects of inactivity can be greatly reduced by fairly modest increases in physical exercise, and this is consistently delivered by urban designs that are mixed use, high density, and walkable. If regular physical activity is the magic bullet to good health, and a walkable city consistently encourages activity, irrespective of expressed preference for exercise, it appears that we should build walkable cities to improve overall health.

Outside the scope of this paper, area that warrants further attention for urban health studies is the effect of natural and green space on people's mental health and well-being. Numerous studies in this area are set out in Bird (2005) which is directly relevant to the form taken by a city and its balance of built/open space. Access to green space is also covered in the Marmot Report (Geddes et al., 2011). Green space has particular relevance to this paper because it can cater simultaneously for recreational and utilitarian exercise, for example a park which incorporates direct walking and cycling routes. Similarly, the reports covered in this study use walkability as a metric and it would be useful to carry out further study on the use of other environmental actors (e.g., pleasure derived from proximity of natural surroundings) though this would be harder to measure objectively than walkability.

This paper has, concentrated heavily on walking, but it is possible that similar relationships exist between the quality of bicycle routes and infrastructure and people's tendencies to cycle. Future studies in the area of healthy urban planning are ongoing and there is significant potential for further insight. Whilst the design and operation of land use evaluation models has the potential to be extremely complicated, it nonetheless appears self evident, from the extensive research covered in this paper, that the promotion of dense, well-connected mixed-use sustainable urbanism should carry significant weight in promoting public health. This is in addition to the environmental benefits that may also be wrought form increasing rates of active travel (Woodcock et al., 2009). Finally, the benefits of active travel extent to pollution reduction and climate change mitigation and these too should be considered in the context of sustainable urban design.

# References

Allison, D. B., Fontaine, K. R., Manson, J. E., Stevens, J., & VanItallie, T. B. (1999). Annual deaths attributable to obesity in the United States. *Journal of the American Medical Association, 282*(16), 1530–1538.

Barton, H. (2009). Land use planning and health and wellbeing. *Land Use Policy, 26S*, S115–S123.

Barton, H., Grant, M., & Guise, R. (2010). *Shaping neighbourhoods: For local health and global sustainability* (2nd ed.). London, UK: Routledge.

Bassett, D., Pucher, J., Buehler, R., Thompson, D., & Crouter, S. (2008). Walking, cycling and obesity rates in Europe, North America, and Australia. *Journal of Physical Activity and Health, 5*, 795–814.

Bell, A. C., Ge, K., & Popkin, B. M. (2002). The road to obesity or the path to prevention: Motorized transportation and obesity in China. *Obesity Research, 10*, 277–283.

Bird, W. (2005). *Natural thinking: Investigating the links between the Natural Environment, Biodiversity and Mental Health*, RSPB. Retrieved from http://www.rspb.org.uk/Images/naturalthinking_tcm9-161856.pdf

Cox, W. (2011). *Urban Transportation Policy Requires Factual Foundations; Heritage Foundation.* Retrieved from http://www.heritage.org/research/reports/2011/02/urban-transportation-policy-requires-factual-foundations

Department of Health. (2011). *UK physical activity guidelines.* Retrieved from https://www.gov.uk/government/publications/uk-physical-activity-guidelines

Ephemeral Scraps. *The quack doctor.* Retrieved from https://www.flickr.com/photos/biomedical_scraps/6860258506/sizes/o/in/photostream/

Frank, L. D., Engelke, P. O., & Schmid, T. L. (2003). *Health and community design: The impact of the built environment on physical activity.* Washington, DC: Island Press.

Frank, L. D., Schmid, F. T. L., Sallis, J. F., Chapman, J., & Saelens, B. E. (2005). Linking objectively measured physical activity with objectively measured urban form. *American Journal of Preventative Medicine, 28*, 117–125.

Frumkin, H., Frank, L. D., & Jackson, R. J. (2004). *Urban sprawl and public health.* Washington, DC: Island Press.

Geddes, I., Allen, J., Allen, M., & Morrisey, L. (2011). *The Marmot review: Implications for spatial planning.* Retrieved from http://www.nice.org.uk/nicemedia/live/12111/53895/53895.pdf

Gill, T. (2008). Space-oriented children's policy: Creating child-friendly communities to improve children's well-being. *Children & Society, 22*(2), 136–142.

Hanlon, P., Walsh, D., & Whyte, B. (2006). *Let Glasgow flourish.* Glasgow, UK: Glasgow Centre for Population Health.

Holtzclaw, J. (1994). *Using residential patterns and transit to decrease auto dependence and cost.* Retrieved from http://docs.nrdc.org/smartGrowth/files/sma_09121401a.pdf

Humpel, N., Owen, N., & Leslie, E. (2002). Environmental factors associated with adults' participation in physical activity. *American Journal of Preventive Medicine, 22*(3), 188–199.

Katzmarzyk, P. T. (2010). Physical activity, sedentary behavior, and health: Paradigm paralysis or paradigm shift? *Diabetes, 59*(11), 2717–2725.

La Citta Vita. *Irving, Texas / Dallas suburb.* Retrieved from https://www.flickr.com/photos/49539505@N04/6044604666/in/photolist-ad9bnQ-mLReY-aDNEN1-adAdZb-9c19NW-bsMMYX-6Zn7D3-bNEeCB-sDb6T-9n37Tq-6wQ7tV-6wQa2H-6wUkqG-6wUijm-6wPUGH-6wQ1dP-6wPX92-6wPCFc-6wPmcx-6wTHLY-6wPTpk-6wU55C-6wTB5W-6wPn3v-6wPpgp-6wTyVu-6wPnPt-6wPrRF-6wPksc-6wPjuR-6wTRGy-6wPYtV-6wU3Ao-6wTAdy-6wU149-6wPXQ8-6wTYdC-acHBe8-7aewjZ-6wTKGq-6wU2JW-c66r3m-7QmhzT-2GGaH-6Le7jP-8mWTJc-8s2onK-7zYDqp-e3Sxp-e3Sxt-4uYUzP

Leyden, K. M. (2003). Social capital and the built environment: The importance of walkable neighborhoods. *American Journal of Public Health, 93*, 1546–1551.

Lopez, R. (2004). Urban sprawl and the risk of being obese. *American Journal of Public Health, 94*(9), 1574–1579.

NICE. (2008). *Public Health Guidance 8: Physical activity and the environment.* Retrieved from http://guidance.nice.org.uk/PH8

O'Toole, R. (2007). *Debunking Portland: The city that doesn't work.* Cato Institute Policy Analysis no. 596. Retrieved from http://www.cato.org/pubs/pas/pa-596.pdf

Putnam, R. D. (2000). *Bowling alone: The collapse and revival of American community.* New York, NY: Simon & Schuster.

Randall, T. A., & Baetz, B. W. (2001). Evaluating pedestrian connectivity for suburban sustainability. *Journal of Urban Planning and Development, 127*(1), 1–15.

Saelens, B. E., Sallis, J. F., Frank, L. D., & Chen, D. (2003). Neighborhood-based differences in physical activity: An environment scale evaluation. *American Journal of Public Health, 93*(9), 1551–1558.

Sallis, J. F., Frank, L. D., Saelens, B. E., & Kraft, M. K. (2004). Active transportation and physical activity: Opportunities for collaboration on transportation and public health research. *Transportation Research Part A, 38*(4), 249–268.

Saunders, L. E., Green, J. M., Petticrew, M. P., Steinbach, R., & Roberts, H. (2013). What are the health benefits of active travel? A systematic review of trials and cohort studies? *PLoS ONE, 8*(8), e69912. doi: 10.1371/journal.pone.0069912

Solomon, C. G., & Manson, J. (1997). Obesity and mortality: A review of the epidemiologic data. *American Journal of Clinical Nutrition, 66*, 1044S–1050S.

The Royal Commission on Environmental Pollution. (2007). *The urban environment – twenty-sixth report.* London, UK: The Stationery Office.

Townsend, P. *Preventative directions for cholera.* Retrieved from https://www.flickr.com/photos/20654194@N07/12699070113/in/photolist-kmb47H-4fdREB-4c4Dq5-8cw89Y-k1AKHL-86aDw4-gXNWaY-a6oayS-boXty6-4ccjpf-dtYair-7oRZ2r-fnGMoA-4aPZmB

Transportation Research Board. (2005). *Does the built environment influence physical activity? Examining the evidence [abstract].* Retrieved from http://onlinepubs.trb.org/onlinepubs/sr/sr282summary.pdf

Van Dyck, D., Deforche, B., Cardon, G., & DeBourdeaudhuij, I. (2009). Neighbourhood walkability and its particular importance for adults with a preference for passive transport. *Health & Place, 15*, 496–504.

Woodcock, J., Edwards, P., Tonne, C., Armstrong, B. G., & Ashiru, O., Banister, D., ... Roberts, I. (2009). Public health benefits of strategies to reduce greenhouse-gas emissions: Urban land transport. *The Lancet, 374*, 1930–1943.

Woodcock, J., Franco, O. H., Orsini, N., & Roberts, I. (2011). Non-vigorous physical activity and all-cause mortality: Systematic review and meta-analysis of cohort studies. *International Journal of Epidemiology, 40*, 121–138.

World Health Organization (WHO). (1947). *Constitution of the World Health Organisation.* Retrieved from http://apps.who.int/gb/bd/PDF/bd47/EN/constitution-en.pdf

## Websites

Active Transport Collaboration, University of British Columbia: http://www.act-trans.ubc.ca

Active Living by Design: http://www.activelivingbydesign.org

British Heart Foundation Statistics Database: http://www.heartstats.org

Change 4 Life: http://www.nhs.uk/change4life/Pages/change-for-life.aspx

Glasgow Centre for Population Health: http://www.gcph.co.uk

NHS Choices: http://www.nhs.uk/Conditions

NHS Livewell: http://www.nhs.uk/Livewell/fitness/Pages/Howmuchactivity.aspx

SMARTRAQ: http://www.act-trans.ubc.ca/smartraq/pages/

University of the West of England, Centre for Sustainable Planning and Environments: http://www.bne.uwe.ac.uk/cep

University of the West of England, The WHO Collaborating Centre for Healthy Cities and Urban Policy: http://www.bne.uwe.ac.uk/who

Walking the Way to Health Initiative: http://www.wfh.naturalengland.org.uk

# Dementia-Friendly Architecture

## Integrating Evidence in Architectural Design

Gesine Marquardt

Faculty of Architecture, Technische Universität Dresden, Germany

**Abstract**

Rising life-expectancy has led to an increased risk of developing dementia. The characteristics of dementia affect many aspects of the individual's life and often lead to institutionalisation. The well-being, functionality, and behaviour of people with dementia can be supported through dementia-friendly design. One of the most relevant aspects is the design of the spatial layout of the environment. It needs to allow for direct visual access to all places relevant for performing activities of daily living. At the same time, spatial designs that are very open and interconnected might account for difficulties in the spatial representation of people with dementia. The need to combine two contrary goals when striving for evidence-based architectural designs for people with dementia constitutes a challenge for architects. The dichotomy is to allow for visual access to all relevant places, and simultaneously, to create boundaries that separate spaces one from another in order to render them architecturally legible.

**Key words:** architectural legibility, architecture, dementia, design, spatial representation

## Facts and Figures on Dementia

The increasing longevity in industrial countries promises a compression of morbidity and the acquisition of several additional years of good health (Christensen, Doblhammer, Rau, & Vaupel, 2009). However, at the same time, the risk of developing dementia increases with age. Experts estimate that 35.6 million people currently live with dementia worldwide. This number could potentially double within the next 20 years to 115.4 million in the year 2050 (Prince & Jackson, 2009). The medical professionals have controversial views on the question of whether dementia is an inevitable process at the end of human life that only the individual's early death may prevent. Also, it is not known why more women than men are affected.

The symptoms of dementia occur slowly over time, affecting: memory, orientation, attention, language, and problem solving (World Health Organisation [WHO], 1992). The most common form is Alzheimer's disease which accounts for 50–75% of the total number of cases (American Psychiatric Association [APA], 2007). In the absence of effective medical therapies for dementia, the individual's quality of life has been focussed on by researchers of various professional backgrounds. Architects, striving for the design of therapeutic environments, are amongst them.

## Framework and Goals of Dementia-Friendly Design

People with dementia are especially subject to their environments. Their well-being, functionality, and behaviour can be supported through dementia-friendly design. The ecological gerontology explains this relationship through established concepts such as the person-environment-fit concept (Lawton & Nahemow, 1973). This concept describes the degree to which a person is compatible with his or her environment; a prerequisite to fulfiling one's full potential. The Environmental Docility Hypothesis, however, indicates that people who are subjected to restrictions on their health or cognitive ability, such as people with dementia, cannot always adapt the environment to their specific needs (Lawton & Simon, 1968). This implies that people with dementia are more dependent on the environmental characteristics of their dwelling. Therefore, their living environment should be designed in such a way that meets with their specific needs and provides sensory stimulation. This way, their well-being, functionality, and behaviour can be positively affected.

Design recommendations and built examples in this field can be found in Brawley (1997), Cohen and Weisman (1991), Diaz Moore, Geboy, and Weisman (2006), and Judd, Marshall, and Phippen (1998). This research suggests that a therapeutic environment is one that has a familiar appearance, personalised spaces, and supports autonomy through adequate lighting and colour-contrast. Furthermore it provides sensory stimulation through views and access to the outside, as well as through natural light entering the building. A therapeutic environment especially fosters social interaction by offering communal spaces of a non-institutional appearance. Figure 1 suggests a dementia threshold that accounts for a diminished adaption scope to environmental press (Gutzmann, 2003). Through a therapeutic environmental design, which incorporates the dementia threshold, the well-being, functionality, and behaviour among people with dementia can be positively affected (see reviews by Calkins, 2009; Day, Carreon, & Stump, 2000; Tilly & Reed, 2008).

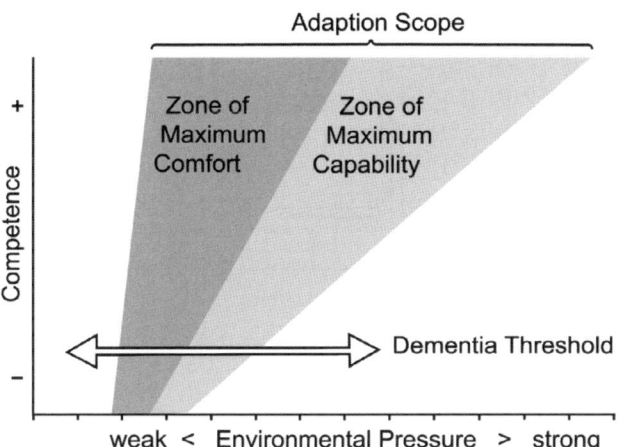

**Figure 1.** Model of the dementia threshold.

# Accommodating Changes in Spatial Representation for People With Dementia

Even though there is a growing body of research on dementia-friendly, therapeutic environmental design, some myths about dementia design still seem to persist. In guidance for Architects, Carers, and Clinicians, floor plan designs in the layout of a continuous loop around an inner courtyard are often recommended. It is also frequently emphasised that the environment should be rendered almost overly accessible. Open floor plans with little spatial boundaries seem to be the recommended design typology of choice for people with dementia. Whilst it is most important for physical accessibility (such as using a walker or wheelchair) that there are no borders, such as thresholds, this may be very different for the "cognitive accessibility" for people with dementia.

In larger spatial entities, such as nursing homes or hospitals, the layout of the circulation system determines whether a space is accessible. All users, but specifically patients, need to reach certain destinations, such as the dining room or the toilet, to maintain their independence, and perform their activities of daily living. Being able to understand how dementia patients follow a route, such as the corridor from their individual room to communal areas, and recognise the destination upon arrival, are essential to successful placement of living and functional rooms and design in general (Brush & Calkins, 2008). Further steps in this process are, as Diaz Moore et al. (2006) pointed out "conditioned by the innate physical and perceptual-cognitive abilities of the person as well as by the spatial and sensory information provided by the environment in which the person finds herself." (Diaz Moore et al., 2006, p. 117).

Left: central corridor          Centre: L-shape,              Right: continuous loop

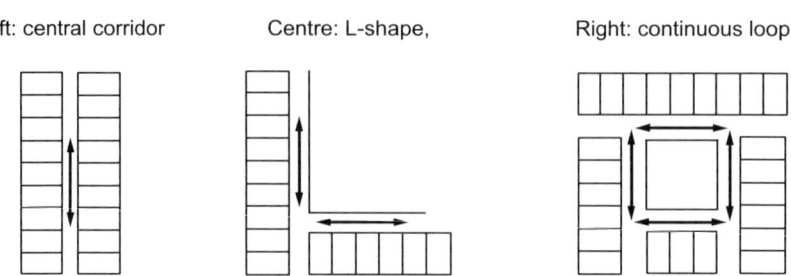

**Figure 2.** Floor plan typologies of nursing homes.

Empirical studies investigating the layout of the circulation system identified typical floor plans which are shown in Figure 2. A consistent outcome of the studies was that direct visual access to relevant places is helpful for the resident's orientation (Marquardt & Schmieg, 2009; Passini, Pigot, Rainville, & Tétreault, 2000; Passini, Rainville, Marchand, & Joanette, 1998).

With a larger number of patients or residents the number of individual bedrooms increases, and thus the corridor necessary for circulation may substantially gain in length. There are controversial results on whether a straight and possibly long corridor has a negative impact on nursing home resident's orientation. The number of studies addressing this matter is limited and the results are conflicting. Some studies support architectural design efforts to avoid straight hallways and double-loaded corridors (Elmståhl, Annerstedt, & Ahlund, 1997; Netten, 1989), with others finding improved orientation in straight layouts. In linear circulation systems, residents are able to find their way better than in any layout that features a shift in direction, such as L-shapes or continuous loops around an inner courtyard (Marquardt & Schmieg, 2009). The continuous loop however, is often discussed as the design of choice for people with dementia. It is supposed to provide an accessible, easily navigable environment which provides freedom for independent mobility. To solve this controversy between architectural practise and empirical research the orientation process of people with dementia needs to be explored (Marquardt, 2011).

The overall decline of spatial orientation and wayfinding performance of people with dementia is caused by their impaired cognitive spatial skills, including mental spatial representation (Liu, Gauthier, & Gauthier, 1991). These internal representations of the environment in one's mind are called cognitive maps, which are a prerequisite to orientate oneself and to the successful locating of places. A cognitive map contains environmental information on places that lie beyond the perceptual range of vision (Kitchin, 1994). The mental visual representations of those objects, places, and routes are produced by an area of the brain called Precuneus. Since it is involved with visuospatial processing and memory it is also called the mind's eye (Fletcher et al., 1995). Since there is an overall decline of cognitive abilities associated with dementia, it is expected that orientation and cognitive mapping, also is limited. It is further hypothesised that the decline in orientation can be ascribed to the fact that the cognitive map deforms and breaks apart. Functional MRI studies of the neural basis of personally meaningful, autobiographical mental visual images have demonstrated a cerebral network including the mind's eye (Donix et al., 2010; Poettrich et al., 2009). These studies showed reductions in the metabolism of the brain, including the area of the Precuneus, the mind's eye. This implies that with advancing dementia, residents may encounter greater difficulties in retrieving a mental visual image of a place that they cannot see, rendering them unable to generate, maintain, and use a cognitive map. The design of circulation systems, highlight the importance of direct visual access to all places relevant to a dementia resident's wayfinding and the imperative to avoid changes in the direction of the circulation system. However Elmståhl et al. (1997) found that a central corridor can have negative effects on the vitality of residents. Therefore, aspects of a therapeutic environment, as outlined in the introductory paragraph, need to be integrated into linear corridor designs.

# Communicating Spatial Information Through Environmental Design

## Enhancing Architectural Legibility

Environments designed for people with dementia provide them with a sense of self, time, and place. They need to be designed in such a way that they communicate information to the person because of their cognitive deficits. People with dementia therefore need to be addressed in various non-conventional ways. Often, goal-oriented verbal communication is no longer possible with non-verbal ways of communication utilised (Vasse, Vernooij-Dassena, Spijkera, Rikkerta, & Koopmansa, 2010). Through the creation of architecturally legible spaces the environment can play an important role in communicating information to the users. A considerate utilisation of colours, materials, lighting, furnishing, etc. informs them about where they are, what the intended use of the space is, and what behaviour is appropriate there. Thus, a small-scale, non-institutional but homelike character and a personalised environment are considered to be a central influencing factor on behaviour (Charras et al., 2010; Garcia et al., 2012; Zeisel et al., 2003).

The importance of an environmental design approach which aims for the creation of non-institutional and architecturally legible spaces for people with dementia has been the subject of research by Charras, Eynard, Viatour, and Frémontier (2011). They postulate the need to design an environment that is considered as the living environment of people that will fulfil their needs and aspirations. They stress the importance of taking into account "... the residents' regional and socio-cultural background in order to provide them with and promote identity, safety, conviviality, social relationships, attachment and respect, intimacy as well as inter-individual differences" (Charras et al., 2011, p. 33).

Studies on wayfinding design define the *legibility* of a setting "... as the degree to which a building facilitates the ability of users to find their way within it" (Weisman, 1981). Even though in designing for people with dementia a broader definition of the term "legibility" is used, creating an architecturally legible environment is also the most important prerequisite for supporting the spatial recognition and representation of people with dementia.

In order for people with dementia to understand the meaning and function of a room it has to be architecturally legible and have boundaries that clearly separate it from other spaces. A study using the architectural methodology space syntax (Hillier & Hanson, 1984), which allows the assessment of the spatial layout of an individual home from the inhabitants' point of view, showed a relationship between the spatial layout of the home and the successful performance of the resident's activities of daily living (Marquardt et al., 2011). Using space syntax it is possible to visualise spatial configurations broken down into components, by representing them as graphs that describe the relative integration and connectivity of convex spaces (in this context: Rooms) within a given system (in this context: The house). A measure of the degree to which a room is connected and integrated into the whole spatial system of the home and how much it is "broken up" into different spaces or rooms can be calculated from the graphs. Figures 3 and 4 show

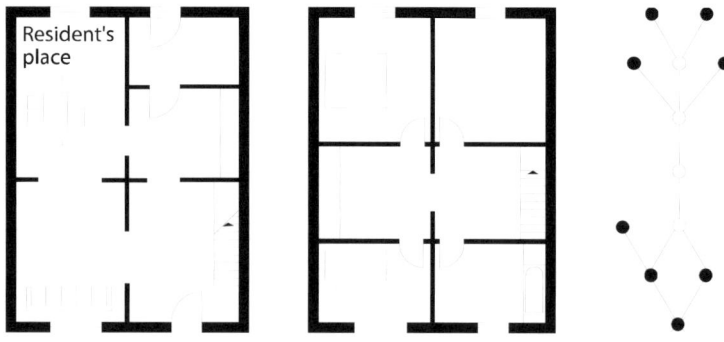

**Figure 3.** Floor plan and resulting graph of a home with a high measure of convexity.

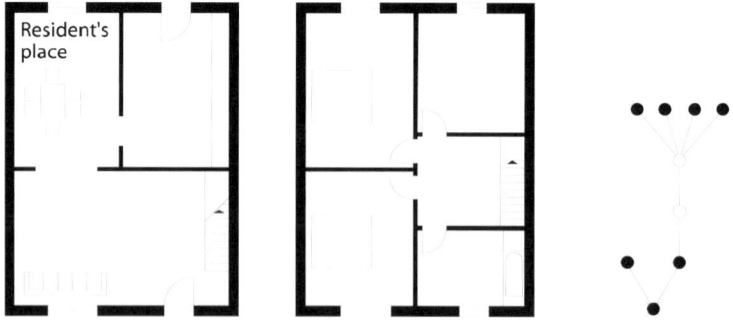

**Figure 4.** Floor plan and resulting graph of a home with a low measure of convexity.

examples of floor plans and the resulting graphs, justified to the place where the resident spends most of their time. White nodes indicate circulation areas and open spaces, black nodes rooms with a function. Figure 3 shows a floor plan with a high measure of convexity, indicating s spatial system which is highly broken up into different spaces. Figure 4 shows the reverse; a floor plan with a rather low measure of convexity, describing a spatial system with the same function, but less different spaces being used to accommodate these functions.

The results of the study discussed imply that spatial systems, that are to a lesser degree broken up, and that feature enclosed rooms with an architecturally clearly legible meaning and function (such as kitchen, hallway, living room) might be better memorised and associated with the spatial layout of the home, resulting in higher independence of a resident with dementia. The reason for this effect may be found in the floor plan designs: Layouts that are very open and interconnected might account for difficulties in both the spatial recognition and spatial representation of people with dementia.

## Integrating Spatial Reference Points

So far, the term *architectural legibility* has been discussed as an important prerequisite for the spatial representation of people with dementia. As the concept of legibility is rooted in wayfinding design, the way in which an architecturally legible environment can support the wayfinding abilities of people with dementia will be explored next.

As outlined before, the ability to generate, maintain, and use a cognitive map is limited in people with dementia. However, the absence of a cognitive map can be partially compensated by the use of other kinds of orientation strategies. People with dementia may orientate themselves allocentrically within their environment, from one decision point to the next, until they reach their desired destination. Providing signposting would seem to be an effective intervention to help residents use this type of strategy to find their way around (Passini et al., 2000). However research suggests that, appropriately designed signs are necessary for this method to be effective. Older adults with cognitive impairments may have poorer sign comprehension and experience difficulties with wayfinding signs that have icons only, whereas text seems to be better understood (Namazi & Johnson, 1991; Scialfa et al., 2008). Studies further suggest that personalisation of visual cues might be a considerable technique to improve the effectiveness of signposting. Personal cues, such as written names, portrait-type photographs of residents as young adults, and personal memorabilia, were positively correlated with residents' ability to locate their room or identify belongings (Gross et al., 2004; Nolan & Mathews, 2004; Nolan, Mathews, & Harrison, 2001).

In summary, cues best come into effect serving as spatial anchor points for allocentric orientation if their function or meaning is legible and of relevance to the residents. It is also important that cues are unique in their design, because differentiation between similar elements becomes increasingly difficult with advancing dementia. Examples of effective cues found in nursing homes are mounted wall displays of historical equipment for household

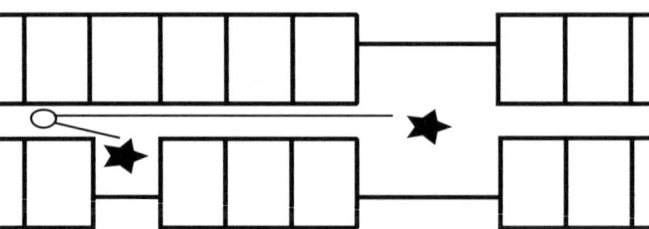

**Figure 5.** Floor plan featuring open spaces to serve as reference points and direct visual access to relevant places.

activities such as washing or tailoring, or historic pictures and paintings of specific regional and cultural origin.

Figure 5 shows a schematic floor plan of a nursing home with resident's rooms to both sides of a central corridor. The straight layout of the circulation system provides visual access, open spaces on both sides of the corridor allow natural light to fall into the building and generate views to the outside. Through their design and function these open spaces need to become meaningful, architecturally legible places which can communicate information about the place to the residents and thus serve as spatial anchor points. Possible designs that could facilitate meaningful wayfinding anchor points are the creation of thematic areas with biographical meaning to the residents that perhaps trigger memories of activities such as housekeeping, gardening, or other activities from their past. Through the articulate use of colour and lighting, architecturally legible, and memorable places that serve as spatial anchor points are generated. However, these features cannot compensate an adverse spatial design (Elmståhl et al., 1997; Marquardt & Schmieg, 2009; Passini et al., 1998, 2000).

## Architectural Implications

### Evidence-Based Design of Environments for People With Dementia

It has been argued that there is a correlation between the architectural design of residential homes and the well-being and behaviours of people with dementia. Therefore, in order to achieve the desired outcomes through design, empirical evidence resulting from research studies needs to be incorporated when designing environments for this specific group. Indentifying and integrating the best available evidence has been central to several fields, predominately to medicine, public health, and nursing for many years. In Architecture, this design approach has been used for about 10 years and is called evidence-based design. It is defined as "... the process of basing decisions about the built environment on credible research to achieve the best possible outcomes" (Levin, 2008). However, not all design decisions can be substantiated by findings from research. Some fields of healthcare design are not actively researched, whilst other areas may only build on studies that lack a robust design that may not be considered rigorous enough. However, the major challenge for the further advancement in the field of evidence-based design is the provision of meta-knowledge (Durmisevic & Ciftcioglu, 2010). The following design recommendations aim at providing aggregated knowledge for the design of dementia-friendly environments.

## Design Recommendations

Integrating evidence in architectural design for people with dementia may provide a challenge for architects. Following the available studies results, they need to accommodate seemingly contrary goals: To allow for visual access to all relevant places, and, simultaneously, to create boundaries to separate spaces one from another in order to render the environment architecturally legible. The following design recommendations build on the evidence presented at this paper.

To arrive at an optimal design solution, the first step should be to fully consider the implications of room layout and the most appropriate shape of circulation system. Direct visual access needs to be established between all places relevant to the activities of daily living for a person with dementia, however, when navigating between larger spatial entities, changes in the direction of the circulation system pose problems for the dementia patient and should be avoided. However, due to the shape or size of the building site or in order to avoid long corridors in units with a higher number of residents, changes in circulation system direction may become necessary and result in floor plan shapes such as an L. If this is the case, direct visual access may no longer be possible and the resident's orientation needs to be supported. Assuming that allocentric orientation strategies come into effect in this layout, a meaningful and memorable reference point needs to be placed at the position where the direction changes. Placing a therapeutic kitchen or dining room at this spot constitutes an excellent reference point that can serve as spatial anchor point. To render it architecturally legible and to create a memorable space it needs to be distinct from surrounding spaces, which can be achieved through designing articulate distinctions in size, shape, colour, and lighting.

Another aspect to be considered in the creation of dementia-friendly environments is the spatial syntax or the degree to which the environment can be broken up into different spaces for dementia patients, with an individually assigned function and meaning. These considerations are rather simple in a private home environment, where every available space can be given a unique function, such as the hallway, kitchen, living room, bathroom, etc. Architecturaly significant designs of residential homes should encompass distinct, meaningful, and well-signed spaces for living, thus supporting residual cognitive maps and spatial representation of people with dementia.

In larger spatial entities, such as nursing homes or hospitals, repetitive elements cannot be avoided: There are several bedrooms, bathrooms, and maybe, even a larger number of dining and other activities rooms. If all these places are distinctive designs from one another, such as decorated doors to the individual bedrooms set in vividly coloured wall recesses, the environment may communicate too much information to the resident, or patient, and thus become confusing. Architects therefore also need to combine spaces with similar function, creating an environment which is broken up to a lesser degree. This way, the homely spatial representation is mediated by intelligent design.

Further, the environment needs to be architecturally legible. The function of rooms and other spaces as well as the behaviour that is expected and appropriate there, need to be made clearly legible. This can be achieved through room size and proportion, as well as the use of materials and furnishings. In this manner, distinctive places which correspond with the spatial recognition of people with dementia are created. In a final step, supportive orientation systems such as signage that can help to further differentiate the spatial environment need to be incorporated in the design.

## Conclusions and Directions for Future Research

Environments for people with dementia require a therapeutic design which provides sensory stimulation, accommodates their specific changes in spatial representation, and communicates spatial information to them. Empirical studies which support a relationship between design features of the spatial environment and behaviour outcomes of people with dementia have been identified. Based on these results, recommendations for a dementia-friendly architectural design have been given. However, further research is needed to better understand the relationship between architecture and the well-being, functionality, and behaviour of people with dementia. Meta-knowledge of research findings needs to be readily available during the design process. Only this way architects will be able to integrate the evidence stemming from research studies into their architectural designs.

Furthermore it is of great importance, not only to integrate the research evidence into the designs, but also to evaluate buildings and environments that are the result of an evidence-based design process. Post Occupancy Evaluations as a methodology of evaluating the success of design criteria may be appropriate for some users of residential homes such as professional staff and family members of dementia patients. This form of data collection and its subsequent analysis could further enhance Architects understanding of the end users in their different capacities. The expected findings would be of utmost value to both the field of evidence-based design as well as dementia-friendly design. In summary, a holistic design approach for dementia-friendly environments, which is based on research evidence, needs to be further developed and the findings continuously evaluated. The application of research findings into "real world" design applications is increasingly important given that we have an ageing population. This article has highlighted the need for a greater scientific understanding of the specific needs of dementia patients and wider research that helps bridge the applicability gap in knowledge, between design professionals and end users.

# References

American Psychiatric Association [APA]. (2007). *Practice guideline for the treatment of patients with Alzheimer's disease and other dementias.* American Psychiatric Publishing.

Brawley, E. (1997). *Designing for Alzheimer's disease-strategies for creating better care environments.* New York, NY: Wiley.

Brush, J. A., & Calkins, M. P. (2008). Cognitive impairment, wayfinding, and the long-term care environment. *Perspectives on Gerontology, 13*(2), 65–73.

Calkins, M. (2009). Evidence-based long term care design. *NeuroRehabilitation, 25*(3), 145–154.

Charras, K., Eynard, C., Viatour, G., & Frémontier, M. (2011). The Eval'zheimer model: Fitting care practices and environmental design to institutionalized people with dementia. *Neurodegenerative Disease Management, 1*(1), 29–35.

Charras, K., Zeisel, J., Belmin, J., Drunat, O., Sebbagh, M., Gridel, G., & Bahon, F. (2010). Effect of personalization of private spaces in special care units on institutionalized elderly with dementia of the Alzheimer type. *Non-Pharmacological Therapies in Dementia, 1*(2), 121–137.

Christensen, K., Doblhammer, G., Rau, R., & Vaupel, J. (2009). Ageing populations: The challenges ahead. *The Lancet, 374*(9696), 1196–1208.

Cohen, U., & Weisman, G. (1991). *Holding on to home. Designing environments for people with Dementia.* Baltimore, MD: John Hopkins University Press.

Day, K., Carreon, D., & Stump, C. (2000). The therapeutic design of environments for people with dementia: A review of the empirical research. *The Gerontologist, 40*(4), 397–416.

Diaz Moore, K., Geboy, L. D., & Weisman, G. D. (2006). *Designing a better day. Guidelines for adult and dementia day services centers.* Baltimore, MD: Johns Hopkins University Press.

Donix, M., Poettrich, K., Weiss, P. H., Werner, A., von Kummer, R., Fink, G. R., & Holthoff, V. A. (2010). Age-dependent differences in the neural mechanisms supporting long-term declarative memories. *Archives of Clinical Neuropsychology, 25*(5), 383–395.

Durmisevic, S., & Ciftcioglu, O. (2010). Knowledge modeling tool for evidence-based design. *Health Environments Research and Design Journal, 3*(3), 101–123.

Elmståhl, S., Annerstedt, L., & Ahlund, O. (1997). How should a group living unit for demented elderly be designed to decrease psychiatric symptoms? *Alzheimer's Disease and Associated Disorders, 11*(1), 47–52.

Fletcher, P., Frith, C., Baker, S., Shallice, T., Frakowiak, R., & Dolan, R. (1995). The mind's eye-precuneus activation in memory-related imagery. *Neuroimage, 2*(3), 195–200.

Garcia, L. J., Hébert, M., Kozak, J., Sénécal, I., Slaughter, S. E., Aminzadeh, F., Dalziel, W., Charles, J., & Eliasziw, M. (2012). Perceptions of family and staff on the role of the environment in long-term care homes for people with dementia. *International Psychogeriatrics, 24*(5), 753–765.

Gross, J., Harmon, M. E., Myers, R. A., Evans, R. L., Kay, N. R., Rodriguez-Charbonier, S., & Herzog, T. R. (2004). Recognition of self among persons with dementia pictures versus names as environmental supports. *Environment and Behavior, 36*(3), 424–454.

Gutzmann, H. (2003). Therapeutische Ansätze bei Demenzen [Therapeutic approaches for dementia] In Therapeutische Ansätze bei Demenzen. In C. Waechtler (Ed.), *Demenzen. Frühzeitig erkennen, aktiv behandeln, Betroffene und Angehörige effektiv unterstützen* [Dementias. Early recognition, active treatment effective support for patients and their families]. Stuttgart, Germany: Thieme.

Hillier, B., & Hanson, J. (1984). *The social logic of space.* Cambridge, UK: Cambridge University Press.

Judd, S., Marshall, M., & Phippen, P. (1998). *Design for dementia.* London, UK: Hawker.

Kitchin, R. M. (1994). Cognitive maps: What are they and why study them? *Journal of Environmental Psychology, 14*(1), 1–19.

Lawton, M. P., & Nahemow, L. (1973). Ecology and the aging process. In C. Eisdorder & M. P. Lawton (Eds.), *Psychology of adult development and aging.* Washington, DC: American Psychological Association.

Lawton, M. P., & Simon, B. (1968). The ecology of social relationships in housing for the elderly. *The Gerontologist, 8*(2), 108–115.

Levin, D. (2008). Defining evidence-based design. *Healthcare Design, 8*(8), 8.

Liu, L., Gauthier, L., & Gauthier, S. (1991). Spatial disorientation in persons with early senile dementia of the Alzheimer type. *American Journal of Occupational Therapy, 45*(1), 67–74.

Marquardt, G. (2011). Wayfinding for people with dementia – A review of the role of architectural design. *Health Environments Research and Design Journal, 4*(2), 22–41.

Marquardt, G., Johnston, D., Black, B., Morrison, A., Rosenblatt, A., Lyketsos, C., & Samus, Q. M. (2011). Association of the spatial layout of the home and ADL abilities among older adults with dementia. *American Journal of Alzheimer's Disease & Other Dementias, 26*(1), 51–57.

Marquardt, G., & Schmieg, P. (2009). Dementia-friendly architecture: Environments that facilitate wayfinding in nursing homes. *American Journal of Alzheimer's Disease & Other Dementias, 24*(4), 333–340.

Namazi, K. H., & Johnson, B. D. (1991). Physical environmental cues to reduce the problems of incontinence in Alzheimer's disease units. *American Journal of Alzheimer's Disease and Other Dementias, 6*(6), 22–28.

Netten, A. (1989). The effect of design of residential homes in creating dependency among confused elderly residents: A Study of elderly demented residents and their ability to find their way around homes for the elderly. *International Journal of Geriatric Psychiatry, 4*(3), 143–153.

Nolan, B. A., & Mathews, R. M. (2004). Facilitating resident information seeking regarding meals in a special care unit: An environmental design intervention. *Journal of Gerontological Nursing, 30*(10), 12–16.

Nolan, B. A., Mathews, R. M., & Harrison, M. (2001). Using external memory aids to increase room finding by older adults with dementia. *American Journal of Alzheimer's Disease and Other Dementias, 16*(4), 251–254.

Passini, R., Pigot, H., Rainville, C., & Tétreault, M. H. (2000). Wayfinding in a nursing home for advanced dementia of the Alzheimer's type. *Environment and Behavior, 32*(5), 684–710.

Passini, R., Rainville, C., Marchand, N., & Joanette, Y. (1998). Wayfinding with dementia: Some research findings and a new look at design. *Journal of Architectural and Planning Research, 15*(2), 133–151.

Poettrich, K., Weiss, P. H., Werner, A., Lux, S., Donix, M., Gerber, J., von Kummer, R., Fink, G. R., & Holthoff, V. A. (2009). Altered neural network supporting declarative long-term memory in mild cognitive impairment. *Neurobiology of Aging, 30*(2), 284–298.

Prince, M., & Jackson, J. (2009). *World Alzheimer Report.* London, UK: Alzheimer's Disease International. Retrieved from http://www.alz.co.uk/research/files/World%20Alzheimer%20Report.pdf

Scialfa, C., Spadafora, P., Klein, M., Lesnik, A., Dial, L., & Heinrich, A. (2008). Iconic sign comprehension in older adults: The role of cognitive impairment and text enhancement. *Canadian Journal on Aging, 27*(3), 253.

Tilly, J., & Reed, P. (2008). Intervention research on caring for people with dementia in assisted living and nursing homes. *Alzheimer's Care Today, 9*(1), 24–32.

Vasse, E., Vernooij-Dassena, M., Spijkera, A., Rikkerta, M., & Koopmansa, R. (2010). A systematic review of communication strategies for people with dementia in residential and nursing homes. *International Psychogeriatrics, 22*(2), 189–200.

Weisman, J. (1981). Evaluating architectural legibility. Way-finding in the built environment. *Environment and Behavior, 13*(2), 189–204.

World Health Organization [WHO]. (1992). *The ICD-10 classification of mental and behavioural disorders: Clinical descriptions and diagnostic guidelines.* Geneva, Switzerland: Author.

Zeisel, J., Silverstein, N. M., Hyde, J., Levkoff, S., Lawton, M. P., & Holmes, W. (2003). Environmental correlates to behavioral health outcomes in Alzheimer's special care units. *The Gerontologist, 43*(5), 697–711.

# Objective and Subjective Impressions of an Environmental Intervention in Dementia Care Homes

Louise Ritchie[1] and Edward Edgerton[2]

[1]Institute of Older Persons' Health & Wellbeing, University of the West of Scotland, Hamilton, Scotland, UK
[2]School of Social Sciences, Psychology Division, University of the West of Scotland, Paisley, Scotland, UK

**Abstract**

The physical environment has been increasingly recognised as an important therapeutic tool in dementia care. The present study involved designing and implementing a simple and "cost effective" intervention in the living areas of dementia care homes, by re-arranging the existing furniture in the room in seven different living areas across three care homes in the West of Scotland. Behaviour mapping was used to assess the behaviours of residents, pre and post intervention, and staff focus groups were held following each intervention. The results demonstrate positive changes in behaviour of the residents, however this was not always reflected in staff members' perceptions of the intervention. The results are discussed in terms of implications for future policy and practice within the design of dementia care homes and implications for integrating the use of environmental interventions with existing policies in dementia care.

**Key words:** behaviour mapping, Dementia, physical environment, staff perceptions

## Introduction

The design of the physical environment is increasingly being recognised as a therapeutic aid in the everyday lives of people suffering dementia. There seems to be a consensus as to which features are useful with regard to design for dementia (Judd, Marshall, & Phippen,

1998). These encompass the idea that homes are small and "home-like" in style with traditional fixtures and fittings that are relevant to the individual/s living there, rooms which have a clear purpose and are legible, appropriate use of signage, landmarks, and colour for orientation and good levels of lighting.

The majority of this research has been carried out in specific areas of care home environments (e.g., bathrooms, bedrooms, corridors) (See Day, Carreon, & Stump, 2000 for review) however, there has been little research that has looked at social or communal spaces within care homes, for example, lounges or day rooms and dining areas. It has been found that whether residents stay in large care homes or in smaller units they are likely to spend a large proportion (between 65% and 72%) of their time during the day sitting in a lounge area (Barnes, 2006). The present research will examine the impact of an intervention which was put in place in seven different dementia living environments with the aim of providing a basis of research to inform future design.

## Design of the Intervention

The intervention was developed based on environmental psychology theories, previous research in dementia care homes and similar environments (e.g., psychiatric geriatric wards). The main principle of the intervention was to create a choice of smaller areas for residents to use that served different purposes by rearranging the existing furniture within the room.

## Theoretical Background to Intervention

Lawton's (1979) Environmental Docility Hypothesis discusses the idea of creating a therapeutic environment for elderly people. The term therapeutic environment is defined by Lawton as a physical and organisational environment that supports the functioning of an elderly person by counteracting the deficits that are associated with growing old in our society. The Environmental Docility Hypothesis posits that "normal" living environments can become increasingly disabling for a person with a disability, especially as that disability worsens. It also states that the "normal" environment can act as a barrier to well-being and independence. This is based on the idea that the environment becomes a stronger determinant of behaviour as personal competence decreases (Lawton, 1990). Lawton highlights that interactions with the environment generally occur on an unconscious basis until some factor changes to disturb the relationship. One factor may be a decline in cognitive function due to dementia. This reduces a person's competence and therefore an environment in which they have previously functioned and interacted well in, could become challenging to the person. On the positive side, Lawton states that small and simple environmental modifications can have a disproportionate strong, positive effect on the well-being and independence of a person with dementia. This view uses environmental design to make up for deficits in personal competence.

The second theory underpinning the research is the Behaviour-Constraint Approach (Proshanky, Ittelson, & Rivlin, 1970). This is commonly used in Environmental Psychology research and focuses more on the environment-behaviour relationship in general rather than on a specific user group like dementia sufferers. Stage 1 is the user perceiving a loss of control over the environment. This perceived loss of control would generally result in negative feelings or discomfort. After numerous failed attempts to regain control of the environment a person may develop learned helplessness. This may have a more pronounced impact on people with dementia as they are more sensitive to the environment and may have less understanding of the control they have of the environment (Judd et al., 1998). Loss of control has been associated with a number of negative behaviours in people with dementia including agitation (Lawton, 1990) and passivity (Colling, 2004).

The intervention employed in this study is designed to provide a choice of areas for the residents to use, therefore giving them a sense of control over how they use their environment, and at the same time, reducing the negative effects of learned helplessness such as agitation and passivity. This will be done by making small, simple changes to the living environment, using the existing furniture in the area to create smaller spaces within the large room which will allow for a choice of activities.

## Previous Research

The literature that does exist on the design of communal areas in dementia care homes focuses mainly on the size of the areas. The general consensus from this is that smaller spaces are better. Schwarz, Chaudhury, and Brent Tofle (2004) found that smaller recreational rooms were used more often than one large room. Staff also commented that the change to smaller rooms had improved staff-resident interaction and that privacy was greater in the new, smaller rooms. Special Care Units (SCUs), for dementia care are smaller than traditional care homes, have smaller rooms and give residents a choice between communal spaces (Calkins, 2001). Smaller units appear to result in less resident agitation and depression as well as more socialising and relationship forming. However, care homes and organisations often do not have the resources to redesign units from one large area to multiple smaller areas. If this is the case it is recommended that the room is reduced into smaller spaces as much as possible using furniture arrangement and dividers (Nazarko, 2006). This recommendation will be integrated into the present research.

The idea of providing a choice for residents is also thought to be important as demonstrated in the behaviour-constraint model above. Barnes (2006) found that daytime location of residents in dementia care homes was associated with quality of life and states that having a choice of different spaces for residents to go to can have a positive impact on quality of life. Calkins (1988) recommends providing areas in which residents can socialise or can just observe others without participating. Lawton (1979) also states that it is important that residents have a range of social and recreational choices available to them. Having a choice of different spaces affording different levels of privacy increases feelings of environmental control and can therefore reduce the associated feelings of negative effect and helplessness. It has also been found that the opportunity to participate in every-day activities and to have opportunities to socialise is something that people with dementia value highly (Phinney, Chaudbury, & O'Connor, 2007).

The aim of this study is to examine the efficacy of the intervention over seven different environments. There are two hypotheses relating to the behaviour mapping data. These are that the intervention will:

- increase positive behaviour
- decrease negative behaviour

It also aims to consult staff members on their views of the intervention. The subjective views of staff members and the results of the objective measure of residents' behaviour will then be considered together for a full analysis of the efficacy of the intervention.

# Methodology

## Design

The research adopted a pre/post intervention design, measuring residents' behaviour for 3 week periods before and after the intervention was put in place. Staff interviews and focus groups were held following the intervention.

## Participants

The seven living environments were contained across three care homes in the west of Scotland. The most recent reports from the Care Commission (now the Care Inspectorate) were obtained to contribute to the background characteristics of the care homes. These reports rate the care homes on a number of dimensions, however for the purposes of this research only the rating of the environment was included. This was rated on a scale of 1–6, 1 being poor and 6 being excellent. Table 1 summarises the main characteristics of each care home.

## Materials

The main method of data collection for the study was based on behaviour mapping. The behaviour coding system in this case was developed using preliminary observations of the

**Table 1.** Characteristics of the participating care homes

|  | Care Home A | Care Home B | Care Home C |
|---|---|---|---|
| Purpose built? | Yes | No | Yes |
| Number of residents | 15 | 30 | 40 (in 4 separate units) |
| Number of living areas | 1 | 2 | 4 (one in each unit) |
| Environment rating from care inspectorate | Average | Poor | Good |

areas being studied and previous research which has used behaviour mapping with a dementia or geriatric-psychiatric population (Cohen-Mansfield, Werner, & Marx, 1989; Devlin, 1992; Ittelson, Proshanky, & Rivlin, 1970). The behaviour coding system developed, had three main behaviour categories which were split into three to four sub-categories of more specific behaviours. These are outlined in Table 2 along with the codes assigned to each behaviour type.

Following the intervention and the completion of the behaviour mapping data collection, a staff focus group was held in order to find out how staff perceived the intervention and its impact on residents. This process was also used to discuss the impact of the specific

**Table 2.** Behaviour coding categories

| Behaviour category | Specific sub-category | Description |
|---|---|---|
| Positive behaviours | Active | Residents are engaged in a specific behaviour, for example watching TV, reading. |
|  | Interaction | Resident is talking to or listening to someone else. |
|  | Content | Resident does not appear to be engaged in any behaviour but appears aware of the surrounding environment and appears happy and not distressed. |
| Negative behaviours | Passive | Resident is not engaged in any behaviour and does not appear to be aware of stimuli in the surrounding environment. Eyes may be glazed, appear withdrawn or head may be facing downwards. |
|  | Agitation | Agitation can be defined as "Inappropriate verbal, vocal or motor activity that is not judged by an outside observer to result directly from the needs or confusion of the agitated individual." |

interventions and any particular benefits or problems the staff observed with them. The focus group was recorded using a digital recorder and transcribed for analysis. These were analysed using thematic analysis.

## Procedure

Each case study followed the same general procedure. Behaviour mapping sessions were held four times a week for 3 weeks pre and 3 weeks post intervention. These were held at different times of the week to cover a range of different time periods. Behaviour codes were used to count the number of times each behaviour type was observed in the area. This was recorded by the observer placing a tick in the appropriate box of the recording sheet for each of the five minute observations. Inter-rater reliability checks were carried out by a second observer who was present at 25% of the observations.

The intervention was put in place following the completion of the pre intervention behaviour mapping; one week was given as a settling in period. An example of the intervention in Care Home A is shown in Figure 1A and 1B. After the completion of the post intervention behaviour mapping, staff focus groups were held with a sample of staff in each unit (although this was scaled down to a number of semi-structured interviews due to lack of availability of staff).

# Results

## Behaviour Mapping

There were two hypotheses addressed in each case study for the behaviour mapping data. These were that post intervention there will be:

- An increase in positive behaviour,
- A decrease in negative behaviour.

### Hypothesis 1: Positive Behaviours
Table 3 outlines the mean behaviour count for each of the positive behaviour categories. From this, it can be seen that hypothesis 1 was fully supported in four of the seven case studies. In case studies 3 and 4, only content behaviour was found to significantly increase post intervention, whilst in case study 7 only active behaviour was found to increase post intervention. This provides substantial support for hypothesis 1, that positive behaviour will increase post intervention.

### Hypothesis 2: Negative Behaviours
Table 4 shows the mean behaviour count for each of the negative behaviour categories. From this, it can be seen that hypothesis 2 is fully supported in studies 1, 2, 4, and 5

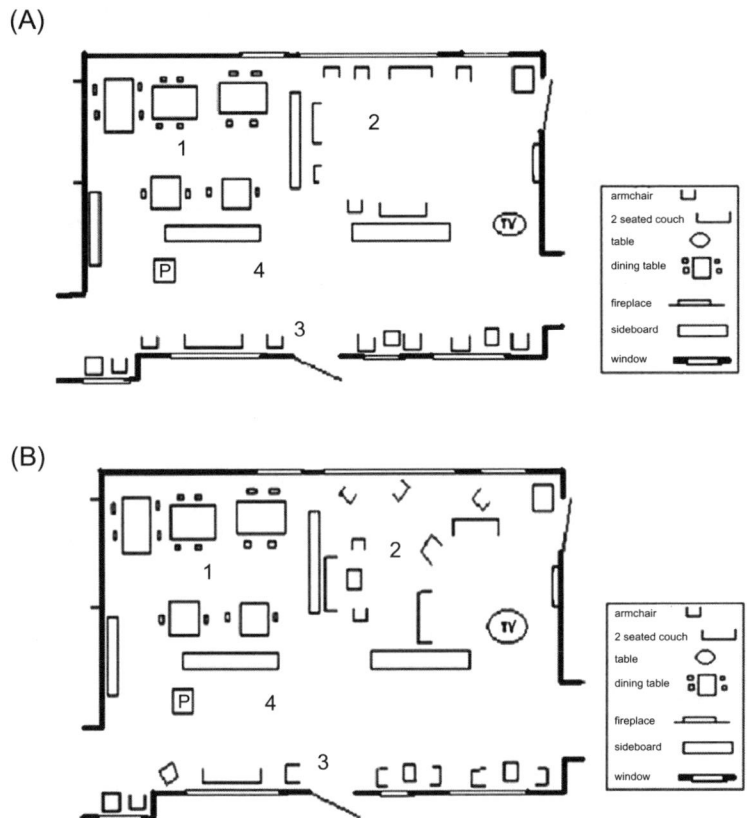

**Figure 1.** (A) Care Home A: pre intervention. (B) Care Home A: post intervention.

**Table 3.** Mean count per 5 min observation of positive behaviour categories

| | Active | | | Content | | | Interaction | | |
|---|---|---|---|---|---|---|---|---|---|
| | Pre | Post | F | Pre | Post | F | Pre | Post | F |
| Case study 1 | 2.17 | 2.28 | 3.84** | 2.54 | 3.24 | 25.579*** | 0.34 | 0.61 | 4.61* |
| Case study 2 | 0.61 | 1.13 | 10.627*** | 1.53 | 2.55 | 44.997*** | 0.20 | 0.34 | 4.746* |
| Case study 3 | 0.28 | 0.41 | ns | 0.51 | 0.84 | 52.479*** | n/a | n/a | |
| Case study 4 | 0.89 | 1.47 | 14.145*** | 1.57 | 1.93 | 14.564*** | 0.25 | 0.38 | 10.28** |
| Case study 5 | 1.2 | 1.38 | ns | 1.7 | 1.93 | 5.564* | 0.51 | 0.47 | ns |
| Case study 6 | 1.16 | 1.5 | 11.519*** | 1.74 | 1.99 | 8.842** | 0.31 | 0.49 | 11.378** |
| Case study 7 | 1.08 | 1.38 | 5.783*** | 1.63 | 1.68 | ns | 0.39 | 0.38 | ns |

$*p < .05$; $**p < .01$; $***p < .001$; $ns$ = not significant; n/a = no sufficient data.

**Table 4.** Mean count per 5 min observation of negative behaviour categories

|              | Passive | | | Agitation | | |
|--------------|---------|---------|-----------|-------|-------|-----------|
|              | Pre     | Post    | F         | Pre   | Post  | F         |
| Case study 1 | 1.68    | 1.14    | 42.145**  | 1.19  | 1.01  | 3.939*    |
| Case study 2 | 0.968   | 0.14    | 247.81*** | 0.48  | 0.08  | 31.694*** |
| Case study 3 | n/a     | n/a     |           | 0.23  | 0.21  | ns        |
| Case study 4 | 0.17    | 0.08    | 12.303*** | 0.26  | 0.14  | 6.036**   |
| Case study 5 | 0.41    | 0.23    | 15.647*** | 0.38  | 0.2   | 8.16***   |
| Case study 6 | 0.24    | 0.17    | ns        | 0.29  | 0.23  | ns        |
| Case study 7 | 0.28    | 0.21    | ns        | 0.32  | 0.17  | 7.26***   |

$^*p < .05$; $^{**}p < .01$; $^{***}p < .001$; ns = not significant; n/a no sufficient data.

and partly supported in study 7 where agitation significantly decreased but passivity did not. Studies 3 and 6 did not provide any support for hypothesis 2 although in the case of study 3, this may be due to an overall low usage of the room in general. Overall, though there is considerable support for hypothesis 2 then there will be a decrease in negative behaviours post intervention.

## Staff Focus Groups and Interviews

The interviews from the staff focus groups and interviews were transcribed and thematically analysed. There were three main themes identified. These were:

- Positive reactions to the intervention,
- Negative reactions to the intervention,
- A resistance to change in the work environment.

Staff from all three of the care homes showed some positive reactions to the intervention. Examples of these are shown in the quotes below:

I think the open window idea, you know that you introduced yourself, people are using the chairs more. Even one resident in particular, who sits in their room a lot, always enjoys coming along and sitting there, definitely. (Care Home A)

You can see how some residents really enjoyed the changes you made. I don't think we realise how much of an effect it can have on them. (Care Home B)

I thought they were really good, especially the window seats. (Care Home B)

During the day a few of them liked sitting looking out of the window. (Care Home C)

I think it looked better as well, rather than having all the chairs sitting in a line, with everyone facing the television. Sometimes they get a bit agitated just sitting in front of the TV all day. (Care Home C)

Within the first theme, staff also identified specific behaviour changes that they had observed which they attributed to the intervention.

Like one lady who normally only speaks to other residents if she's shouting at them, she was sitting in the group of chairs at the window chatting away nicely to other ladies. She seemed to be having a great time. (Care Home B)

The two-seater over at the wall with the table and other chairs, two residents sat there for ages and we gave them tea and cakes and stuff and I think they felt as if they were out somewhere. They liked that. It was different, rather than them just sitting all separate. (Care Home C)

Whilst there were positive reactions to the intervention, staff also perceived some specific problems with the intervention. In general, these were practice related in that the staff perceived the intervention prevented them carrying out an aspect of their job as easily as they had previously. In most cases this referred to moving and handling issues.

When you're using hoists and stand aids for some of the residents you've not got enough room to move about. You know you do not need to keep asking people to move or change where they are comfortable, sort of thing. You can just get in and out without upsetting everybody else. (Care Home A)

It was a bit difficult to get residents in and out the room so we had to move chairs occasionally but we always tried to put them back in the right place. (Care Home B)

The changes in Unit 4 I thought were a bit cramped, you could not get the equipment that we use through, wheelchairs, stand aids, hoists, and we had to move a chair. (Care Home C)

The final theme, resistance to change, was only identified in the focus group in Care Home A. This theme suggested that the change was not welcome in the care home as the staff felt that they knew the residents better and how to address their needs.

They wander, they used to just wander round the room but now they wander round the chairs. We try to put the chairs as close to the wall as possible you know but at an angle so they cannot get past. It means that nobody's getting disturbed and no-one's falling over them, it's practical.

Dementia's an illness and once they're used to their environment to change that environment actually does not help them.

They get used to their way about and ups and downs. They know where everything is ... and if you were to change that in anyway, that automatically can change their mind pattern and it can change their behaviour.

Obviously I understand that people are trying to improve the quality of life for dementia patients without looking at the whole thing; they think automatically oh I'll give them this but they are not looking right into it. The more you put in front of someone with dementia the more confused they become and that does not help. It might not sound right but basic living makes it a lot easier for them. It makes it more complicated by trying to put things in place, it just complicates it more.

The three themes identified in the staff focus groups will be revisited in the discussion section and discussed alongside the objective behaviour measures.

## Discussion

From the behaviour mapping data, there was at least some support in all seven case studies for hypothesis 1, that there would be an increase in positive behaviour post intervention. This indicates that the intervention in each of the case studies was successful in encouraging positive behaviours such as watching TV, looking out the window, social interactions, content behaviour, and other behaviours such as reading, playing games, or purposefully walking. This was an aim of the interventions, in that it was designed to enable residents to engage in more activities (such as watching TV). It has been found that residents with dementia place great importance on being able to engage in everyday activities (Phinney et al., 2007). These results are similar to that found by Devlin (1992) where the introduction of low dividers into a psychiatric day room resulted in more positive use of the space. It may also reflect an increase in the perceived control of the environment as residents have an option of where to sit and can move to avoid stressors in the environment.

Similarly, there was a lot of support from the behaviour mapping data for hypothesis 2, that there would be a decrease in negative behaviour post intervention. From this, it can be concluded that the intervention was successful in reducing the amount of negative behaviours displayed in the area, including passive behaviour and agitation. This may reflect the finding from Calkins (2001) that agitation in people with dementia is reduced in smaller units and smaller group numbers. Although this research did not architecturally reduce the size of the living area, it did create smaller areas out of one large area. This highlights the fact that simple changes can be made to existing environments and yield positive changes in residents' behaviours. This supports the recommendation from Nazarko (2006) that it is important to do all that can be done to break up large living spaces into smaller areas.

When comparing the behaviour mapping results with the staff focus groups, there were a number of similarities between the objective and subjective measures. Both the behaviour mapping results and the staff focus groups highlight the positive impact the intervention had, showing an increase in positive behaviours within residents.

Staff members were able to identify particular changes in residents' behaviours, for instance an increase in residents interacting with each other. In contrast, when considering negative points of the intervention, the care home staff identified more problems than the behaviour mapping results suggest. There were some specific problems highlighted in certain environments by the behaviour mapping data, e.g., in case study 3, where there were no significant changes in behaviour. This was attributed to the existing physical features of the room (poor lighting, limited windows, and location in the care home) resulting in an overall low usage of the space before and after the intervention. Conversely, the staff in all care homes voiced negative concerns about the intervention. These were mainly related to the intervention in some way preventing the staff from doing their job as they had done previously. For example, the previous furniture arrangement allowed staff to use moving and handling equipment in the living area easily, whilst the new arrangement meant that they had to move furniture in order to get the equipment in.

The discrepancies between the behaviour mapping results and the staff views highlight the importance of considering the needs of all users of the environment before implementing design interventions. This is especially important in healthcare environments such as dementia care homes as the care staffs' opinions are very important in the success of any intervention. Previous research has highlighted differences in perceptions of the environment, between both staff and residents (Passini, Pigot, Rainville, & Tetreault, 2000) and also between different types of staff groups (e.g., nursing and administration staff) (Shattell, Andes, & Thomas, 2008). This was evident in the current study as, despite the success of the intervention shown by the behaviour mapping data, the intervention was not kept in place in any of the case studies. Ultimately, the staff has control over the environment, so alter it to make their working environment as straightforward as possible.

In summary, this paper has two separate outcomes. Firstly, the objective behaviour data demonstrates a successful intervention across a number of different dementia living environments. This shows that small, simple interventions can have a positive impact on the behaviour of people with dementia in a care home environment as suggested by Lawton's environmental docility hypothesis (1979). It should be noted however that the intervention was more successful in some of the case studies than others, and future research should attempt to take into account subtle differences between care environments. Secondly, the research highlights the importance of consulting staff when designing the intervention as from the objective impression of the intervention was positive, whilst the subjective impression from the staff had mixed views. These results have important implications for future practice and policy making, stressing the importance of considering the needs of all users in future design interventions in dementia care homes. As this study highlighted the differences in needs of the staff and residents from the environment of the care home it may be that future research needs to investigate ways in which to enable staff members to understand and make changes in the environment to benefit residents. By supporting staff members to do this it gives control of the environment to the staff. As discussed previously, control is a major aspect in the environment-behaviour relationship. If this improves staff perceptions of the environmental changes it may mean that successful environmental interventions such as the one in this study become a permanent feature in the care home environment.

This research is an important starting point for the increase of high quality, empirical research within the field of dementia-friendly environments and environmental psychology. As dementia becomes more prevalent in our society it is important that this strand of research is continued for the following reasons. Firstly, to create dementia-friendly environments that enable and support people with dementia whilst helping family members and care staff to provide a good standard of care. Secondly, upon dissemination of this research and research like this it raises awareness and increases understanding of the disorder and the disabling nature of its symptoms.

# References

Barnes, S. (2006). Space, choice and control, and quality of life in care settings for older people. *Environment and Behavior, 38*, 589–604.

Calkins, M. P. (1988). *Design for dementia: Planning environments for the elderly and confused.* Owings Mills, MD: National Health Publishing.

Calkins, M. P. (2001). Special care units and the environment: Advances of the past decade. *Alzheimer's Care Quarterly, 2*(3), 41–48.

Cohen-Mansfield, J., Werner, M. A., & Marx, M. S. (1989). An observational study of agitation in agitated nursing home residents. *International Psychogeriatrics, 1*(2), 153–165.

Colling, K. B. (2004). Caregiver interventions for passive behaviours in dementia: Links to the NDB model. *Aging Mental Health, 8*(2), 117–125.

Day, K., Carreon, D., & Stump, C. (2000). The therapeutic design of environments for people with dementia: A review of the empirical research. *The Gerontologist, 40*(4), 397–416.

Devlin, A. S. (1992). Psychiatric ward renovation: Staff perceptions and patient behaviour. *Environment and Behaviour, 24*, 66–84.

Ittelson, W. H., Proshanky, H. M., & Rivlin, L. G. (1970). A study of bedroom use on two psychiatric wards. *Hospital and Community Psychiatry, 21*, 25–28.

Judd, S., Marshall, M., & Phippen, P. (1998). *Design for dementia.* London, UK: Hawker Publications.

Lawton, M. P. (1990). Residential environment and self-directedness among older people. *American Psychologist, 45*(5), 638–640.

Lawton, P. (1979). Therapeutic environments for the aged. In D. Canter & S. Canter (Eds.), *Designing for therapeutic environments: A review of research* (pp. 233–276). London, UK: John Wiley & Sons.

Nazarko, L. (2006). Creating the ideal home for people with dementia. *Nursing and Residential Care, 8*(5), 221–223.

Passini, R., Pigot, H., Rainville, C., & Tetreault, M. H. (2000). Wayfinding in a nursing home for advanced dementia of the Alzheimer's type. *Environment and Behavior, 32*(5), 684–710.

Phinney, A., Chaudbury, H., & O'Connor, D. L. (2007). Doing as much as I can do: The meaning of activity for people with dementia. *Aging and Mental Health, 11*(4), 384–393.

Proshanky, H. M., Ittelson, W. H., & Rivlin, L. G. (Eds.). (1970). *Environmental psychology: Man and his physical setting.* New York, NY: Rineheart and Winston.

Schwarz, B., Chaudbury, H., & Brent Tofle, R. (2004). Effect of interventions on a dementia care setting. *American Journal of Alzheimer's Disease and Other Dementias, 19*, 172–176.

Shattell, M. M., Andes, M., & Thomas, S. P. (2008). How patients and nurses experience the acute care psychiatric environment. *Nursing Enquiry, 15*(3), 242–250.

# Environmental Perception, Behavior, and Place-Identity

# A Customisation of Urbanites

## Boosting Place-Identity

### Lineu Castello

Federal University of Rio Grande do Sul (UFRGS), Porto Alegre, Brazil
UniRitter-Mackenzie Universities, Porto Alegre, Brazil and São Paulo, Brazil
CNPq (Brazilian National Research Council), Brasilia, Brazil

**Abstract**

The paper addresses the creation of invented places and their influence on people-environment behaviour, focusing on place-identity. It begins with a brief reconsideration of multidisciplinary understandings of place-identity and an examination of the involvement of planners in the design of places, moving on to investigate the adaptation of urban dwellers to new morphological creations – new places – and their impact on human behaviour. It then considers the creation of new forms of identity being developed amongst today's urbanites in relation to their environment. Changes in place-identities are appreciated through new methodological insights that highlight customisation of their mutual global-local and local-global interaction. The study finally focuses on the consequences for environment-behaviour studies, evaluating variations in relations between place-identity and urban morphologies; urbanity patterns; customised appropriations; and sustainability opportunities.

**Key words:** invented places, place-identity, research links

## Introduction

More than seven billion people live on this planet today. Most of us live in urban environments. Therefore, we are urbanites. An urbanite is a person located in or characteristic of a city or city life. Urbanites are increasingly exposed to new values and visions in the contemporary public realm and are therefore open to customisation through new behaviour. Customisation, one should recall, means making something according to requirements or responding to specific circumstances.

As we critically rethink developments in planning and design and constantly reassess today's built and natural environments, the progress of research in environment-behaviour studies indicates that urban life is also susceptible to extraordinary changes, which is a point rarely taken into account at the field's academic conferences. Urban life actually progresses through change, and the existence of new phenomenological manifestations in person-environment interactivity must be acknowledged, even more so if *place* becomes the key issue. Human beings have an innate disposition for engagement with different spots interspersed in their overall living space, and for selection of a few for attribution of the idiosyncratic *meaning* of *place*, "(...) those units of experience within which activities and physical form are amalgamated: places" (Canter, 1977, p. 1).

Place is a particular spatial quality – a qualified space, in fact – recognised in the environmental sciences as a psychophysical theoretical construct. The characteristics of a place – which can be material and non-material, subjective and objective, inherent or acquired – comprise what can be said to constitute the *place's identity*. This author's field of urban-architectural studies concentrates on the study of places. Among other topics, it is currently involved in deeper examination of two crucial components officially adopted in the field's professional practices, those of employing the policies and practices of placemaking and placemarketing.

# A Symposium on Place-Identity

Place-identity was the subject of a specific Symposium presented at the 22nd International IAPS Conference in Glasgow in June 2012. The Symposium S15 "Place-Identity Research Issues" focused on the relationship between place-identity research issues and their actual and possible impacts on design practice and policy. In addition to our own presentation of the paper "A Customisation of Urbanites" at the Symposium, studies were also presented by Aleya Abdel-Hadi ("Place-Identity Research Issues – Impact on practice and policy"), Mario Paris ("Place-making and Artificial Identity: The example of Superplaces"), and Eman El Nachar ("Place-Identity: An integrative dimension in housing policy").

# Place-Identity: A Multidisciplinary Understanding

Place-identity is a concept that cuts across a number of different disciplines, which allows for differing interpretations that vary according to the original bias of the particular discipline. In urban planning, for example, place-identity is commonly accepted as one of the three components selected by Kevin Lynch (1968, p. 8) as the fundamental determinants of an environmental image (the other two being structure and meaning). In urban design, the British team of architect-planners led by Matthew Carmona, firmly believes "(...) that people need a sense of identity, of belonging to a specific territory and/or group"

(Carmona et al., 2003, p. 97) and illustrates this sense of identity in a specific territory – a place – through the classic cataloguing of *place-insideness* and *place-outsideness* put forward by the geographer Edward Relph (1976) in his earlier studies about place and placelessness. It was also Relph who consciously observed that "Identity of place is as much a function of inter-subjective intentions and experiences as of the appearances of buildings and scenery, and it refers not only to the distinctiveness of individual places but also to the sameness between different places" (Relph, 2007, p. 103). From a psychological point of view, Gabriel Moser (2005, p. 477) had previously remarked that a "(...) way in which place has been related to identity is through *place-identity*, as a specific aspect of identity comparable to social identity". Sociologists are extremely keen on providing vivid narratives portraying place-identity. Focusing on New York's "death and life of authentic urban places," Sharon Zukin, for instance, complains that "One neighbourhood after another had lost its small scale and local identity", adding, "I do miss the look and feel of neighbourhoods whose diversity was tangible in the smells and sounds of ethnic cooking" (Zukin, 2010, p. x). These in themselves offer two admirable images of place-identity, but the portrayal extends even further with her introduction of the French term *terroir*, which denotes the spatial features granted to local foodstuffs (say) by the natural characteristics of a particular place.

The literature about *place* has also evolved to produce a considerable body of multidisciplinary research. Titles generally envisage the *making* of places, often focusing on them in two forms: unplanned and created. Our own research work acknowledges two tenuously differentiated types of place, naming them *spontaneous* and *invented*. Although naturally amalgamated, these two typologies leave room for the addition of two explicit terminologies: places of urbanity and places of cloning (Castello, 2010). Spontaneously generated places are called *places of urbanity* and invented places (i.e., those that try to clone the urbanity found in the spontaneous ones) are said to be *places of cloning*. Our hypothesis is that places of cloning can generate real places of urbanity.

Public spaces in cities today reflect the needs and aspirations of individual communities and of society at large. However, the society of which we are currently a part is different; it is a society of information technology, a condition that enables this society

> [...] to be singled out in relation to others. Firstly, because it is a society occupying a new type of world, an urbanised world. Secondly, because besides being urbanised, it is also a globalised world. (...) Thirdly, because it is a society which is for the first time translating into real terms the shift from the old economy of production into the new economy of consumption (Castello, 2010, p. xv).

In view of changes occurring in contemporary societal behavioural patterns, *changes* in the *types* of places demanded by this society for the enactment of its daily existential practices can also be expected.

This is of course only an assumption, but as such it will pervade the whole of the present document. Such clarification seems necessary here because this idea is sometimes regarded as somewhat provocative, especially in more conservative settings, having already caused minor discomfort on occasions. This is mainly due to the fact that it upsets the balance of some of the more crystallised understandings surrounding the concept of place and the understanding of place-identity. On more than one occasion audiences have reacted with some annoyance when presented with these new places, complaining that they are more than anything typically *non-places* (using the term coined by the anthropologist Marc Augé). Our interpretation sees them as *new* places rather than non-places, and as such, created to meet the requirements of a *new* society. Indeed, it is never too late to emphasize that it is ultimately *people* who decide *what is* or *what is not a place* and definitely not an intellectual aristocracy taking upon themselves the role of teaching people the ideas they have developed about place. Because that is probably just what they have done: developed ideas about it, rather than *experiencing* the new manifestations of urbanity, which they look on with perplexed eyes, outraged by a phenomenon which they still cannot fully grasp.

## *Born to be Wow!* The Practice of Placemaking and Placemarketing

A quick glance at the research linking theoretical progress to professional practice indicates that places are actually planned, designed and evaluated in response to the desire to create a dynamic empathy with users. Consequently, current (post) modern understanding of place, within present realms of (post)modern societal mores, can be accepted to involve a degree of *change in people's behaviour*, which as a result will often call for a *change in people's frame of mind*. In other words the insertion of invented places into traditional environments may lead to a subtle degree of *customisation*.

When coming across this "born to be wow!" advertisement amidst the daily bombardment of media messages, our immediate response led to the world of invented places, recalling the power of (some) invented places to fill people's imaginations with elements of the "anaesthetics of the architectural culture" (Leach, 1999) that invariably endow place with *wow* features in the built environment today, that is, "wild" impressive images. This might in some way explain why some scholars look on invented places with angry antagonism. However, as theoreticians who also work as practitioners have observed, such as Jan Sircus, who worked "(...) as an architect and as a senior Disney 'Imagineer'" (Carmona & Tisdell, 2007, p. 102), "Many interpretations of place might not work for the cultural élite, who demand authenticity, but most places, real or invented, have a pop-culture audience (...). People enjoy both, whether, its place created over centuries, or created instantly" (Sircus, 2007, [2001], pp.126–127).

## Situating Local Place-Identity Within a Global Perspective

One of the typical manifestations of invented places is the insertion of "prettified" images of places for a competitive use of "urbanity" – that unique quality that cities present to their citizens in terms of communication and sociability – as a tool for attracting people and entertaining them in a wide range of iconic places. Empirical research demonstrates that stimuli influencing human experiences in the built environment, usually employed at the macro levels of urban planning policies, are increasingly being adopted on the level of local projects, allowing the presence of global influences to operate in definition of local place-identities. The literature contains interesting research input that can provide guidance for new methodological insights in the area. Three of these will be highlighted in this paper, namely those dealing with changes (i) in the control of land; (ii) in people's behaviour; and (iii) in the uses of vacant land. Each gives rise to new lines of research, dealing as they do with a whole new set of investigative directions, and will therefore be approached individually. Examination of morphological changes attributed to land control will be addressed first, studying the pattern and creation of the fragments introduced into consolidated urban morphologies by invented places. Secondly, the changes in urbanity patterns attributable to the invention of new places will be investigated. Thirdly, the new manifestations introduced by the use of the edges of places and buffer zones in loose spaces nearby and the variations that eventually accrues.

It is our understanding that place-identity is being customised on a local level within a global perspective. It can therefore be assumed that transactions between local *urbanites* and the *built environment* designed under global incentives would tend to become customised.

## Identity and Morphology

One of the major criticisms of the creation of invented places relates to negative effects on the morphology of the consolidated urban fabric, with their insertion often involving discontinuities. According to a British journalist in the United Kingdom "(...) what is increasingly common is the creation of open-air property complexes which also own and control the streets, squares and open spaces of the city. Like Docklands, (...) new places have been created in these former industrial areas (...)" (Minton, 2009, pp. 15–18). Her research indicates that new invented places can create extended urban fragments. This type of morphological configuration has been recorded by several other researchers. One such, with a different scope but providing revealing insights, has been put forward by the research team organised by Kevin Thwaites, also in Britain, which states that a very distinctive phenomenon is being displayed through what they call "transitional edges" (Thwaites et al., 2011). These "transitional edges" establish an interface between built form and open space in urban environments and "(...) are often the focus of social activity and interaction which is not planned but spontaneous and which in many instances are shaped by such social activity" (idem p. 2). Morphologically, a transitional edge may take the form of what the authors call a "segment," an interim part that represents a place in its own identity. These edges are usually "(...) formed from the overlapping of two adjacent spaces and as such possess characteristics that appear as a continuity of both, making a place with its own particular qualities (...)" (Thwaites et al., 2011 p. 6). The resulting configuration

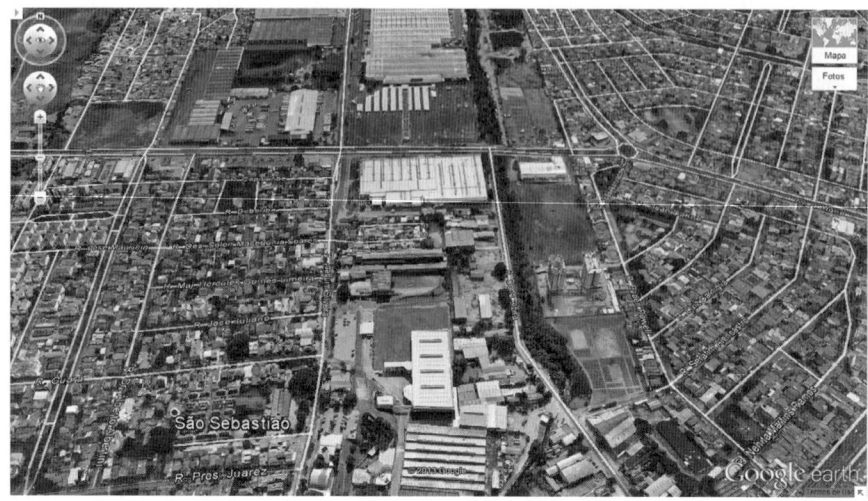

**Figure 1.** Porto Alegre. Turbulent changes in morphological identity. (Map data: Google Earth @ 2013)

reveals different indentations in the fabric, which the authors refer to as "types of segments" (in terms of urban morphology).

Another impressive change introduced by the insertion of invented places can be exemplified in our home city of Porto Alegre in Brazil. Important mixed-use developments are causing severe disruptions to the local traditional fabric of the city, substantially altering the morphology of delineated blocks, obstructing several streets, interfering with local traffic flow and changing the previously consolidated perception of local place-identity. One such fracture can be seen in Figure 1.

Incidentally, in terms of urban design these conditions are said to be the cause of a worrying consequence typical of contemporary urbanisation, which is the urban typology known as the *fragmented metropolis* (Shane, 2011).

## Identity and Urbanity

Urbanity experienced in invented places is subject to variations according to the new identity that starts to "impregnate" the place. The urbanity in these areas may become different from that encountered in spontaneously created places (Castello, 2011b). One famous example can be provided by the widespread provision of new urban shopping malls sprouting up in cities all over the world. The amazing effects introduced by certain malls are leading to an undeniable boost in the perception of urbanity enjoyed inside them. Indeed "(...) certain aspects of urbanity that until recently were the exclusive privilege of the old core cities (...) [are] made possible by the site-unspecific reproduction of "urban" outdoor space inside air-conditioned indoor megaspaces" (Ruby, 2002, p. 24). Taking into account the management and control strategies practiced in such places – both existing and invented –, they can become decisive for the development of urbanity. Security strategies, or rather the *perception* of security strategies, for instance, are much more related to urbanity than might at first be imagined. The extreme care paid to security issues in invented places – a quality often advertised in their placemarketing – can lead to changes in people's behaviour in the newly invented places. It is increasingly acknowledged (albeit indirectly) that "there are psychological dangers (...) in creating places which have too much security and as a result are too safe and too controlled". In the end, they "(...) remove personal responsibility, undermining our relationship with the surrounding environment and with each other and removing the continual, almost subliminal interaction with strangers (...)" (Minton, 2009, p. 33). One surprising by-product of this is that people become more frightened when having to confront unforeseen situations that arise unexpectedly in their daily urban life. In other words, people get used to enjoying urbanity without worrying about security.

Contrasts in the enjoyment of urbanity can be observed in Figures 2 and 3. Figure 2 shows the relaxed (though controlled) urbanity enjoyed in an up-market shopping mall in Stratford (suburban outer London). Figure 3 depicts the urbanity experienced at Camden Lock (local inner London), likely to be accompanied by clear concerns about lack of security.

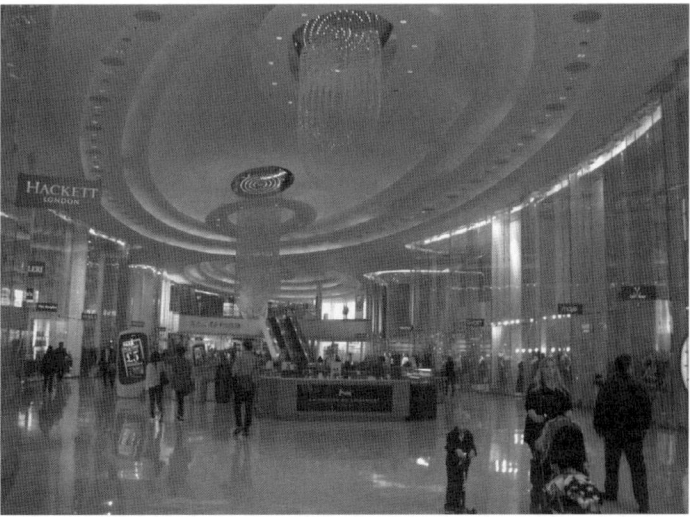

**Figure 2.** Stratford Westfield mall. Changes in urbanity identity.

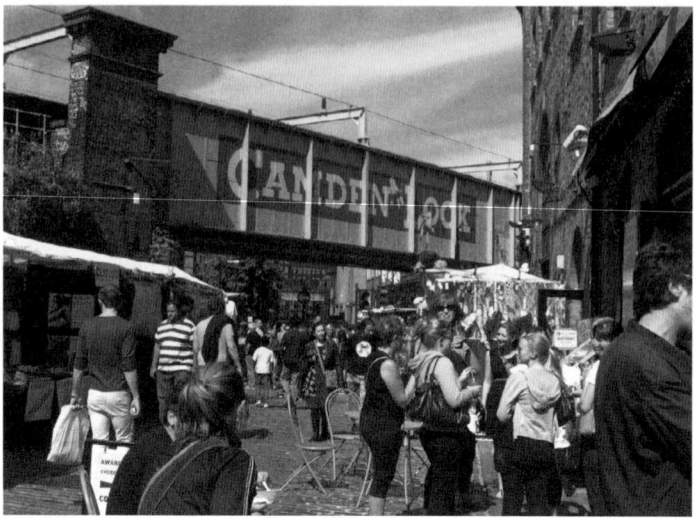

**Figure 3.** London, UK: Camden Lock. Changes in urbanity identity.

## Identity and Appropriation

Recent studies argue that people are appropriating the loose spaces of cities and attributing original uses to them. People appropriate loose urban space "to relax, to protest, to buy and sell, to experiment and to celebrate" (Franck & Stevens, 2007, p. i), and the term "loose space" means a space outside the fixed or primary use it was originally intended for, such as a sidewalk used for the exchange of goods and services, or a brownfield site used as a skateboard area. Bearing this in mind we recently raised the idea of "PlaceLeaks" at the IAPS Korean Regional Symposium, which discusses the occurrence of an overspill of "(...) energies (human, social, economic, cultural, experiential, and so forth) normally concentrated in places, "percolating" to the immediate edges of that place" (Castello, 2011b, p. 3), hence setting up new informal places of urbanity in the surrounding interfaces. PlaceLeaks therefore refers to transitional spaces located comfortably on the edges of contemporary urban interventions and mainly linked to mega-intervention operations. Many of them involve the simultaneous creation of *transitional edges* (Thwaites et al., 2011) located precisely at their interface with the urban fabric, offering supporting energy seen as suitable for the stimulation of new social experiences.

This would apply to many placemaking and placemarketing tactics that include the dramatic insertion of iconic buildings into traditional environments, generally from the hands of today's so-called "starchitects"; or to the re-urbanisation of old disused areas, such as the redevelopment of brownfield sites. This latter case is exemplarily illustrated

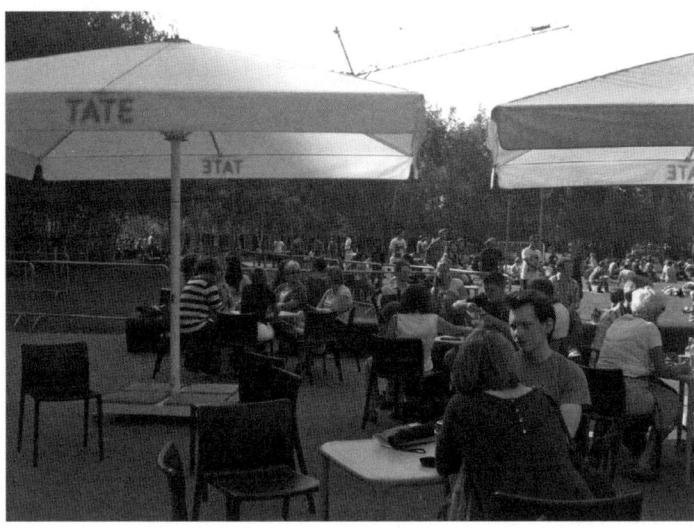

**Figure 4.** London, UK. Leakage of Tate Modern energy spreading across the whole vicinity.

by London's Tate Modern Gallery, designed by the Swiss architects Herzog and de Meuron, whose remodelling of the former Bankside power station has been extraordinarily successful both as a cultural icon and as a place of urbanity, welcoming five million visitors each year. Over and above this, the buffer zone at the edge of the project is experiencing unexpected public appropriation (as seen in Figure 4), pointing to spontaneous and energetic social interaction created from the Tate's leakage of energy, allowing people to express their enjoyment of a place shaped by social forces.

## Identity and Sustainability

Finally, it is worth mentioning another viewpoint here, in which this whole discussion of place can be significantly associated with the quest for more environmentally sustainable development. This issue is convincingly addressed (Castello, 2011a) in a paper recently presented at the International Conference on Green Buildings and Sustainable Cities in Bologna (Italy), albeit in front of a sceptical audience formed mainly of engineers. The paper's topic concerns the assumption that extensive anthropical development of natural environments in actual urbanisation has led urban sustainability to develop a crucial interface that *bridges the behavioural and ecological sciences*. This paper accordingly discusses (i) planning actions for halting urban sprawl, which includes the reuse of

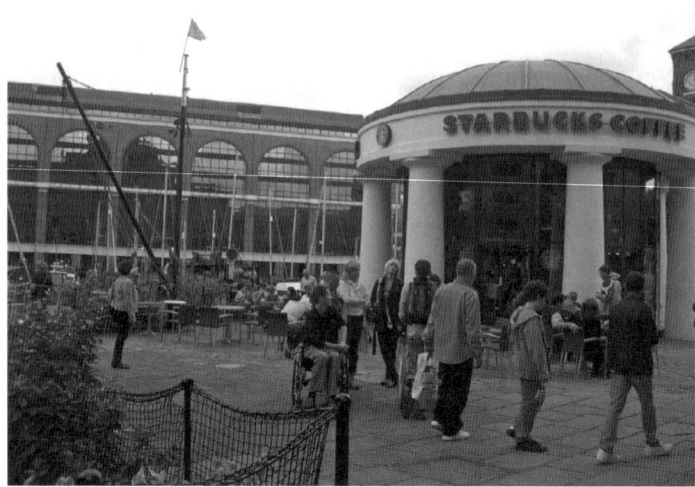

**Figure 5.** London, UK: St. Katherine's Docks. The neighbourhood has been "Starbucked."

abandoned inner-city brownfield areas; (ii) the creation of places imbued with symbolic meaning, such as the reuse of strategic cultural heritage elements; and (iii) a tactical combination of both, encouraging the invention of places in historic brownfield sites. All in all, the concept of urban sustainability can no longer be assumed to be focused solely on *greenfields*, but must allow for the incorporation of other "shades," like the inclusion of *brownfields* at the heart of the concept. Figure 4 provides an illustration of this, showing the creation of a new place in an old brownfield area bursting with identity; similar observations can almost be made of old industrial areas in general, such as St Katherine's Docks in central London, which has been converted into new "mixed use" developments (Figure 5).

## Conclusion

To sum up, it seems likely that urbanites and certain spaces of the cities they inhabit can become closely related; urbanites are used to allocating their symbolic spatial attachment to specific urban spaces they recognize as places; such places become particularly distinguishable among the undifferentiated territorial extent of the rest of the city because they are said to have acquired identity.

Figuratively speaking, one can imagine a sort of *a customisation of urbanites* occurring in contemporary places. This hypothesis, though necessarily disturbing, implies that when design practices and policies are appropriately managed they can effectively influence – and act upon – people-environment transactions between urbanites and their places. Bombarded by the spectacle of carefully designed and managed invented places, urbanites tend to become responsive to the experience of a different kind of urbanity. That is to say, they tend to grow *accustomed to a sort of branded urbanity*, an urbanity progressively inserted into their behavioural patterns through the contemporary practices of placemaking and placemarketing.

One striking consequence of these discussions is the formulation of a further – and unusual – conjecture; that *urbanites react to customisation*. Urbanites customise (so to speak) global issues, as they become accustomed to perceiving them. People react by "imprinting" local identity profiles on places constructed under global directives. Human urbanites practice social customisation and invent new uses for loose spaces. Moreover, they create "PlaceLeaks" alongside their valued places. Although demanding constant monitoring through empirical research, recognition of these new manifestations points to methodological innovations for more relevant urban-architectural goals, aimed at the enhancement of social and environmental achievements through design. This is new!

And more than just new, it supports the need for a full exploration of the inter-relationships between research, policy and practice, to address their likely convergence. Architects "(...) strive towards new figures in which to accommodate public life, emphasize existing forms in which public life continues to take place, or search for new approaches to changing public practices" (Avermaete et al., 2009, p. 11). In this light, the ideas expressed in the paper addressing the occurrence of "PlaceLeaks", in which practitioners avoid the introduction of disruptive aberrations on the margins of their interventions and allow for a freer and more fluent person-environment congruence, stimulate the genesis of new public places alongside the existing repertoire of places. The conference theme of *Planning, Design, and Evaluation in Human Environments* acquires new possibilities in terms of "gluing" the fragments derived from contemporary urban configuration "(...) where multiple urban actors were free to build their fragmentary, utopian designs" (Shane, 2011, p. 203), whose theoretical foundations were established by pioneer architects such as Kevin Lynch and Gordon Cullen.

# References

Avermaete, T., Havik, K., & Teerds, H. (Eds). (2009). *Architectural positions. Architecture, modernity and the public sphere*. Amsterdam, The Netherlands: SUN Publishers.

Canter, D. (1977). *The psychology of place*. London, UK: Architectural Press.

Carmona, M., Heath, T., Oc, T., & Tiesdell, S. (2003). *Public places. Urban spaces*. Oxford, UK: Architectural Press.

Carmona, M. & Tiesdell, S. (Eds.). (2007). *Urban design reader*. Oxford, UK: Architectural Press.

Castello, L. (2010). *Rethinking the meaning of place. Conceiving place in architecture-urbanism*. Farnham (London), UK: Ashgate.

Castello, L. (2011a). A browner shade of green. *Procedia Engineering, 21*, 319–324.

Castello, L. (2011b). Invited symposium. Placeleaks. A passage to place. In *Proceedings of IAPS Network Symposium 2011* [CD-Rom]. Daegu, S. Korea: IAPS-CSBE and Housing Network.

Franck, K. A., & Stevens, Q. (Eds). (2007). *Loose space. Possibility and diversity in urban life.* Abingdon, UK: Routledge.

Leach, N. (1999). *The anaesthetics of architecture.* Cambridge, MA: The MIT Press.

Lynch, K. (1968). *The Image of the city.* Cambridge, MA: The MIT Press.

Minton, A. (2009). *Ground control. Fear and happiness in the twenty-first-century city.* London, UK: Penguin Books.

Moser, G. (2005). Place-identity. In R. W. Caves (Ed.), *Encyclopedia of the city* (pp. 477–478). New York, NY: Routledge.

Relph, E. (1976). *Place and placelessness.* London, UK: Pion.

Relph, E. (2007). On the identity of places. In M. Carmona & S. Tiesdell (Eds.), *Urban design reader* (pp. 103–107). Oxford, UK: Architectural Press.

Ruby, A. (2002). Transgressing urbanism. In J. Brouwer, A. Mulder, & L. Marz (Eds) *TransUrbanism* (pp. 16–31). Rotterdam, The Netherlands: V2/NAI Publishers.

Shane, D. G. (2011). *Urban design since 1945 – A global perspective.* Chichester, UK: Wiley.

Sircus, J. (2007 [2001]). Invented places. In M. Carmona & S. Tiesdell (Eds) *Urban design reader* (pp. 126–129). Oxford, UK: Architectural Press.

Thwaites, K., Romice, O., Porta, S., Mathers, A., & Simkins, I. M. (2011). Invited symposium. Transitional edges. Towards a better balance of form, place and understanding in urban design. In *Proceedings of IAPS Network Symposium 2011* [CD-Rom]. Daegu, S. Korea: IAPS-CSBE and Housing Network.

Zukin, S. (2010). *Naked city. The death and life of authentic urban places.* New York, NY: Oxford University Press.

# Young People's Attachment to Place

Maria Nordström

Stockholm University, Sweden
Swedish University of Agricultural Sciences, Alnarp, Sweden

## Abstract

Childhood places and childhood experiences are often in focus when adults look back and remember places of emotional importance to them. Such places remind them of where they belong, eliciting feelings of attachment. Depending on where they have grown up and their relationships with their families, such feelings seem to differ and are stronger in people with families that were emotionally involved in the physical environment where they have lived, than in people with families without such involvement. In this paper the reason for the difference in emotional engagement with the physical environment is interpreted to depend on the individual person's early experiences and seen as related to attachment behavior in childhood, in which relationships with parents play a decisive part. Place attachment is hypothesized to be strong in individuals with parents emotionally involved with the physical environment where the family has lived and where the individual grew up. This hypothesis is tested in a study, analyzing expressions of wishes for places to live in by young people in two different physical environments in Sweden, the countryside and the big city, with a special focus on adolescents. Adolescence is a period of development when the individual comes to value their previous experiences in new and interesting ways, with consequences for their adult life. During adolescence cognitive achievements become prominent in the young person's attitudes to their environment as well as a new social interest. However, it is also a time of great emotional importance given the fact that the individual is now becoming a person in their own right, establishing their emotional independence and reconsidering, but perhaps not changing the attachment to their childhood places. The background to the hypothesis presented in this paper is a model for a developmental theory of place attachment.

Key words: place attachment, childhood experiences, developmental changes, urban and rural environments

## Place Attachment and Attachment Theory

Place attachment is a concept of long and high standing in environmental psychology (Scannell & Gifford, 2010). The interest of environmental psychologists in the concept has to do with the implication, as stated by Low and Altman in an early paper (1992, p. 6), that "the primary target of affective bonding of people is to environmental settings themselves." However, in the same paper, Low and Altman also made it clear that "a number of scholars indicate how attachment to places may be based on or incorporate other people – family, friends, community, and even a culture" (p. 9). In an effort to combine both the environmental aspect suggested by the concept and its social aspects, Morgan has outlined a developmental theory of place attachment (2010). Morgan's model for a developmental perspective on place attachment can be seen as a reaction to the fact that since the late 1980s "most investigations of the relationship between place and identity have relied heavily on adult focused, cognitive and social frameworks, largely ignoring psychobiological developmental processes, as though place attachment arrives fully formed in adulthood" (Morgan, 2010, p. 14). A developmental perspective offers a way to view the interdependence of environmental aspects with social aspects as it appears in the young individual's experiences. Morgan refers to two motivational systems in the child: (1) that of attachment-affiliation and (2) that of exploration-assertion, which alternate satisfying the individual's need for safety and security by seeking the physical proximity of the parent, the "attachment figure", with satisfying the child's curiosity and need for exploration on their own. The two motivational systems, according to Morgan, form a "sequence/which/results in a to and fro movement between attachment figure and environment" (Morgan, 2010, p. 15). This sequential behavior, which has been characterized as an "attachment-exploration balance" by Bell and Ainsworth (1972), can be observed during all childhood, modified and developed due to the child's growing cognitive and social capacities and new experiences. Sequential behavior in children has been observed in their recurring physical movement to go away from and return back to their home and it has been interpreted as a way to establish a relation with the environment as well as create a notion of their home as a distinct place.

When children start exploring areas away from home, they expand their physical home range successively and stepwise (Gaster, 1995). Leaving home to explore the unknown is a challenge to children and helps them learn about the environment as well as about their own environmental competence (Harloff, Lehnert, & Eybisch, 1998; Moore, 1990). Morgan suggests that it is the interdependence of the two motivational systems, the exploration-assertion system and the attachment-affiliation system, which is the reason why place attachment is emotionally so strongly anchored in the individual, combining their experiences from physical exploration into the environment with their experiences of safety and trust, granted by the attachment figure and their family, in that physical environment. Attachment behavior changes character during childhood and adolescence due to developmental changes in the individual, but as has been pointed out by Allen and Manning (2007), attachment behavior remains operative all life: "Although safety and survival obviously retain their primacy across the life span, on a practical basis, by adolescence the number of situations in which proximity to an attachment person is required to maintain safety and survival has become vanishingly small. This is not to say that the attachment system does not remain operative" (p. 29).

Researchers working in the footsteps of John Bowlby, who formulated the theory of attachment in human relations, showing how attachment behavior during the first year of the child focused on a specific mother-figure (1958, 1969), point out the defining characteristics of attachment. One characteristic of the phenomenon is persistence, which has to do with the fact that attachment "does not wane through habituation" (Weiss, 1991, p. 67). Weiss underlines that "continuing separation from an attachment figure produces pining which abates only slowly and imperfectly. Should inaccessibility of the attachment figure be fully accepted, the result, for an extended interval at least, is not cessation of pining but rather the incorporation of pining in an outlook of despair", meaning that attachment to a person, once established, remains unaltered and sometimes unalterable. The individual does not seem to be able to exchange one attachment figure for another.

It is the hypothesis of this paper that because the attachment behavior of the child takes place early in life and in a specific physical environment, this environment becomes the place of attachment for the child and that just as with the specificity of the attachment figure this environment cannot be replaced by any other for the child. It is here assumed that this is the defining characteristic of place attachment in children and young people and that the place to which the individual is attached, is unique because at the heart of place attachment are specific physical experiences combined with the emotional experiences with specific attachment figures.

With the emphasis on young children's concrete ways of establishing a relationship with place, as well as with an attachment figure, the aim of this paper is to illuminate the quality of persistence in attachment during childhood and youth, without suggesting that to adults, with more flexible ways of understanding and reacting to the environment, place attachments should be seen as static. Brown and Perkins point out that "Transformations in place attachment occur whenever the people, places or psychological processes change over time" (1992, p. 284). In an overall general theoretical framework for place attachment, suggested by Scannell and Gifford, three dimensions of importance to understand place attachment are the following: person, psychological processes and place (2010). The developmental approach in this paper along with the focus on the child's perspective, suggest that the most relevant dimension of Scannell and Gifford's framework is that of psychological processes and more specifically those referring to expressions of feelings and affect.

## Attachment During Adolescence

When the individual child grows up and enters adolescence, the manifestation of their attachment to the place of their childhood comes to the fore, especially if the adolescent has to leave the place to get educated and to earn a living elsewhere. A three-year longitudinal study of youth in rural USA about mental health and occupational choice showed how emotionally hard it was for the youth who decided to move away to do so, while the youth who decided to stay were emotionally better off, despite the fact that the prospects for them of finding jobs and earn a living in the home area were bad (Elder, King, & Conger, 1996). The researchers' assumption was that cognitive development would make it easy for young people to make a choice about their future chances of getting a job and thus to decide where to live. The reason for making the study longitudinal was that the researchers expected changes in the relationships of the young people to their parents as the young people grew older, and in their identity processes making them emotionally more independent and socially more open to people beyond the family. They found that 75% of the youngsters in 8th grade wanted to live near their parents, while three years later in 11th grade only 50% of the young people wanted to do so. The researchers were surprised to find so many of the young people wishing to remain. In the whole group of children the researchers identified three patterns characterising the attitudes of the children to changing places and moving away. One pattern, a stay pattern, was evident in those students who remained attached to their families during the three year period and were committed to living close to their families and remaining in their childhood community. Another pattern, a leave pattern, was of students who were planning to move away from the area, committed to leave their families and childhood communities behind. Finally, a third pattern, a conflict pattern, was of students, who changed their notions during the three year period of the study from first having been committed to leaving the area but later changing their ideas and choosing to stay in the area. Students with a stay pattern had a less promising academic record, less educated fathers and were not inclined to see the job market as a problem.

The youth intent on staying reported better mental health than the two other groups. Staying in the region, however, implied a possible future risk for them, which could put them under socioeconomic stress, something which in turn might affect their family attachment. "Economic hardship tends to weaken ties to parents", Elder, King, and Conger point out (p. 400). The youngsters with a leave pattern, the group intent on leaving high school and their childhood environment and with good prospects of succeeding academically and eventually professionally, were not as well off psychologically and this was also the case for the students in the conflict group. Eventually the leave group may find compensation later on in life, the researchers speculate, trading short term distress at youth for long-term gains.

This interesting study shows that to leave their parents, their community and the environment where they have grown up, comes at a cost to young people and that this is not an easy step to take, however promising the future might seem. The well-being of the group of young people with a stay pattern reflects the emotional importance to young people both of the relationship to the physical place where they grew up and to their parents.

A limited Swedish study can add some more light to this interdependence of parents and place for children's place preferences (Trondman, 2000). A questionnaire about their ideas for a future place of residence was distributed to two groups of children living in a small rural town One group of children was middle class with parents working as civil servants and without any tradition of living in the town or belonging to the environment, while the other group was working class and firmly rooted in the town for generations. Trondman, a sociologist, found that the working class children saw themselves as less inclined to leave the rural town than the middle class children, even though a growing number of working class children, as they grew older, stated that they would move away. However, there were clear differences between the children with an attachment to the place and those without. This difference, Trondman concluded, had to do with the fact that middle class children were taught by their parents, themselves lacking an attachment to the place, to be prepared to move away for education and work and to be ready to "take off" as soon as opportunities presented themselves (Trondman, 2000, p. 73). The important addition to Trondman's conclusion from the perspective of environmental psychology is that the place as well as the parents should be seen as important to the place attachments shown by the working class children, making their decision to move away so much more difficult than for the children without such an attachment, as Elder, King, and Conger showed in their study. What is shown by both Trondman and Elder, King and Conger is that individuals' attachment to place is not a rational matter, dominated by cognitive thinking, but linked to the individuals' emotional dependence on and relationships with their families and their life together in the specific physical environment where the individual has grown up.

## Expressions of Place Preferences by School Children Living in Different Swedish Environments

In a follow-up to a comprehensive study on children's environmental conceptualization seen from the perspective of developmental psychology, in which the conceptualization was interpreted in analyses of written essays by children 8 to 17 years old (Nordström, 1990), essays were collected to find out how children's different environmental backgrounds might be reflected in such essays. The reason for doing this follow-up study was a finding in the first study of a small sample of essays, written by countryside children, which were clearly deviant from the essays by the majority of children, who were urban and middle class. In the first study three different cognitive developmental patterns were found, one for children aged 8–12, another for children 13–15, and a third pattern for children 16–17 years old. In the follow-up study this developmental pattern was used to collect essays by children aged 10, 15 and 18 years. Twenty essays by school children in each age group were collected, making a total of 120 essays (Nordström, 2000a, 2000b). One group was living in a remote area of the Swedish countryside and the other group was living in Sweden's capital city, Stockholm. Stockholm is the most prosperous area of the country, while the rural area, from which the countryside children were selected, the southeastern corner of Sweden, is an area with little economic development and with bad prospects for work. The essays were content analyzed in the same way as in the first study.

The instruction to the school children, who wrote their essays in the manner of traditional school compositions, was that they should write what the title, "This is how I would like to live", made them think of as they heard the title from the person giving them the instruction to write the essay. No other instructions were given to the school children, which makes it possible to understand the essays in psychological terms as an expression of free association to the theme of the essay.

In the following, the content analyses of the essays by each age group will be presented and the similarities and differences of the essays by the urban and the rural children will be described. The essays written by the 10-year old countryside children show an intense physical engagement with the environment and often too with persons of the family and friends in their community. The school children write about what they do, what places look like where they like to be and they describe the look of the houses where they live. Nature is present in many essays and especially the boys describe sensual qualities experienced by them when in contact with nature: "There is a meadow close to our house. It is very nice on warm summer nights, especially when the grass has been mowed down." Another boy of the same age writes that he would like to live "close to a calm river. I would look at the river and fish in it." Comparing the essays by the countryside children with those by the urban children, an environmental engagement similar to that of the young countryside children was not found. The urban children write about imagined places, places that they once had visited or where they had spent their holidays, but not about places or their homes in their everyday environment. They present ideas about places, some of which are highly imaginative like "living on the moon" and "in a rocket in the sky", rather than their own experiences of specific places.

A common pattern in the essays by the 15-year old children living in the same remote countryside as the 10-year old children is that they imagine that they will move away for a while and live in different circumstances from now but that later on, with a family of their own, they will return to live a life similar to the one they now live and know well. They do not demonstrate a wish to look out for different and unknown experiences. Two girls even express wishes to continue to live as they now live, in a way similar to that of the 10-year old children. One of the girls enumerates in the manner of an inventory the animals on her parents farm, where she now lives, as well as the different buildings on the farm, what the dwelling-house looks like and what plants and trees there are in the garden. This essay portrays a person anchored in present time and in the place of her childhood. The other girl starts her essay by declaring that "I want to live just as I now live." She too enumerates what kinds of animals there are on her parents' farm but she also describes a bit of the country-side landscape: "there is a river near-by and small roads with gravel, not asphalt", the last comment seems to indicate that lacking asphalt roads is a good thing. The ending of the essay reads: "My father has taught me how to drive a tractor so sometimes I am the one who is out in the fields driving, plowing or harrowing the fields."

Neither of these girls seems to anticipate breaking away from their family to settle anywhere else as of now, and, in particular, the girl, who takes pride in being able to help her father in the work on the farm, driving the tractor, seems to envision staying on the farm to work there. In the terms of Elder, King, and Conger, these girls can be said to display a stay pattern in their plans for the future. Other children in this countryside group indicate that breaking up from home will be complicated. The reader gets the impression that the children hesitate to pronounce their own wishes. They write that they like living as they do at home and they describe the houses where they live, sometimes with a modest alteration, gently expressed here by one girl: "If I could change one thing in our house that would be that I do a door with a proper lock." She concludes her essay by writing that "It does happen sometimes that I want to live at the outskirts of our village, in the countryside with a lot of animals and a forest nearby with hardwood trees, where you can go horse-riding." At the very end of her essay, she finally expresses her wish: "a big nice house with a whirlpool bath!" Wishing for a life of one's own, meaning breaking away from one's parents and the childhood environment, is clearly not an easy matter.

The urban 15-year old school children do not mention their parents with the exception of one boy, who wants to leave the city to settle in the countryside, from where his family comes, and one girl, who mentions that she is pleased to live as she now lives, in the apartment of her parents. The remaining urban children mention and describe instead the material character of their wished for dwellings, most often flats, and they indicate where they want these to be located, all in big cities, some of which are foreign cities, choices which might stem from ideas or from something they have heard about, meaning that these children appear to be open to novelty and the unknown.

The essays by the oldest group of the rural students, 18 years of age, doing their last year of school, show interesting changes from the essays by the 15-year old students. Nobody writes that they will keep on living as they now do, i.e., to live with their parents, and parents are not mentioned. No one writes about living in the countryside. When they mention their childhood places they do so to motivate their choices of qualities in their projects for the future. They want to find houses with similar qualities to what they have been used to during their childhood. Creating a world of their own, then, does not mean that they want to leave behind the qualities that they have experienced as young persons. One countryside boy writes that he wants to live as he always has done "apart from the fact that I live in the city." Another boy states that he would like to live somewhere "where I feel welcome and at home." The rural 18-year old students clearly have accepted the fact that they will have to move away from their childhood environment to find a job. They will choose a city not too far away from their parents or they will find a second home in the countryside to keep contact with their places of attachment and with their families. They express a sensibility to the environmental qualities of where they will live and express the need of having to counteract the disturbing and hectic qualities of urban living which they anticipate and which they express some anxiety about. The general impression from the essays by the rural 18-year old students is that their childhood environment still plays an important role in their lives. The essays by the urban 18-year old students are more disparate in character than those by the rural students. There are a few essays in which childhood environment experiences stand out as important but most essays express no specific wishes for a place to live in and some students seem to be at a loss what to wish for. An echo from the essays by the youngest urban essay-writers, the 10-year old ones, can be found in the urban 18-year-old ones' wishes to live "in the middle of a desert", "in hotels" or "in a more harmonious society." Among the urban youth is a boy with a countryside background, something which he admits does influence his desire to move away from the big city to settle in a small community similar to the one where he grew up. He stresses that his family is what is most important to him.

## Conclusions From the Study

Summarizing the result of the study by analysing the essays by the 10, 15 and 18-year old school children, it is clear that the rural children at all ages express a feeling of what can be called an attachment to place. With single exceptions, no such expressions were found in the essays by the urban school children. The rural children mention more environmental qualities than the urban children and they express personal experiences more than the urban children, whose essays have an abstract quality because they are dominated by ideas rather than experiences. Another difference between the two groups is that the rural school children more often mention their families and their friends than the urban school children. A conclusion of the study is that environment to the rural children seems to be more of a reality than for the urban children, indicating that the urban children do not seem to have attachments to places in the way that the rural children seem to have. The differences found between the school children at all three levels of development indicate that the school children's wishes for a place to live in is an expression of a real psychological difference between the two groups.

## Final Remarks

Place attachment is perhaps a phenomenon most easy to recognize in the adult person as they give evidence of it when making a choice where to live, when a choice is possible to make. When individuals have not been able to make such choices or when disruptions in their place attachments occur, people have shown depression-like psychological reactions (Brown & Perkins, 1992; Fried, 1963; Matt, 2011), attesting to how fundamental place attachments "are to the experience and meaning of everyday life" (Brown & Perkins, 1992). In this paper an effort has been made to try to understand place attachment in young people by studying children's changing notions of place as they grow and reach adolescence from a developmental perspective. The hypothesis put forward about place attachment, as related to the inseparable experiences in the young child of both places and parents according to the developmental theory proposed by Morgan, seems to be supported by the analyses made of Swedish school children's wishes for a place to live in. The analyses show that when children grow up in an environment where the physical environment is accessible and used by them and their parents, the attachment of the children to their parents and to the environment is more clearly pronounced than when children grow up in a place where there is no such environment at hand. In many countries today, processes of urbanization are taking place at high speed. Sweden is the country in Europe where urbanization is most rapid and Stockholm is a city with exceptionally quick and dense building, resulting in housing environments with few outdoor places accessible for children and their parents to use. The main conclusion from this study is that when the physical environment is accessible and used by children and their families, it makes it possible for them to get emotionally involved with the places where they live and the physical environment is therefore of great emotional value. This environmental value should be taken into account by politicians and planners as they decide on and plan housing areas and physical space.

# References

Ainsworth, M. D. S. (1989). Attachments beyond infancy. *American Psychologist, 44*, 709–716.

Allen, J., & Manning, N. (2007). From safety to affect regulation: Attachment from the vantage point of adolescence. *New Directions for Child and Adolescent Development, 117*, 23–39.

Bell, S. M, & Ainsworth, M. D. S. (1972). Infant crying and maternal responsiveness. *Child Development, 43*, 1171–1190.

Bowlby, J. (1958). The nature of the child's tie to his mother. *International Journal of Psycho-Analysis, XXXIX*, 1–23.

Bowlby, J. (1969). *Attachment and loss. Vol. 1: Attachment*. New York, NY: Basic Books.

Brown, B. B., & Perkins, D. D. (1992). Disruptions in place attachment. In I. Altman & S. M. Low (Eds.), *Place attachment. Vol. 12: Human behavior and environment. Advances in theory and research* (pp. 279–304). New York, NY: Plenum Press.

Elder, G. E. Jr., King, V., & Conger, R. D. (1996). Attachment to place and migration prospects: A developmental perspective. *Journal of Research on Adolescence, 6*(4), 397–425.

Fried, M. (1963). Grieving for a lost home. In L. J. Duhl (Ed.), *The urban condition* (pp. 151–171). New York, NY: Basic Books.

Gaster, S. (1995). Rethinking the children's home-range concept. *Architecture & Comportement/Archtitecture & Behaviour, 11*(1), 35–41.

Harloff, H. J., Lehnert, S., & Eybisch, C. (1998). Children's life world's in urban environments. In D. Görlitz, H. J. Harloff, G. Mey, & J. Valsiner (Eds.), *Children, cities, and psychological theories. Developing relationships* (pp. 55–84). Berlin, Germany: Walter de Gruyter.

Low, S. M., & Altman, I. (1992). Place Attachment. A Conceptual Inquiry. In I. Altman & S. M. Low (Eds.), *Place attachment. Vol. 12: Human behavior and environment. Advances in theory and research*. New York, NY: Plenum Books.

Matt, S. J. (2011). *Homesickness: An American history*. New York, NY: Oxford University Press.

Moore, R. C. (1990). *Childhood's domain. Play and place in child development*. Berkeley, CA: MIG Communications.

Morgan, P. (2010). Towards a developmental theory of place attachment. *Journal of Environmental Psychology, 30*, 11–22.

Nordström, M. (1990). *Barns boendeföreställningar i ett utvecklingspsykologiskt perspektiv/Children's Conceptions of how they would like to live. A developmental psychology perspective*. Gävle, Sweden: Statens Institut för Byggnadsforskning.

Nordström, M. (2000a). *Känslan för platser. En jämförande utvecklingspsykologisk studie ab barns och ungdomars värdering av fysisk miljö i Sverige och Frankrike, Del 1: Landsbygdsbarn* [Sense of place. A comparative-developmental psychology study of how children and youth value their physical environment in Sweden and France. Part 1: Countryside Children]. Stockholm, Sweden: Kulturgeografiskt seminarium 1/00, Stockholm University.

Nordström, M. (2000b). *Rummet som plats. En jämförande utvecklingspsykologisk studie ab barns och ungdomars värdering av fysisk miljö i Sverige och Frankrike, Del 2: Stadsbarn* [A space to live in. A comparative-developmental psychology study of how children and youth value their physical environment in Sweden and France. Part 2: City Children]. Stockholm, Sweden: Kulturgeografiskt seminarium 1/00, Stockholm University.

Scannell, L., & Gifford, R. (2010). Defining place attachment: A tri-partite organizing framework. *Journal of Environmental Psychology, 30*, 1–10.

Trondman, M. (2000). Att flytta eller stanna, det är frågan. Om barns och ungdomars föreställningar om att vilja bo kvar i Hällefors eller att flytta [To move away or to stay. About children's and youth's notions about remain in Hällefors to move away]. In G. Graninger, G. Blücher, & L. Nyström (Eds.), *Vi flytt nu. Om befolkningsflyttningarna i Sverige*. Karlskrona, Sweden: Vadstena Forum.

Weiss, R. S. (1991). The attachment bond in childhood and adulthood. In C. Murray Parkes, J. Stevenson-Hinde, & P. Marris (Eds.), *Attachment across the life cycle* (pp. 66–76). London, UK: Routledge.

# Urban Parks in Curitiba, Brazil

## Visibility and Permeability Analyses of Internal and External Configurational Properties

Renato Tibiriçá de Saboya, Sofia Arrias Bittencourt,
Mariana Colin Stelzner, and Vera Helena Moro Bins Ely

Architecture and Urban Design Department, Federal University of Santa Catarina,
Florianópolis, Brazil

**Abstract**

Visibility and permeability are important factors shaping architectural spaces. In this paper, we analyse patterns of visibility and permeability integration and their relation to patterns of movement and co-presence in an urban park in Curitiba – PR. A theoretical and methodological difficulty emerged concerning the formal definition of barriers to physical permeability, since many spatial elements cannot be considered as actual barriers to movement, but are perceived as such to varying degrees of intensity. To examine these subtleties, several alternative descriptions of barriers were tested and compared against observed patterns of movement and co-presence, gathered in on-site observations. The analyses showed that the internal configuration of the park and its relation to the street grid in which it is located, can influence the use and distribution of activities. The results also show that subtle barriers like curbs and benches can also strongly affect the way the park is used, with global integration values being more successful in predicting density of appropriation than pure visibility measures. Nevertheless, there is evidence that visibility levels influence the behaviour of vulnerable groups, driving them away from areas with low visibility.

**Key words:** integration, permeability graphs, space syntax theory, urban parks, visibility graphs

## Introduction

Green urban areas contribute to the qualification and function of city spaces. In addition to active and passive leisure they: provide ornamentation and a sense of identity to neighbourhoods or even entire cities, promote social interaction, create local microclimates, and contribute to environmental preservation and biodiversity. Parks contribute to the integration and leisure of its users, providing spaces for several activities. The possibilities of engaging in active and passive activities make parks one of the most democratic spaces available today. This democratic trait stimulates the co-presence of people from different social backgrounds, races, cultures, and origins, which allows their interaction or, at least, mutual consideration and awareness of one another and of social diversity.

However, for this experience to be fulfilled, the spatial organisation of the park must be adequate to facilitate its comprehension and use. In the same way, their integration into the urban tissue must encourage their appropriation by encouraging the flow (especially of pedestrians) towards the inside portions of the park and, if possible, connection to important sections of the city.

The design, configuration, orientation, and relationship of the parks features may also have a significant role to play in users' patterns of behaviour (Alexander, Ishikawa, & Silverstein, 1977; Gehl, 2011; Jacobs, 1961). This paper seeks to use a central urban park in Curitiba, Brazil as a specific case study to explore its defined properties. Specifically it addresses the parks internal configuration in relation to its immediate surroundings, focusing on the spatial patterns, visibility, and permeability. It also examines the link, if any, between the park characteristics and the way they relate to movement and co-presence patterns observed empirically. In order to do this, we use the concepts and tools of Space Syntax Theory (Hillier & Hanson, 1984; Turner, Doxa, O'Sullivan, & Penn, 2001). Space Syntax theory allows the topological configuration of an environment to be considered in relation to its independent component variables. In the context of this study, Space syntax is particularly useful in describing and analysing patterns of designed space. The underlying theory seeks to address: How can we measure the configurational properties of spatial systems? What is the role of configuration in movement, co-presence, and higher order social phenomena? (and) What is the nature of the relationship between social organisation and spatial configuration?

## Hypotheses

The study has an exploratory nature. Nevertheless, there are some underlying assumptions providing guidance to research efforts that may be seen as hypotheses:

- Areas with more visibility and visual integration are more heavily used than areas with low visibility and visual integration.
- The structure of barriers to movement creates spaces with more or less physical

integration, which in turn leads to more or less appropriation, respectively.
- Elongated areas tend to have more movement of people, whereas more convex areas tend to be used by people in static activities.
- Areas with less visibility tend to drive off people in more vulnerable groups: especially women and children.

## On Visibility and Permeability

The interplay between space visibility and accessibility is one of the most important tools available to designers when thinking about and organising architectural space (Koch, 2010). These aspects often interact in complex ways in order to: elicit meanings, suggest patterns of behaviour, create opportunities for interaction, express different values, and so on.

Areas which can be easily seen tend to be used more frequently. That presumably happens because people would be able to: (a) see that it exists as opposed to spaces which cannot be easily seen and may go unnoticed by those unfamiliar with the place, (b) see what is happening in it, which in turn may act as motivation for joining these activities (Gehl, 2011; Jacobs, 1961), and (c) estimate its safety in terms of the degree to which it can be surveyed by people in adjacent areas. Moreover, the mere possibility of seeing a space brings it "closer" to one's subjective world and tends to make it more present in his or her daily thoughts and decisions[1] (Kahneman, 2011). In addition, areas that can be seen from many other locations provide constant information to the observer as to where he or she is and therefore can be used as reference points in a complex environment. This makes the task of moving through space less demanding from a cognitive effort perspective:

> If we hold length constant and break the same length of line into segments and connect them at angles which prohibit continuous visibility [. . .], we do not add significantly to the energy effort required to move along it, but we do add greatly to the informational effort required. (Hillier, 2003, p. 2–3).

Visibility, therefore, is a vital component of legibility. On top of this cognitive function, highly visible spaces are often the site where special architectural elements are located, such as monuments and important religious and civic buildings. Likewise, other meanings can be suggested by the manipulation of visibility levels: spaces with high visibility tend to be associated with importance, distancing, power, formality, legibility, collectivity, publicness, sacredness, and uniqueness. Conversely, low visibility spaces are usually

---

[1]    Kahneman (2011) explains this phenomenon from the standpoint of cognition in what he calls the "what you see is all there is" effect.

perceived as being introverted, secretive, auxiliary, regular, private, and ordinary. Nevertheless, the fact that not all spaces with high or low visibility elicit the kinds of meanings outlined above shows that there are other factors interacting with visibility in order to accomplish them. Among these factors are: size, colour, cultural background, local history, and the relations established to the surroundings. In addition to these factors, accessibility afforded by the design and location of the park in conjunction with transportation links to it are also important factors. Also among them is the accessibility afforded by a space, understood as the ease with which it can be physically reached.

The relationship between visibility and accessibility is neither simple nor direct. The physical distance of an element, for example, when combined with high visibility may reinforce the meaning of distance in a symbolic or social hierarchy. In this regard we may think of Greek temples or Brazilian colonial churches located on hills, removed from the everyday activities of the city but constantly visible during the movements of daily life. This asymmetry may also be used to explain functional requirements, as it happens with a stage: despite being highly visible, its accesibility is very limited.

We therefore have a range of possible meanings associated with the combinations of high and low visibility in conjunction with high and low accessibility:

- High visibility/high accessibility: functional and visual reference point, collective, public, formal, civic, extroverted, powerful.
- High visibility/low accessibility: symbolic reference, important, powerful, distant (in a social scale), sacred, exposed.
- Low visibility/high accessibility: secondary, auxiliary, ordinary.
- Low visibility/low accessibility: low importance, service-related, individual, private, introverted, distant (both physically and in a symbolic sense).

## Method

The research begun with a comparison of two parks, Passeio Público and Bosque João Paulo II, and how their insertion into the urban fabric affected their use by the population. After the initial thoughts to compare different park locations it was evident the extent and depth of the variables contained in the research warranted the use of a more focused approach. The use of space syntax to investigate the relationship between visibility and accessibility and patterns of movement and co-presence is complex and therefore considered an appropriate method. Nevertheless, we felt the need to deepen the analysis in order to investigate in more detail the internal configuration of the park and the relationships among visibility and accessibility as explored briefly above, as well as observed patterns of movement and co-presence. Therefore, we selected one of the parks as a case study, Passeio Público, to carry out the new set of analysis described in this paper.

A description of users' appropriation of the park was initially explored. This involved recording the users' location on a typical day on video and converting it to points in a Geographic Information System (GIS) as a "snapshot" of users locations. In addition information regarding their age group, gender, and the type of activities (static or dynamic) they were engaged in were recorded. With this data, an appropriation density raster layer was generated on the GIS using a Kernel Algorithm and an 18 m radius.[2]

The park morphology and configuration and, more particularly its visibility and accessibility patterns, were analysed by means of Space Syntax methodological instruments mainly through isovists, two-dimensional polygonal representations of the visible area from a particular point (Benedikt, 1979; Hillier, 2007; Hillier & Hanson, 1984). The isovist size gives an approximation of the visual control of a location. The process describes, in a quantitative manner, the number of other points it can see as well as its visual prominence by indicating the quantity of points from which it can be seen. This is the first measure used in the analysis and is also known as "visibility connectivity," since every point in an isovist is considered connected to each other in a graph and, in a raster layer, the number of points corresponds to its area.

Integration was used to capture the degree to which each space is close to every other space in the system.[3] Regarding isovists, the integration measure corresponds to the inverse of the minimum number of "topological steps" necessary to reach every other point in the system. Points in space connected to each other, within the context of an isovist, are considered 1 topological step apart. Hence, "Global Integration," (also known as Rn) is inversely proportional to the quantity of changes in direction from a given point in space, needed to reach every other point. It therefore "[...] provides useful information about the number of decisions people will have to make to reach a destination point" (Kalff et al., 2012, p. 12). Integration using isovists may be calculated using eye-level barriers or "knee-level" barriers, the latter being referred to as "permeability" analysis, since it fundamentally deals with barriers to movement and not visibility.

In order to generate the syntactic map, a fundamental input is the system of barriers and permeability. With regards to visibility, barriers are evident enough, especially in a nearly flat terrain as in the case with Passeio Público. The barriers to movement, on the other hand, are a little trickier to assess. The Space Syntax Theory is usually applied in larger scale analysis and therefore limits the inclusion of barriers to clear-cut boundaries between public and private realms, such as buildings and walls. Nevertheless, in the microscale adopted for this study, waist-level obstacles may be considered barriers, although they could be transposed if needed. Even more ambiguous is the barrier effect posed by plant beds. In some cases their transitions to the park's paths were very subtle, with virtually no difference in height.

---

[2]   Alexander et al. (1977) argue that this is the maximum radius within which people can interact satisfactorily in public spaces.

[3]   For more details on the measure of spatial integration and the concept of "closeness" as put forward by the Space Syntax, please refer to Hillier et al. (1987) and Hillier and Hanson (1984).

In order to account for these subtleties, as well as evaluate different ways of modelling the system of barriers and permeability, four alternative descriptions were tested:

- Description 1 considered only barriers to visibility, such as walls, and dense vegetation.
- Description 2 added permeability barriers that don't necessarily block visibility, like lakes and fences.
- Description 3 took into consideration all barriers from descriptions 1 and 2 and added knee-level barriers such as benches and handrails.
- Description 4 included, below knee-level elements, notably plant beds.

Because of space limitations, the maps presented on this paper refer only to descriptions 1 and 4 (Figure 1).

## Results

Figure 1 shows a simplified map of the park. It is located in the central area of Curitiba and its interface to the urban fabric is mediated by four entrances, since the perimetre is constituted by fences that provide visibility but not permeability to movement.

## Visibility Maps

The first map in Figure 2 depicts actual barriers to visibility, such as walls, buildings and dense vegetation (see Figure 1). It shows that the most visible areas are the corners, which is a usual outcome in this kind of map. These high visibility areas coincide with bus stops and main park entrances. This shows coherence in their location, if the goal was to make them easily visible and found by pedestrians from the surrounding streets. These high visibility areas fade smoothly to a medium level at a central area of the park (in light grey in Figure 2) which also happens to be the most intensely used. Low visibility areas are mostly confined to the east portion, because of a large vegetation mass acting as a visual barrier.

Although the inner park may be considered to be visually integrated to the outside area as it can be seen from the outside, it is not completely physically integrated. This happens because the outer fence poses no barrier to visibility, but prevents movement in all but a few entrance points along the edge of the park. This condition allows outside pedestrians to have a good visual grasp of its interior, which may act as a stimulus for going in and spending time in it. Nevertheless, if they choose to go in, they have to reach very specific access points. This can be partially overcome by the current location of the entrances that

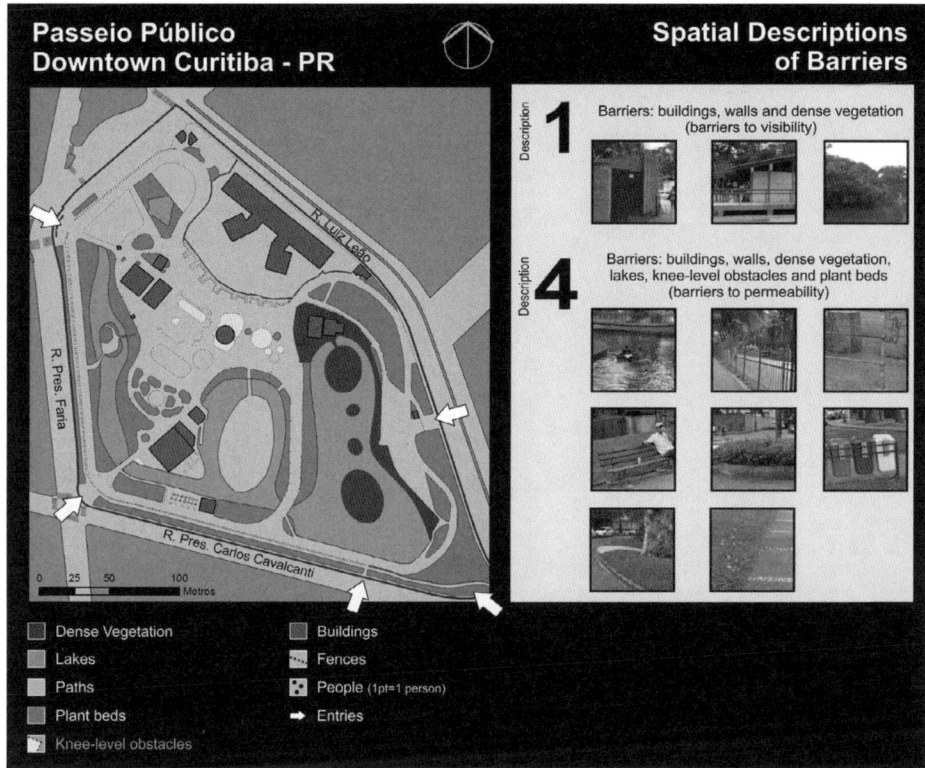

**Figure 1.** Passeio Público's plan and spatial description of barriers to visibility and access.

try to take advantage of the pattern of movement from the outer grid, but it is clear that a more permeable boundary would tend to improve the park's overall accessibility. This is one of the main factors influencing the spatial configuration and perception of the park, since it creates a marked difference between visibility and permeability patterns. We will explore this aspect in more detail below.

On the second map of Figure 2, which excludes the surroundings, it is possible to observe the internal organisation of the park without the interaction with the outside. There appears to be a large central area with high visibility, which is also related to the two main entrances of the park (on the west portion) and the area with the highest presence of users. On the other hand, we note that the area with the lowest degree of visibility is also the portion with correspondingly lower presence of users. Because of this, users approaching the park from the east are offered a very low visual appreciation of the park. This undermines the cognitive incentive that could exist if its inner spaces and other attractive features were seen by passersby.

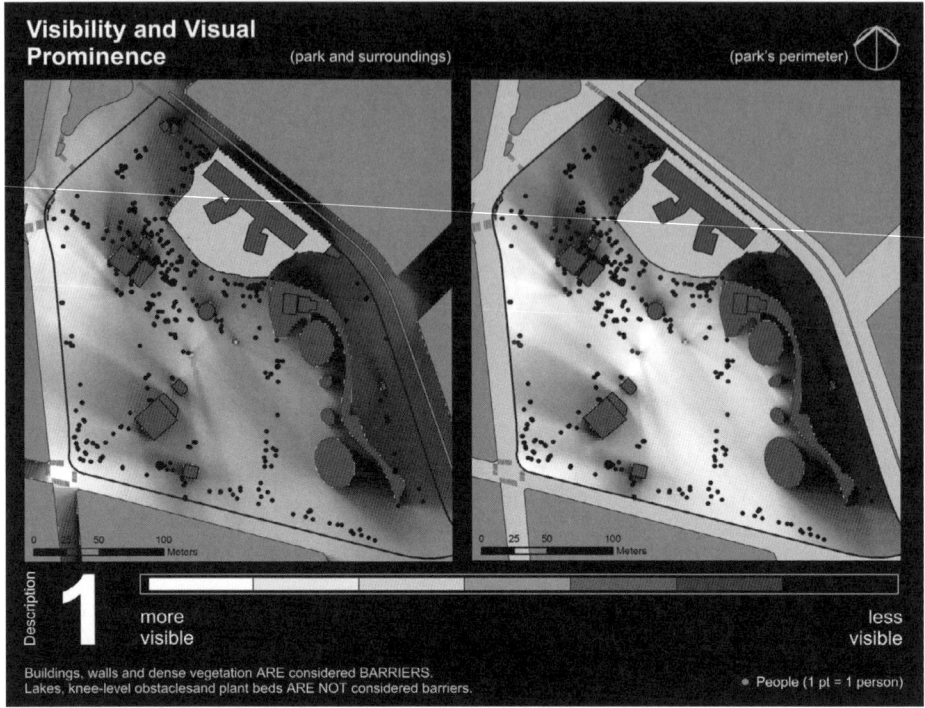

**Figure 2.** Description 1: Visibility analysis. Users are represented by black dots.


## Permeability Maps

The following maps depict permeability patterns with a description that encompasses the largest range of barriers (description 4). The objective here is to evaluate how much the "virtual barriers" influenced movement patterns and stationary activities.

With the addition of barriers that allow visibility but block movement, the difference in integration levels between inside and outside becomes steeper. It becomes clear that the outer fence has a significant impact on the integration levels inside the park with regard to permeability patterns. With entries restricted to a few points, the park becomes a separate space. The obvious restrictions in access act as a barrier to user flow through the park and impose longer metric and topological distances. Even though some entrance points coincide with areas of higher values of permeability on the outside, they are mostly on the west portion. Through-movements are thus impaired by the lack of more directly connected entrance points on the east portion.

The inclusion of lakes as barriers, emphasised by dense vegetation, had the effect of highlighting the segregation between the east and southeast portion. In this instance, the lack of physical permeability and visual connectivity reinforced each other to create a more segregated area in comparison to the rest of the park. Correspondingly, this part of the park seems secondary in relation to the more central areas, resulting in many users not aware of its affordances.

The park's permeability decreased, with the addition of grass lawns surrounding the park in great extensions, separating it from the surrounding area. The spots with higher permeability were the pathways close to most of the facilities and the one that connects to exits. The east portion of the park was the most segregated, consistent with the observation of pedestrian flows.

When considering plant beds as an obstacle to movement in the inside of the park only, the map showed some integrated lines connecting the middle of the park with the exits, especially the west one. This is also a characteristic verified during the on-site observation, with a large flow of pedestrians entering from the west.

Generally, the most integrated areas according to the syntactic analysis actually corresponded to those most intensely used. However, the integration analysis, considering only the park's perimetre and disregarding its surroundings, showed more similarity to the park's appropriation. This highlighted the axis that connects the west entrance to the park's centre, which was the portion most appropriated by people. This area is simultaneously highly integrated and visible, which corroborates the initial assumptions. On the other hand, the east segregated portion (in dark grey, Figure 3) shows a much smaller appropriation density, as intuitively expected. Apparently this higher similarity achieved by the perimetre-only simulation is due to the segregated nature of the park, with its outer fences and few entry points that minimise the influence of external configurational characteristics on inner activities.

Some specific points challenged the predictions of our configurational analysis. The first one is situated on the extreme north portion of the park, where there is some gymnastics equipment. Despite being situated in a "corner," slightly segregated, it presented high appropriation levels. Another, perhaps surprising, area that demonstrated a highly segregated space but nevertheless high appropriation levels was a small board games area situated on the south side of the park. These points show the importance of some activities as attractors, and the level of complexity involved in their choice.

## Activities and User Profiles

Description 4 permeability map was intersected with the users and their different profiles (Figure 4). This was developed in order to evaluate different levels of appropriation according to gender and activities.

The first two hypotheses to be verified were (a) if areas with low visibility and permeability levels drove off people in more vulnerable groups (especially women and children)

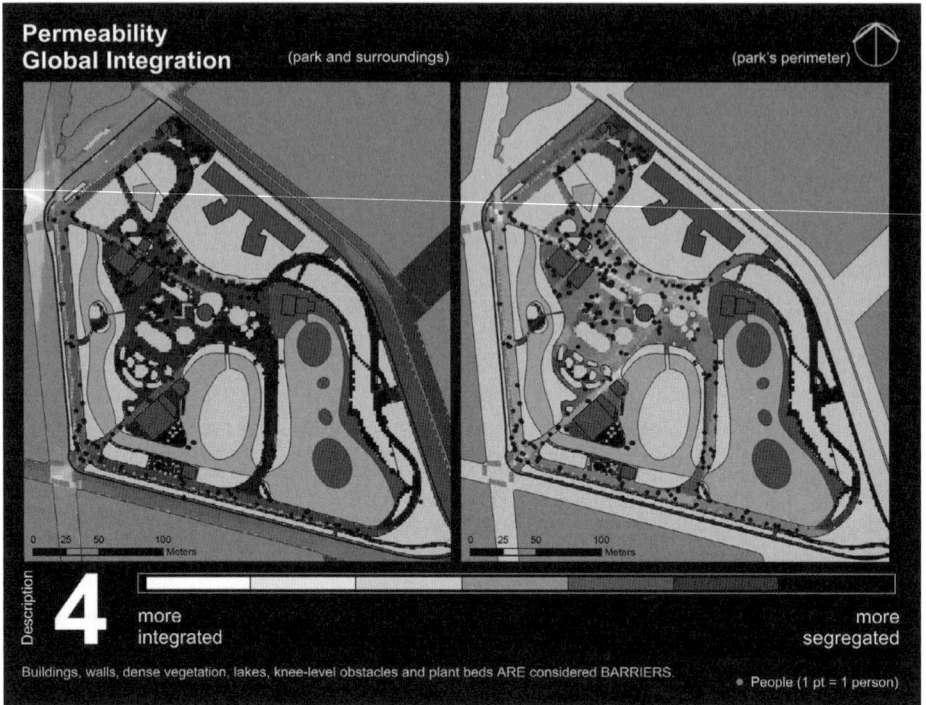

**Figure 3.** Description 4: Integration analysis.

and (b) if mothers with their children tend to choose places with low permeability and locate themselves in visible and integrated areas.

Considering description 4 and surrounding areas, it is possible to depict an equal quantity of men and women around the park, with more concentration on integrated areas. However, on the east and less visible portion of the park it is noticeable there was a greater presence of men than women. The converse happens on the central portion of the park, where there is a higher concentration of women.

On the first case, the overlapping of the east portion with the area of lowest permeability and visibility is a possible reason for both its low usage and even lower presence of female users. The second case has two possible causes: The central area is a convex space with low permeability, next to high permeability pathways and where it is located the park's playground. The high percentage of women in this particular space could be due to its location and permeability, or by the equipment in it or more likely the combination of both.

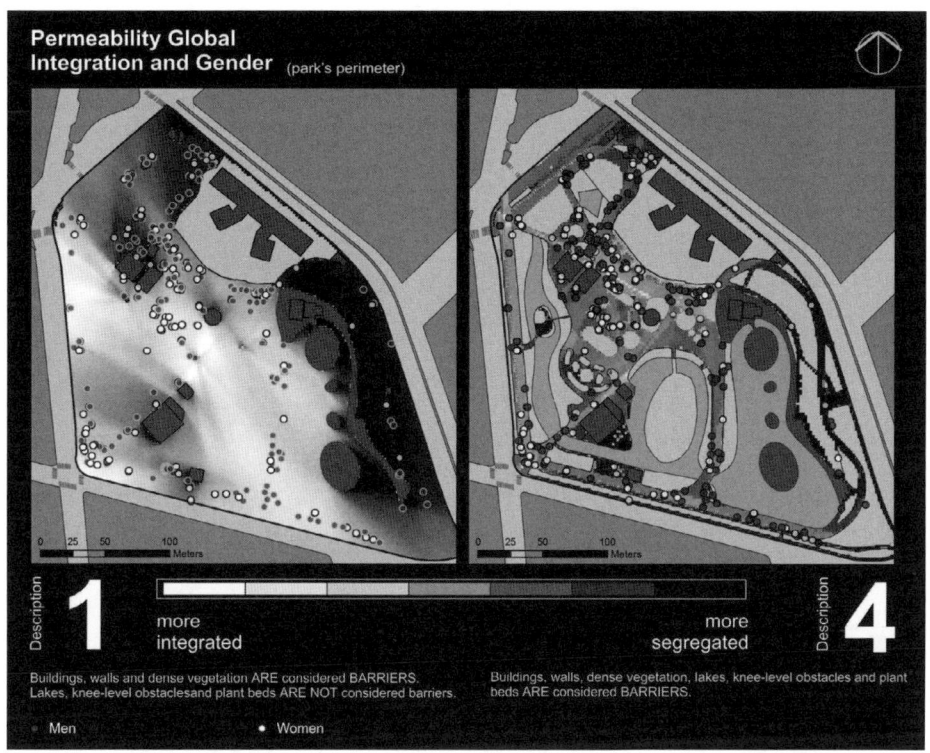

**Figure 4.** Comparison between permeability integration and gender, without surroundings.

With respect to the distinction between movement and static activities, Figure 5 shows that people in movement tend to concentrate on linear paths, as expected. Moreover, corroborating the previous findings, the most intensely used spaces for movement activities are the most integrated lines. In contrast stationary activities tend to concentrate on more convex spaces. Nevertheless, the most used convex spaces were those that were adjacent to the most integrated linear spaces.

Another finding is that there are a lot of situations in which stationary activities happen in linear spaces. It suggests both a potential conflict and possible complementary relationship. For instance, people passing by may conflict with stationary ones if there is not enough room for both activities to occur simultaneously. But if treated in a sensitive manner, these activities may complement each other, given that people like to interact with

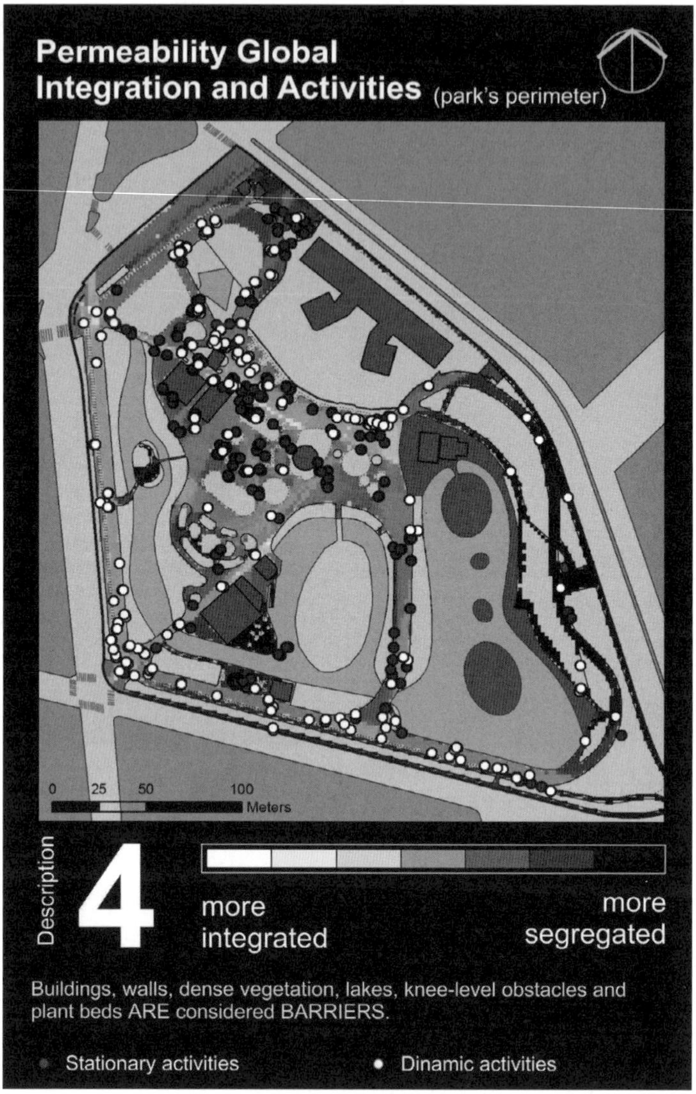

**Figure 5.** Comparison between permeability integration and type of activities, with surroundings.

each other even in passing. It therefore requires that linear spaces, and particularly the most integrated ones, have adequate width and adjacent spaces for stationary activities like sitting, reading, talking, or just observing the landscape.

# Conclusions

The results help corroborate Space Syntax findings on how spatial configuration influences appropriation patterns, especially by determining the degree of influence that barriers and permeability as well as their arrangement have on the park's appropriation. The models generated through Space Syntax correlated well to the on-site observation, even without taking into account other aspects such as: The attractions inside and outside the park, the residential or built density of the surroundings and the park's relationship with other green areas. All of this leads to the conclusion that space configuration is a highly influential factor on user appropriation patterns throughout the park.

That being said, description 1, which depicted only visibility barriers, showed a very poor ability to predict user's distribution. Integration, on the other hand, showed more accurate results when other relevant barriers were added to the map. This suggests that visibility in itself is not the main aspect when it comes to understanding appropriation patterns. The interrelationship of field visions, represented by isovists integration, is what seems to be the key to understanding them, since integration maps were significantly more accurate than pure (local) visibility analyses.

Two remarks must be made, though. First, "fields of vision" are in fact fields of vision and free movement, in the sense that they reveal what a pedestrian can see but also that they allow him or her to become aware that there are no barriers preventing him from moving in any direction inside any given isovist. We can therefore see that visibility and permeability work in a deep symbiotic way and that any separation, even for analytical purposes, presents ontological problems. Secondly, a close examination of visibility, integration, and appropriation density patterns shows that, although areas with highest appropriation density did indeed coincide with the most integrated areas according to description 4, these areas were not the ones with higher overall visibility. However, areas with low visibility did show correspondingly low levels of appropriation. This suggests that there may be a "visibility threshold," below which spaces are considered too dangerous or are not considered at all because they are not sufficiently seen by users. Above this threshold, spaces are in principle able to attract users; however, the analyses carried out in this study suggests that this happens mainly to those areas which are adjacent to, and directly visible from, the high integration areas.

Another relevant finding was the influence of visually permeable elements that could be perceived as subtle but important barriers to movement (description 4), such as different ground coverings. After adding these elements as barriers, the integration map became more similar to the real pattern of users. In fact, the performance of the models improved with each new addition of elements as barriers, going from: visibility barriers through permeability barriers, knee-level elements, and ground coverings. Each new type of barrier added a higher degree of correspondence to observed patterns.

Therefore, the study acknowledges the importance of elements considered secondary on the appropriation of open spaces. Benches, half-height vegetation, and several other ordinary elements in urban parks are relevant not only because of their supportive role, but also because they can influence how people perceive spatial configuration, and thus should be carefully considered when designing public spaces.

Furthermore, this validates the potential value of Space Syntax in design processes. It could be used to explore different scenarios and understand the possible consequences of choices made in the design, especially regarding their shape and spatial layout. The importance of analysis such as these lies in their role as preliminary testing tools, particularly when initial design schemes are being tested. Unlike other mathematical and computational simulations that demand a lot of detailing in order to yield relevant results, Space Syntax models can be built with very few details at the early design stages, providing important information that could potentially influence the design outcomes. Moreover, it can be easily comprehended by non-architectural audiences, by its intuitive colour-scheme,[4] thus offering a viable tool to participatory processes and collective decision-making.

# References

Alexander, C., Ishikawa, S., & Silverstein, M. (1977). *A pattern language: Towns, buildings, construction*. New York, NY: Oxford University Press.

Benedikt, M. L. (1979). To take hold of space: Isovists and isovist fields. *Environment and Planning B: Planning and Design, 6*(1), 47–65. doi: 10.1068/b060047

Gehl, J. (2011). *Life between buildings: Using public space*. Washington, DC: Island Press.

Hillier, B. (2003, June). *The architectures of seeing and going: Or, are cities shaped by bodies or minds? And is there a syntax of spatial cognition?* Paper presented at the 4th International Space Syntax Symposium, London, UK.

Hillier, B. (2007). *Space is the machine*. London, UK: Space Syntax.

Hillier, B., & Hanson, J. (1984). *The social logic of space*. Cambridge, UK: Cambridge University Press.

Hillier, B., Hanson, J., & Graham, H. (1987). Ideas are in things: An application of the space syntax method to discovering house genotypes. *Environment and Planning B: Planning and Design, 14*(4), 363–385. doi: 10.1068/b140363

Jacobs, J. (1961). *The death and life of great American cities*. New York, NY: Vintage Books.

Kahneman, D. (2011). *Thinking, fast and slow*. New York, NY: Farrar, Straus, and Giroux.

Kalff, C., Kühner, D., Senk, M., Conroy-Dalton, R., Strube, G., & Hölscher, C. (2012, January). *Turning the shelves: Empirical findings and space syntax analyses of two virtual supermarket variations*. Paper presented at the 8th International Space Syntax Symposium, Santiago, Chile.

Koch, D. (2010). Architecture re-configured. *The Journal of Space Syntax, 1*(1), 1–16.

Turner, A., Doxa, M., O'Sullivan, D., & Penn, A. (2001). From isovists to visibility graphs: A methodology for the analysis of architectural space. *Environment and Planning B: Planning and Design, 28*, 103–121.

---

[4]   Due to technical constraints, the illustrations are provided here in black and white.

# Degrees of Environmental Diversity for Pedestrian Thermal Comfort in the Urban Continuum

## A New Methodological Approach

Carolina Vasilikou and Marialena Nikolopoulou

Centre for Architecture and Sustainable Environment (CASE), School of Architecture, University of Kent, UK

**Abstract**

This study presents the application of a new methodological approach that assesses the impact of local urban design on the development of a comfortable thermal microclimate at street level for pedestrians. In designing connected street patterns as social places that enhance permeability, a certain degree of complexity seems to be necessary to provide different degrees of environmental diversity, and freedom of choice. These concepts have been found to critically effect the thermal sensation and microclimatic perceptions of pedestrians and consequently their use of public space. Pedestrian movement is addressed through a dynamic methodology of sequential environmental analysis and the assessment of variations in the thermal sensation of users through "microclimatic walks." This approach could lead to a greater understanding in patterns of use, pedestrian experience, and behaviour. Identifying degrees of diversity in different urban geometries, along street networks (with more realistic forms found in dense city centres), could give significant results relating to spatial preferences and frequentation patterns of pedestrians on a daily basis and between seasons.

**Key words:** environmental diversity, microclimate, pedestrian thermal comfort, urban continuum, walking

## Introduction

Outdoor thermal comfort has become an increasingly important field of research for urban design and planning (Ng, 2012). The main benefit of investigating the impact of climatic forces in spaces between buildings is the anthropocentric approach that transforms urban design practise into knowledgeable art, destined for and developed by the experience of people. The purpose of this paper is to reintroduce the users perspective into this area of research which has to date been exclusively expressed by professional design expertise. Research that managed to quantify the empirical and qualitative results of architectural observation and urban design projects has, until recently shown that "the environmental conditions imposed on people using open spaces may improve or ruin their experience of them" (Nikolopoulou & Lykoudis, 2007, p. 3691; Nikolopoulou et al., 2004). So, the environmental parameter may become a determinant factor for the comfort and experience of outdoor users. However, the prevailing environmental conditions in turn are largely determined by the urban morphology of the spaces and climate of the place. The way to address the missing link between urban morphology, urban microclimate and people's comfort and experience in open spaces, forms the main topic of this paper.

Studies in the urban and environmental design of open spaces seem to show, that depending on their form and shape, spaces have a variety of microclimatic characteristics. Focussing on the thermal microclimate, two levels of differentiation can be made: inter and intra thermal diversity. Inter thermal diversity relates to the range of climate conditions recorded between spaces with different architectural and geometric descriptors. Intra thermal diversity relates to climatic differences between points within the same urban space (Sinou, 2004). This evidence for environmental diversity has instigated numerous studies investigating the different thermal sensations that can be recorded in various spatial configurations (Steemers & Steane, 2004).

Urban design and transport studies have established the importance of thermally comfortable outdoor spaces used by pedestrians walking (Lenzholzer & Koh, 2010; Nikolopoulou & Lykoudis, 2007; Sauter & Wedderburn, 2008). This is perhaps a particularly important issue in urban design, as pedestrian movements in the urban continuum is the most widespread mode of transport and forms a crucial link between inter-modal transfers and helps fulfil utilitarian and recreational trips (Sauter & Wedderburn, 2008). The benefits of successfully designed spaces enhance the quality of place, economic vitality, and liveability of cities.

It is generally recognised throughout the European community, particularly in developed historical cities such as Copenhagen, Amsterdam, Vienna Barcelona, and Rome, that attracting visitors is one of the keys to developing and maintaining a vibrant community. Pedestrianisation is a part of significant developments in the walking environment and culture in these cities helping to change the urban landscape. Along with the use of the bicycle, these city centres focus on the quality of ambient environments, that lack of vehicles and enhanced outdoor use can bring to their public spaces. The "quality of urban space" becomes paramount for any city's global image and economic development

(Bosselmann, 2008). One way this quality can be achieved is through the understanding of the thermal comfort and experience of pedestrians as they move through the urban continuum of streets and squares, in order to fulfil both utilitarian and recreational needs.

## Thermal Comfort in Outdoor Urban Spaces: The Need for a New Methodological Tool

In 2004, an urban design tool was developed through the Rediscovering the Urban Realm and Open Spaces (RUROS) project. The research initiative brought together eight European universities and Research Centres, with the aim to carry out an integrated analysis of the urban environment taking into consideration the needs of the users of open spaces. This approach involved the application of multiple methodologies such as: monitoring of microclimatic conditions, field surveys with questionnaire-guided interviews with the public, statistical analysis, evaluation of the environmental performance of urban textures, comfort mapping, social study of open spaces, and design guides and proposals. One of the main outcomes of the RUROS project is the combined analysis of the physical environment (microclimate, thermal, visible and audible comfort, urban morphology, etc.) with the users' requirements and satisfaction. This approach was one of the first to involve the user in evaluations of the microclimate and comfort conditions, in a real-world setting. It has been shown that although microclimate is not always a determining factor for comfort, it remains a very important parameter (Sarkar, 2003).

The discussion on the relationship between microclimate and the quality of open spaces in urban environments started almost four decades ago. Urban theorists from both sides of the Atlantic, such as Jacobs (1969) and Gehl (1987), have emphasised the significance of climatically controlled outdoor space via their empirical observations. In doing so they make direct reference to urban textures and spatial enclosures of historic European cities. Adopting a more hands-on approach, Bosselmann and colleagues (Bosselmann, Arens, Dunker, & Wright, 1990) investigated the urban microclimate of "downtown" San Francisco in relation to the urban morphology of the city and particularly its tall buildings. Subsequently, in 1995, an "urban design study" was published in the Journal of the American Planning Association (Bosselmann & Arens, 1995), analysing the effect of future development in Toronto's central area on street-level conditions of sun, wind, and thermal comfort. These examples of previous research serves to highlight there is a body of research that spotlights the urban microclimate to varying degrees, however "modern cities have rarely been shaped by a concern for a comfortable outdoor climate (for pedestrians)" (Bosselmann & Arens, 1995, p. 227). Given the changes to many urban landscapes throughout Europe it is perhaps time for a new body of research on the thermal environment of urban spaces.

In a collective needs-perspective publication, scholars from around the world advocated for improved planning and management of large cities incorporating the use of climate-conscious urban design (Mills et al., 2010). Focussing on climate concerns in urban design, the paper provides a synopsis of the tools employed, from the perspective of the building group level, to achieve outdoor comfort. These include: the outline of spaces between buildings, materials and surfaces, street dimensions and orientation, guidelines for density, height of buildings, uses, and green spaces. Mills et al. (2010) point out the significance of

> planning and design practitioners to be aware of the consequences of urban planning and design decisions [. . .]. Such information would include climate related issues of comfort [. . .]. In this vein, there is an onus on planners to incorporate the views of the local residents on quality of life issues, which perforce includes environmental factors. (p. 235)

In summary, three main knowledge gaps can be identified, which the methodology presented here aims to cover: (1) no research on long-term thermal comfort assessment was done extensively in the field of outdoor thermal comfort research, (2) no consistent urban climate and outdoor thermal comfort research was conducted with the focus on the activity of walking, the most wide-spread and sustainable mode of transport, and (3) no research exists on the spatial and thermal perception of people moving in the urban continuum and the way it may influence their outdoor thermal comfort.

## Pedestrian Movement

Pedestrian movement is circulation, which apart from the purely physical activity of getting from one place to another, permits economic, social, and cultural exchange. The purpose of walking is multi-faceted, with potential to create numerous *by-products of movement* (Hillier, 1996) or for other optional activities to take place. Both utilitarian and recreational activities can be distinguished as: necessary, optional, and social, according to Gehl (1987, 2010). Each activity is ruled by a goal and categorised into groups: resting, playing, gathering, or passing by (Yan & Kalay, 2004). Walking can also be either a single-goal activity or part of a sequence of different activities (sitting, standing, and walking). Types of social activities that include walking are: gaming, talking, and passing by.

There are detailed tendencies that govern individual's behaviour when walking in the urban continuum: edge effect, attraction effect, distance effect, and group effect. These effects describe people's tendency to walk along edges in large spaces (distance to building edges), the influence of aesthetically stimulating elements in the surrounding space, preference of shortest path, distance from walkers-by (separation), speed, skip steps, acceleration, and crossing patterns (alignment), the effect of other people in binding together spatially (cohesion), and shading provision (Lam, 2011). However, the effect of microclimates has not been included. In this research the comfort effect is defined as a function of thermal sensation and outdoor thermal comfort.

In contrast with vehicular movement, pedestrians can only adapt to the circulation facilities provided for them by the urban morphology and architectural arrangement of spaces. In this context, walking satisfies the need for the smallest scale of transport and gives pedestrians the capability for flexible and adaptable (small scale) movements. People's activities on foot involve a substantial amount of meandering, sudden changes of direction, and stop-and-go movements. The way pedestrians behave when walking depends largely on the urban setting, the attractiveness of the place, and other environmental factors. People often walk consciously or unconsciously along places, where it is attractive and comfortable, be it in the shade in summer or choosing a route with other people. The environmental, thermal, visual, and acoustic conditions that prevail in different spaces, could play a significant role in the duration of pedestrian activity outdoors, their experience and perception of comfort, and their choice to move freely. According to Shaftoe (2008, p. 59), "unless we are sitting, lingering, or loitering, we generally experience the environment as we move between places." And goes on to emphasise the input an urban designer could have when improving an existing space or designing a new one: "assuming we want people to have positive aesthetic experiences, we should optimise surface treatments, microclimates, and gradients to provide the best sensory experiences" (p. 59).

The way pedestrians experience the thermal environment outdoors is based largely on the sensory cues they pick up during their movement in the urban continuum. The physical experience of walking relies on the sensory realm, thus determining the comfort and satisfaction pedestrians derive from it (Middleton, 2010). The comfort requirements in urban walkways can be evaluated as physical, psychological, and physiological (Sarkar, 2003). These comfort types can be evident in different scales, and also in macro and/or micro conditions. Some of the widely accepted evaluation criteria of comfort levels for pedestrian circulation in urban networks are the urban morphology of the walkways. This encompasses: geometrical dimensions and characteristics, opportunities for diverse usage with simultaneous enhancement of social interaction, comfortable walking surface, provision of seating, and protection from adverse weather conditions (Whyte, 1980). In her report during the 2003 annual meeting of the Transportation Research Board (USA), Sarkar emphasises the fact, that in order to promote walking as a year-round activity in the circulation network, the microclimate conditions of different urban spaces need to be addressed. For example, "extremely windy or sunny conditions need to be tempered by some moderating influences" (Sarkar, 2003, p. 14). The impact of the physical environment on pedestrian comfort is coupled by the psychological effect that walking can have on pedestrians. The ability to maintain desired walking speed and the ability to participate in various pedestrian activities are two main parameters of pedestrian thermal comfort.

Microclimatic conditions also seem to have a crucial impact on the psychological effect of walking in the urban continuum (Lenzholzer, 2010; Nikolopoulou, 1998). The psychological implications of pedestrians and their behaviour outdoors have been examined in various research such as: the seminal editing work of Proshansky (1970) and David Stea (1970) in his chapter on Space, Territory, and Human Movements. Stea's research stresses: the importance of variability, the need for change, for variety in what might be termed the stimulus field and concludes that the intuitions of the designer are frequently inadequate to cope with the subtle contributions of the designed built environment to user behaviour. Environments built with no consideration of pedestrian movement patterns can lead to potentially conflicting movements and can discourage walking.

## Pedestrian Thermal Comfort

The complexity of walking in the urban continuum could be translated in the multi-sensory experience it provides to the pedestrian. A change in one aspect or quality of the environment, inevitably affects our response to, and perception of, the whole environment (Fitch, 1970, p. 76). However, in order to analyse the experience of the pedestrian in a research project, one has to focus on each sense separately. Although the "problematic nature of privileging one sense of another" (Middleton, 2010, p. 582) has already been pointed out and taken into account in this research, focussing on one aspect of the environmental conditions outdoors provides a valuable understanding of the processes of pedestrian thermal comfort. Research related to the sense-scape of outdoors urban spaces have focused mainly on the visual quality of the designed environment, along with other studies about the sound and olfactory experience (Henshaw et al., 2009; Payne, 2010). The thermal sensation and comfort of people using outdoor spaces, although a growing field of research, remains under-researched. Sense-scape research has tended to focus on "snap shots," in a specific time and space, of the urban user experience and comfort states. Previous research has not tried to link measurement of senses, in a continuous basis, between nodal points of the urban landscape. This gap in research informs the current research paper, on variation of thermal experience between connected urban spaces during the consistent movement of the pedestrian. This type of research is different from previous research and therefore requires a fresh look at methodological measures of investigation. This is the main aim of this paper.

Previous studies on thermal sensation and perception have tended to focus on the microclimatic conditions prevailing in a set of different spaces that may be in the same urban quarter or area, but are usually discontinuous, located in separate areas, or of certain typology (Ali-Toudert, 2005; Johansson, 2006; Lenzholzer, 2010). Sensory studies often derive conclusions by applying "sense-walking" techniques. This consists of participants consciously walking and recording their sensory experience usually with regards to the visual, acoustic, and olfactory environment around them. However, the effect of thermal conditions and their variation on pedestrian experience has not been investigated. This is mainly due to the complexity and multidisciplinary nature of thermal comfort studies.

## Environmental Diversity in the Urban Continuum

The urban context offers a rich and diverse environment that influences both the way we utilise urban spaces (movement, sequence, and activity) and our perception of thermal, acoustic, visual, and olfactory stimuli (Steemers & Steane, 2004). This research contributes, in the first instance, to the vast field that studies the environmental diversity in urban spaces. The main aim of the research is to investigate and analyse the relation between urban morphology, microclimate, and thermal comfort in outdoor public space, focussing on in-situ dynamic measurements.

In the built environment, microclimatic parameters such as temperature, light intensity, and wind speed vary instantaneously as part of every day/normal condition. These variations, mainly influenced by the urban morphology, could potentially influence the thermal and visual comfort of pedestrians. The outdoor public spaces that this research is concerned with are public urban voids, that is, the streets, squares and spaces with vegetation. More importantly, the study focusses on the sequence of streets and squares in the formation of the urban continuum and the real-time pedestrian walking experience in it.

The variation in spatial configurations of public spaces may cause significant differentiation of the microclimatic parameters, such as radiant temperature, relative humidity, and wind speed. These modifications have future design implications and may be able to have an influence on the health and thermal comfort of pedestrians. The quality and intensity of each activity (social or individual) may be influenced by the level of thermal discomfort experienced by pedestrians when they are exposed to the microclimatic conditions, specific to a given place (Givoni, 1998).

The aim of this research is to show the variability of the thermal environment in the urban continuum and evaluate the conditions of thermal comfort for people walking. In doing so it is intended to identify opportunities of adaptation to the changing conditions of the thermal environment. This way the understanding of the environmental diversity in the urban continuum and its implication, in terms of thermal comfort for pedestrians, will allow architects, urban designers, policy makers, and users to perceive outdoor public spaces in all their dynamic and complex nature, including the human parameter in the design decision process.

## A New Methodology Defining Dynamic Thermal Comfort for Pedestrians

Fieldwork measurements of microclimatic parameters were developed by combining two different approaches: dynamic and static. The dynamic approach is based on the values of microclimatic parameters during movement through an urban route explored by the researcher. This analysis was undertaken with the help of portable climatic measurement equipment (*Thelonius* portable weather station, C.A.S.E, University of Kent). The approach consists of complementing the dynamic measurements of environmental parameters by controlling specific factors of influence with an observation matrix. The matrix allows the researcher to form a subjective judgement on the quality of urban and thermal environmental characteristics of the pedestrian route. In fact, the data from the fixed points of measurement along the route form an integral part of the dynamic measurement, although they have been recorded in a static position. This approach (Potvin, 1997) was selected as the closest possible real-time simulation, of the walking activity in the urban continuum that would allow simultaneous climatic measurements. This approach is important in order to ensure stability for the sensors that measure the desired data.

Sense-walking techniques bring a qualitative backdrop to this research and include the organisation of surveys that take place in a given route, by people walking and completing a structured interview. As the focus of this study is the identification of the thermal environment of people's perceptions as they walk in the urban continuum, this new methodology is defined by the author as *thermal walks*. During a thermal walk, participants are consciously engaged in understanding and sensing those climatic conditions around them, relating to the thermal environment. Their thermal sensation is recorded with the help of a structured questionnaire that corresponds to predetermined fixed points of measurements and comparison along the given route.

Every methodological tool presented above is designed specifically to analyse the complexity of sequential movement. Serial Vision is a measurement tool developed by Gordon Cullen in his seminal work *The Concise Townscapes* (1961) and adopted in this research. This tool is one of the first methodological approaches to analyse movement in the built environment, visually. The sequential analysis of thermal walks is a technique that this research pilots. It is specifically used to add thermal aspects to the existing body of research on visual, acoustic, and olfactory measurement of urban pedestrians' environmental experience.

The fieldwork was based on two case studies, in the city centres of major European cities (Figure 1). In each case study, a total of six points of measurement were selected in order to provide comparative data on urban public spaces. Each focus point of measurement is characterised by a distinct morphological structure: in particular its exposure to sun, the nature of materials that define the space and the height of the surrounding buildings, etc. This varied selection of focus points is specifically to create a significant spatial diversity, but more importantly to show the effect of this diversity on the fluctuation of the thermal environment.

## Perceived Variation of the Thermal Environment

The groups of participants on the thermal walks consisted mainly of people working in the area, researchers, and general inhabitants of the city. The participants were given a short brief, prior to the thermal walk, on the nature of the research.

The survey was completely structured and prearranged with people from a wide range of backgrounds and age. Each participant gave consent, prior to participating in the research. In the structured questionnaire, the participants were asked to concentrate on the variations that might occur between different points of the walk, in terms of their thermal sensation, preferences, and characteristics of the space around them.

The questions used to record the thermal sensation of participants focussed on defining a thermal sensation at the starting point as a base line. As participants walked on to the

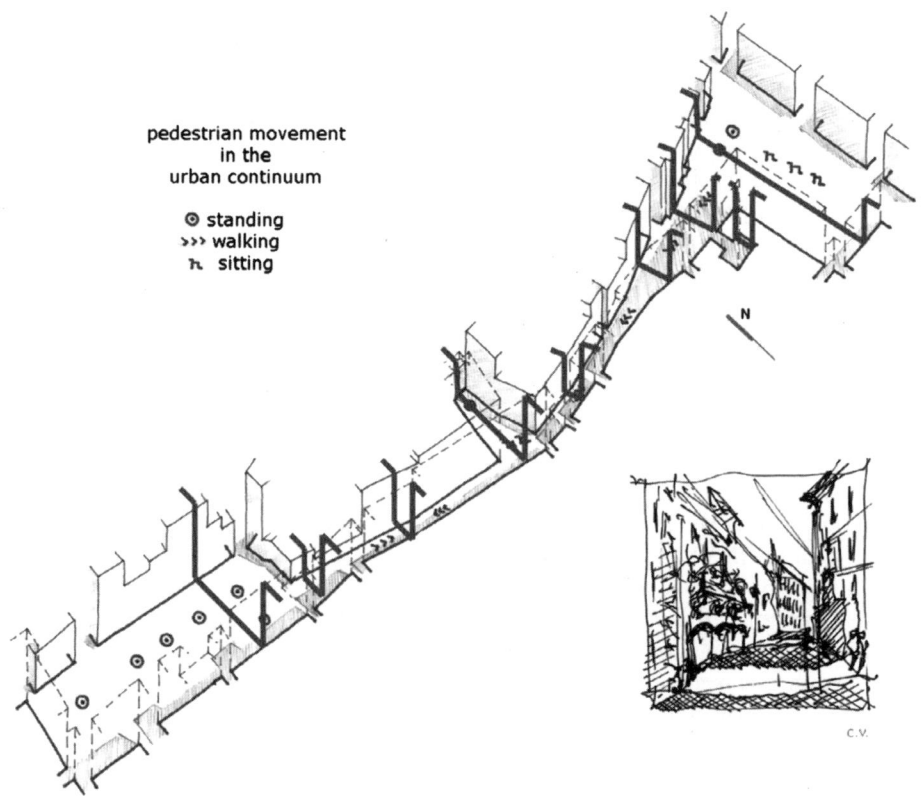

**Figure 1.** The sequential representation of urban spaces in a streets-and-squares network in the city centre of Rome, Italy.

next points of the route, measurements were taken for comparison with new thermal feelings to previous ones. The re-iterative nature of the process at each measurement point in the thermal walk, provided a platform for consistency and reliability.

Below follow some representative questions of the questionnaire:

- How do you find the thermal environment in this precise moment?
- Do you find this: uncomfortably cold, uncomfortably cool, comfortable, uncomfortably warm, uncomfortably hot?
- Do you sense any variation with regard to your previous sensation at this precise moment? – Colder, cooler, neither cool nor warm, warmer, hotter.
- Do you find this new sensation: uncomfortably cold, uncomfortably cool, comfortable, uncomfortably warm, uncomfortably hot?

Each point of evaluation was prearranged and situated in specific spaces, such as: in an open square, in the middle of a narrow street, or adjacent to a small *largo* (small, enclosed square). The participants recorded their evaluations using a 5-point scale, close ended questions with multiple choices and open ended questions. Their responses in relation to the perception of variation (5-point scale) gave a measure of: whether participants were able to identify a specific change in the thermal conditions and define its quality, whether the change was positive or negative, and cooler or warmer respectively. This may be regarded as participants' perceived variation or the ability of pedestrians to identify consciously a change in the thermal environment during their activity and to give a qualitative attribute to this change.

## Conclusions

The study of the relation between the urban morphology, the microclimate, and thermal comfort for pedestrians as they move in the urban continuum, is a study of complexity in the fourth (thermal) dimension. The important number of environmental and personal variables requires the combinations of many methods: measurement of microclimatic conditions, observation and in-situ matrix, and sense walking techniques. It is this approach that distinguishes the current research as different and new.

Urban microclimate research is complex and often difficult to measure and interpret. Adding a "thermal" dimension to the exiting visual, acoustic, and olfactory research can only enhance the knowledge of urban design. Further analysis that will quantify this differentiation using climatic simulation is currently under way. Predicted climatic models, based on the complex urban morphology under consideration should be compared with the findings of the primary fieldwork. Further conclusions will provide a detailed understanding of the perceived variations in the thermal experience of pedestrians walking in a complex urban continuum.

This paper presented the methodological tool of thermal walks, developed to address the study of environmental diversity and pedestrian thermal comfort in the continuum of complex urban spaces. The fieldwork initial results show a tendency for pedestrians to consciously perceive and identify variations of microclimatic conditions whilst walking. Participants seemed to associate climatic variables with specific urban spaces along their given walking route. Initial findings suggest that thermally pleasant spaces do not share a specific geometric characteristic and may vary between seasons. This builds on current urban design research concerning the sense-scape of pedestrians and contributes to the understanding of the ways people perceive the thermal environment outdoors.

The new methodological approach proposes combining techniques that may provide a holistic view of pedestrians' thermal experiences, in a dynamic analysis of real-world design schemes. The understanding of the environmental diversity in the urban continuum and its implication in terms of thermal comfort for pedestrians will allow architects, urban designers, policy makers, and users to perceive outdoor public spaces in all their complex nature. The most significant input of applying this method to further research consists in providing design guidelines that take into account the dynamic comfort of people walking, and thus promoting sustainable modes of transport. One of the main contributions includes the incorporation of the human parameter in the design decision process and the understanding of the spatial preferences and frequentation patterns of pedestrians in the urban continuum on a daily basis and between seasons.

# References

Ali-Toudert, F. (2005). *Dependence of outdoor thermal comfort on street design in hot and dry climate.* Freiburg: Berichte des Meteorologischen Institutes der Universität Freiburg, Nr. 15. (PhD Thesis, Diss-Freidok).

Bosselmann, P. (2008). *Urban transformations: Understanding city form and design.* Washington DC: Island Press.

Bosselmann, P., & Arens, E. (1995). Urban form and climate. *Journal of the American Planning Association, 61,* 226–241.

Bosselmann, P., Arens, E., Dunker, K., & Wright, R. (1990). Sun, wind, and pedestrian comfort: A study of Toronto's central area. Toronto, Canada: Planning & Development Department. Retrieved from: http://escholarship.org/uc/item/0165c77h

Cullen, G. (1961). *The concise townscape.* Oxon, UK: Architectural Press.

Fitch, S. (1970). Experiential bases for esthetic decision. In H. M. Proshansky (Ed.), *Environmental Psychology: People and their physical settings* (pp. 76–84). Dumfries, NC: Holt McDougal.

Gehl, J. (1987). *Life between buildings.* Copenhagen, Denmark: Danish Architectural Press.

Gehl, J. (2010). *Cities for people.* Washington DC: Island Press.

Givoni, B. (1998). *Climate considerations in building and urban design.* New York, NY: Wiley.

Henshaw, V., Adams, M., & Cox, T. J. (2009, August). *Route planning a sensory walk: Sniffing out the issues.* Paper presented at the Royal Geographical Society Annual Conference, University of Manchester, UK.

Hillier, B. (1996). *Space is a machine.* Cambridge: Cambridge University Press.

Jacobs, J. (1969). *The death and life of great American cities.* New York, NY: Modern Library Edition.

Johansson, E. (2006). Influence of urban geometry on outdoor thermal comfort in a hot dry climate: A study in Fez, Morocco. *Building and Environment, 41,* 1326–1338.

Lam, F. G. (2011). *Simulating the effect of microclimate on human behavior in small urban spaces* (Unpublished doctoral dissertation). University of California, Berkeley.

Lenzholzer, S. (2010). Immersed in microclimatic space: Microclimatic experience and perception of spatial configurations in Dutch squares. *Landscape and Urban Planning, 95,* 1–15.

Lenzholzer, S., & Koh, J. (2010). Immersed in microclimatic space: Microclimate experience and perception of spatial configurations in Dutch squares. *Landscape and Urban Planning, 95,* 1–15.

Middleton, J. (2010). Sense and the city: Exploring the embodied geographies of urban walking. *Social and Cultural Geography, 11*(6), 575–596.

Mills, G., Cleugh, H., Emmanuel, R., Endlicher, W., Erell, E., McGranahan, G., Ng, E., Nickson, A., Rosenthal, J., & Steemers, K. (2010). Climate information for improved planning and management of mega cities (needs perspective). *Procedia Environmental Sciences, 1,* 228–246.

Ng, E. (2012). Towards planning and practical understanding of the need for meteorological and climatic information in the design of high-density cities: A case-based study of Hong Kong. *International Journal of Climatology, 32,* 582–598.

Nikolopoulou, M. (1998). *Thermal comfort in outdoor urban spaces*. University of Cambridge (PhD Thesis).

Nikolopoulou, M. (coord.), Kofoed, N., Gaardsted, M., Scudo, G., Dessi, V., Rogora, A., ... Avdelidi, K. (2004). *RUROS: Rediscovering the urban realm and open spaces*. Athens: CRES Edition. Retrieved from http://alpha.cres.gr/ruros/

Nikolopoulou, M., & Lykoudis, S. (2007). Use of outdoor spaces and microclimate in a Mediterranean urban area. *Building and Environment, 42*, 3691–3707.

Payne, S. (2010, April). *Urban park soundscapes and their perceived restorativeness*. Paper presented at the Institute of Acoustics & Noise in the Built Environment, Ghent.

Potvin, A. (1997). *Movement in the architecture of the city: A study in environmental diversity* (Unpublished doctoral distribution). University of Cambridge.

Proshansky, H. M. (1970). *Environmental Psychology: People and their physical settings*. Dumfries, NC: Holt McDougal.

Sarkar, S. (2003, June). *Qualitative evaluation of comfort needs in urban walkways in major activity centers*. Paper presented at TRB Annual Meeting, Washighton DC, US.

Sauter, D., & Wedderburn, N. (2008, May). *Measuring walking: towards internationally standardised monitoring methods of walking and public space*. Paper presented at 8th International Conference on Survey Methods in Transport, Annecy, France.

Shaftoe, H. (2008). *Convivial urban spaces: Creating effective public spaces*. London, UK: Earthscan.

Sinou, M. (2004). *Thermal diversity of semi-enclosed urban spaces* (Unpublished doctoral dissertation). University of Cambridge, Department of Architecture.

Stea, D. (1970). Space, territory and human movements. In H. M. Proshansky (Ed.), *Environmental Psychology: People and their physical settings* (pp. 37–42). Dumfries, NC: Holt McDougal.

Steemers, K., & Steane, M. A. (2004). *Environmental diversity in architecture*. Oxon, UK: Spon Press.

Whyte, W. (1980). *The social life of small urban spaces*. New York, NY: Project for Public Spaces.

Yan, W., & Kalay, Y. E. (2004). Simulating the Behaviour of Users in Built Environments. *Journal of Architectural and Planning Research, 21*(4), 371–384.

# Influence of Chromatic Complexity and Coherence on Evaluation of Urban Scenes

Natalia Naoumova

Architecture and Urban Planning Department, Federal University of Pelotas, Brazil

## Abstract

The aim of this paper is to investigate the relationship between aesthetic appreciation of urban scenes and different levels of chromatic complexity and coherence. It is also to understand the perceptions of urban environments by individuals from different cultural backgrounds (Russian and Brazilian). The investigations are based on scenes from historical buildings in the city of Pelotas, Brazil, with results indicating that colour contributes to the assessment of coherence and complexity of scene by means of chromatic attributes. Scenes with moderate level of complexity tend to be positively evaluated and preferred, while scenes with low and high level of complexity tend to be negatively evaluated. The study suggests mixtures of old and new buildings can be considered coherent by participants if they have a unified style of colouration, that is overall tone of the facades related to the lightness value of colour and contrasts among used chromatic combinations.

**Key words:** environmental perception, urban heritage, urban polychromy

## Introduction

This paper discusses the aesthetic quality of the historic centres related to the polychromy of the urban environment. It is based on the principle that the particular character of the city is formed not only by exceptional architectural monuments, but also the common sets of buildings aggregated from different periods of the past, that represent the accumulated knowledge, habits, and experiences arising from its creators and users. In these buildings, colours are used to communicate information at a visual or symbolic level: about the function of the building, to convey the status of its residents, and to express custom or attract attention (Hope & Walch, 1990). These buildings form the living environment of the city, whose base is in the practice of dwelling.

Empirical evidence suggests that colour can significantly: increase the prominence of buildings, reduce or alleviate the sense of variety and visual coherence of the urban space, and contribute to the proper perception of social ranking and originality of the architecture (Lancaster, 1996). Through colours, historical buildings can also acquire specific symbolic value and thus contribute to the formation of the identity of the built environment further highlighting their historical and cultural character (Lenclos, 1999; Naoumova, 2009).

Recent empirical studies suggest that colours have a strong influence on mental health and psychological state of individuals as well as the obvious aesthetic influences (Beach, Wise, & Wise, 1988). The spontaneous development of the chromatic environment via repainting of buildings and increase in the level of complexity lead to the emergence of new aesthetic standards and cause inevitable transformation of the original polychromy. Furthermore, it is argued that the increase of the complexity and exaggerated sensory-motor stimulation of the human body, caused by greater commercial availability and flexibility in the use of colour, modify not only the visual capabilities, but also the most comprehensive evaluative and perceptual capacities of man in relation to environmental aesthetic qualities (Toska, 2002; Ünver & Öztuk, 2002).

In this context studies on the psychology of colour become interesting for urban planners for several reasons. One of the most important aspects of colour is the perceptual properties and the aesthetic qualities of colour that are closely linked with people's preferences and the public well-being in general. Colour selection therefore takes on greater significance in the design process as it is linked to a wide range of psychological perceptions and emotions. Researching the underlying reasons for individuals' appraisals behind judgments like, beauty and feelings of pleasantness can in turn suggest chromatic strategies and lead to planning principles that enhance a range of districts.

The aim of this study is to investigate the relationship between aesthetic appreciation of urban scenes with older buildings of varying architectural styles incorporating such factors as the presence of different levels of chromatic complexity and coherence in those scenes. In addition the study and comparison of urban environment perceptions by individuals of different cultures and backgrounds is carried out. After realising the need for planning recommendations that enable chromatic improvements in historic areas, it is also intended to study:

- How the increase in complexity of the urban environment and the intensity of chromatic changes affect the perception of the urban scenes.
- Which buildings are perceived as coherent in the scenes of different levels of complexity and chromatic variation?
- What is the affective relationship in the perception of sets of buildings with different colours?

## Theoretical Assumptions

Studying perceptions of aesthetic quality in urban environments is a complex process which requires the use of different methodologies. Theoretical concepts in environmental perception were therefore drawn on as well as previous research methodologies on empirical aesthetics utilised by Nasar (1998), Stamps (2000), and Purcell (1984a). The concept of aesthetic response is based on the idea that the perception of the visual quality is a psychological construction that involves assessments made by people. These evaluations have a connection (i) with the environment and (ii) with the feelings of individuals in relation to environmental peculiarities. The evaluation of the first type is called *cognitive and perceptual judgment* and consists of the immediate reaction and subsequent act of assigning value. The evaluation of the second type is called *emotional* and refers to the change in the psychological state of a person, resulting in a triggered feeling/response (Nasar, 1997).

Previous research highlighting the dimensions of aesthetic responses and preferences in the urban environment suggests that pleasantness, attractiveness, and familiarity are prominent components. The analyses of evaluations on urban scenes encompass two groups of factors, including both *formal* and *symbolic variables*.

The *formal variables* related to the physical characteristics of the stimulus can be observed in any chromatic composition. The colours of a building can be described in terms of simple and isolated dimensions: hue, clarity, saturation, having a certain amount of colours, proportion of the coloured areas, contrasting or harmonious hue combinations, and a specific juxtaposition on the surface of the facade. It is also possible to make a synthetic measurement. It is possible to talk, for example, about the rhythm and hierarchy of colours, or the dominant typology and chromatic range present in the composition. Thus, the participation of the colour in the process of immediate perception (see Gestalt) plays an important role in the formation of the features related to the feelings of affection, such as coherence and order, among others (Janssens, 2001).

In responses about the colours of the buildings, people often mention chromatic harmony and point out that the colours should be organized among themselves by some kind of order (Burchett, 2001; Ou & Luo, 2006). Judd and Wysezcki (1975) argues that chromatic harmony is directly connected with individual preferences or likes and dislikes. In urban scenes, we search for such organisation which may be considered harmonious by people. In this study, *order* and *complexity* were taken as synthetic characteristics of the urban environment and used for the study of scenes with different types of buildings from the perception and evaluation of individuals.

## Method

To investigate the influence of *order* and chromatic *complexity* in the evaluation of the urban scenes, the historic centre of the city of Pelotas, Rio Grande do Sul, Brazil, was examined. Urban scenes, with buildings of different styles, were classified into three complexity levels and within them the three most significant scenes were chosen. The colour control was performed through the System of Colour References – Natural Colour System (NCS).

The first scene represents *higher complexity*. In this scene the buildings painted in colours with high saturation are predominant. In terms of lightness, there were three buildings with light walls and four with darker tones. In terms of hue, five buildings were painted in a colour range of pink and reddish tones; one building had beige and green hues and another blue and green. To sum up, the scene is characterised by the smallest formal and stylistic difference among buildings and greater colour difference with variations in lightness.

The second scene has *low complexity*. The facades have more homogeneity of colours and there are no highly saturated paintings. In terms of lightness, six buildings have light shaded painting and one building presents a dark tone. In terms of hue, there are four neutral colours, beige and grey, one painted in green, and one in pink. Among the seven buildings under review, there are four historic ones, but only two facades feature sophisticated detailing (compatible with the facades of scene 1). In short, the scene presents greater formal and stylistic difference among buildings and smaller colour difference.

The third scene is characterised by a *medium level of complexity*. It presents buildings painted with saturated and neutral colours alternately. The facades are more homogeneous in terms of detail and style. However, the scene has significant chromatic differences. In terms of lightness, there are three gloomy buildings and five light ones. Considering hue, there are buildings painted in green, blue, orange, beige, and red, with two facades having different shades of yellow and two are greyish. Thus, the scene has smaller formal difference among the buildings, but higher colour difference with alternated position and lightness's (Figure 1).

The selected urban scenes were analysed taking into account three aspects connected with aesthetic evaluation: *pleasantness*, *order (coherence)*, *and attractiveness* (understood as *catching visual attention*). Affective characteristics of the scene such as a feeling of *relaxation* (calm – exciting) as well as sympathy connected to the feeling of safety (*friendly – aggressive*) were analysed. We also sought to understand whether the formal features related to the *chromatic complexity* of the scene, specifically: (1) *the amount of different colours*, (2) *the saturation of the predominant colours*, (3) *the contrast among colours of buildings in the scene,* interfere in the evaluated aspects. The analysis of all the issues mentioned was compared between the two groups of participants with different cultural backgrounds, Brazilians (74 college students, among them 20 architecture majors) and Russians (32 college students, among them 10 architecture majors). Questionnaires consisted of simple and multiple choice questions based on the photographic representation of the urban scenes as shown in Figure 1. The data obtained were analysed by means of non-parametric statistics methods recommended for small samples (Siegel & Castellan, 1988).

## Scene 1 High Complexity

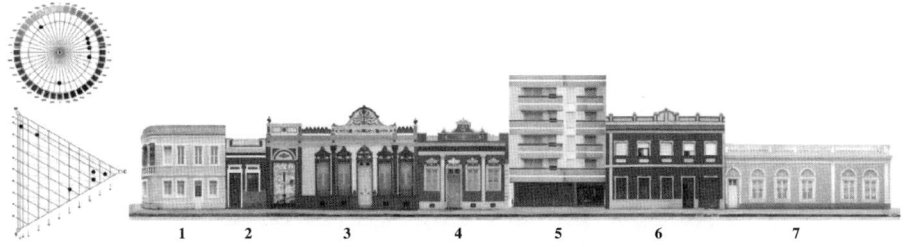

| Number of building ▶ | 1 | 2 | 3 | 4 | 5 | 6 | 7 |
|---|---|---|---|---|---|---|---|
| Dominant color | pink | red | white | red | beige | blue | pink |
| NCS code | S1010-Y70R | S2075-Y70R | S0500-N | S1085-Y90R | S1005-Y20R | S4050-B | S1010-Y80R |
| Details color | white | white | wine color | white | green | green | white |
| NCS code | S0502-Y | S0502-Y | S1575-R10B | S0505-G80Y | S2020-G60Y | S1020-G20Y | S0500-N |

## Scene 2 Low Complexity

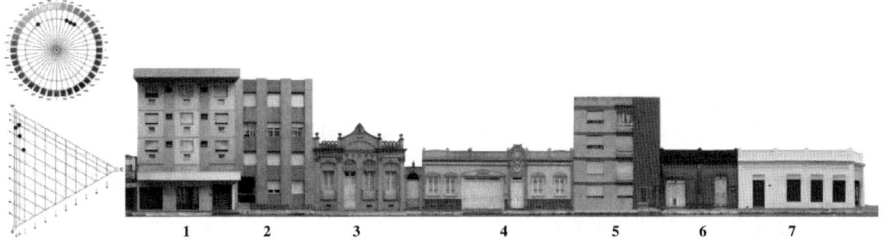

| Number of building ▶ | 1 | 2 | 3 | 4 | 5 | 6 | 7 |
|---|---|---|---|---|---|---|---|
| Dominant color | green | gray | beige | beige | pink | gray | white |
| NCS code | S0510-G30Y | S3020-R70B | S1005-Y30R | S2005-Y20R | S2005-Y40R | S9000-N (2) | S1500-N (1) |
| Details color | green | grey | beige | brown | brown | gray | white |
| NCS code | S3010-G60Y | S2502-G | S1005-Y30R | S5040-Y50R | S5040-Y70R | S9000-N (2) | S1500-N (1) |

**Figure 1.** Characteristics of urban scenes analysed in this study.

Scene 3 Moderate Complexity

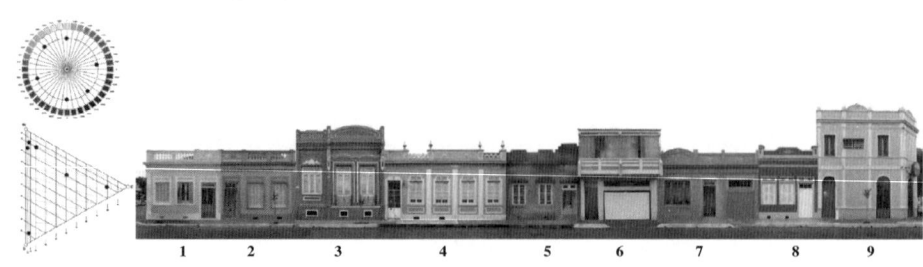

| Number of building ▶ | 1 | 2 | 3 | 4 | 5 | 6 | 7 | 8 | 9 |
|---|---|---|---|---|---|---|---|---|---|
| Dominant color | beige | yellow | blue | green | gray | beige | orange | red | green |
| NCS code | S1502-R50B | S1080-Y | S2040-B | S1010-G | S9000-N | S1002-Y50R | S1080-Y | S1080-Y90R | S1010-G50Y |
| Details color | white | yellow | white | white | gray | white | orange | white | white |
| NCS code | S0500-N | S1040-Y | S0500-N | S0505-G50Y | S9000-N | | S1080-Y | S0502-Y50R | S1005-G20Y |

**Figure 1.** Continued.

# Results

## Pleasantness Analysis of the Urban Scenes

In the evaluation of the scenes in terms of *pleasantness* (comparing frequencies of positive and negative indications), there was agreement between the two groups of participants (Brazilian and Russian). Scene 3 (with moderate complexity) was indicated as the most pleasant one and scene 2 (with low complexity) as the least pleasant one in both groups. However, the intensity of the assessments was different, the Russians appreciated scene 3 more intensely (65.6%), and the Brazilians appreciated scene 2 less, characterising it as *unpleasant* and *very unpleasant* with higher numbers of nominations (41.9%) (Table 1).

## Assessment of the Coherence and Attractiveness of the Urban Scenes

The points of *coherence* and *attractiveness* were analysed based on two opposite variables. In relation to *coherence* the participants were asked (1) if the colours in the urban scene are disordered and (2) if the relations among the colours are harmonious. With reference to attractiveness the participants were asked (1) if the colours in the urban scene are monotonous and (2) if the colours are interesting and varied.

In general, familiarity did not affect the assessment of the level of disorder of the scenes in terms of frequencies of positive indications (Table 2). However, it is interesting to note that according to the Mean Rank values, the two groups evaluated the disorder of

**Table 1.** Pleasantness rating of the three scenes by the two groups of participants

| Scale used for evaluation | Urban scene evaluated | | | | | |
|---|---|---|---|---|---|---|
| | Scene 1 | | Scene 2 | | Scene 3 | |
| | Brazilian | Russian | Brazilian | Russian | Brazilian | Russian |
| Very pleasant and pleasant | 33 (44.6%) | 14 (43.7%) | 15 (20.3%) | 8 (25%) | 42 (56.8%) | 31 (65.6%) |
| Neither pleasant nor unpleasant | 20 (27,0%) | 9 (28,1%) | 28 (37.8%) | 14 (43.8%) | 14 (18.9%) | 7 (21.9%) |
| Unpleasant and very unpleasant | 21 (28.4%) | 9 (28,1%) | 31 (41.9%) | 10 (32.2%) | 17 (24.3%) | 4 (12.5%) |
| Total | 74 (100%) | 32 (100%) | 74 (100%) | 32 (100%) | 74 (100%) | 32 (100%) |
| Mann–Whitney mean rank* | 53.43 | 53.67 | 55.3 | 49.34 | 55.39 | 49.13 |
| Asymp. Sig. (2-tailed) | ns | | ns | | ns | |

*The lower the mean rank value (Mann–Whitney $U$ test) of *pleasantness*, the more positive is the assessment. *ns* = not significant.

the scenes in a different sequence order. Scene 2, with neutral colours and low complexity, was rated as more disordered in the opinion of the Brazilians in comparison with the opinion of the Russians. It seems that the presence of saturated colours in scenes 1 and 3 made them more organised visually to the Brazilian group of responders.

The mean rank values of harmonious relationship among colours indicated differing results between the two cohorts. In scene 2 with neutral colours and low complexity the Russian cohort judged it as more harmonious whereas the Brazilian cohort judged the more colourful scene 1 as more harmonious.

In terms of coherence of urban scenes under review, both cohorts measured similarly in indicative frequencies, on scene 1 which had more complexity and disagreed on scene 2 which had less complexity.

The scene 1 was evaluated as disorganised and less harmonious by most participants in both groups. But the second one the Russians gave a more positive evaluation on the basis of harmony of colours and less positive by the Brazilians, suggesting that there are major discrepancies between groups in the evaluation of the scenes with low complexity and neutral colours. These results support the theoretical assumption (e.g., Purcell, 1984b; Purcell & Nasar, 1992) that discrepancies in the evaluation of the urban scenes may occur when people are exposed to different environmental patterns.

Focusing on monotony and interest as sub components of attractiveness, this research found that in most cases there was significant agreement between the two culturally different groups.

The similarity in evaluation of *attractiveness* suggests that this characteristic is more related to the formal chromatic attributes of the scenes and reflects the immediate perceptive experience of the participants. The discrepancies that occurred were caused by the influence of familiarity of the Brazilian with the more colourful urban environment. For example, in the evaluation of the *interest* and *variety*, the Brazilians considered scene 2 with neutral colours much less interesting than the Russians (Mann–Whitney $U$, Asymp. Sig. = 0.029) (Table 3).

## Assessment of Symbolic Features of the Urban Scenes

The emotional assessment of colours in the urban scenes was measured via the use of two affective scales: (1) *calm – excited* and (2) *friendly – aggressive*. The first evaluation aimed to investigate the visual potential of the chromatic activity of the scene and the second any connection with the sense of security.

Both Brazilian and Russian cohorts indicated scene 1, with high complexity, as *more exciting* than scenes 2 and 3 with low and medium complexity. Over 70% of participants in each group reported that feeling. The significant differences between the groups occurred in the perception of scene 2. More than 80% of the Russians indicated this scene as *calm* and *very calm*, however, less than half of the Brazilians (48.6%) had the same feeling. Projection of the opposite sensation occurred in scene 3 with medium complexity. Although in both groups there was a considerable amount of neutral indications (*neither*

**Table 2.** Perception of order/coherence of urban scenes analysed by using the two components *disorder* and *harmonious relationship among the colours*

| Disorder | Urban scene evaluated | | | | | |
|---|---|---|---|---|---|---|
| | Scene 1 | | Scene 2 | | Scene 3 | |
| | Brazilian | Russian | Brazilian | Russian | Brazilian | Russian |
| Strongly agree and agree | 38 (51.3%) | 17 (53.1%) | 22 (29.7%) | 6 (18.8%) | 28 (37.8%) | 7 (21.9%) |
| Neutral | 11 (14.9%) | 4 (12.5%) | 12 (16.2%) | 4 (12.5%) | 13 (17.6%) | 8 (25.0%) |
| Desagree and strongly desagree | 25 (33.7%) | 11 (34.4%) | 40 (54.1%) | 22 (68.7%) | 33 (43.6%) | 17 (53.1%) |
| Total participants | 74 (100%) | 32 (100%) | 74 (100%) | 32 (100%) | 74 (100%) | 32 (100%) |
| Mann–Whitney mean rank* | 53.64 | 53.17 | 51.04 | 59.19 | 51.24 | 58.73 |
| Asymp. Sig. (2-tailed) | ns | | 0.077 | | ns | |

| Harmonious Relationship | Urban scene evaluated | | | | | |
|---|---|---|---|---|---|---|
| | Scene 1 | | Scene 2 | | Scene 3 | |
| | Brazilian | Russian | Brazilian | Russian | Brazilian | Russian |
| Strongly agree and agree | 24 (32.5%) | 9 (28.6%) | 27 (37%) | 16 (50%) | 27 (36.5%) | 13 (40.6%) |
| Neutral | 8 (10.8%) | 6 (18.8%) | 17 (23.3%) | 9 (28.1%) | 13 (17.6%) | 9 (28.1%) |
| Desagree and strongly desagree | 42 (56.8%) | 17 (53.1%) | 29 (39.7%) | 7 (21.9%) | 34 (46%) | 10 (31.2%) |
| Total participants | 74 (100%) | 32 (100%) | 74 (100%) | 32 (100%) | 74 (100%) | 32 (100%) |
| Mann–Whitney mean rank* | 53.59 | 53.28 | 56.05 | 46.03 | 55.35 | 49.22 |
| Asymp. Sig. (2-tailed) | ns | | ns | | ns | |

*Notes.* Disorder = The scene is confused and disordered, the building colours do not match each other. Harmonious relationship = The scene is harmonious; there is sufficient relationship among the colours of the buildings. *The lower the mean rank value, the *more disordered* is the assessment of the scene and the *more harmonious* is the assessment of the scene. *ns* = not significant.

**Table 3.** Perception of attractiveness of urban scenes analysed by using the two components *monotony* and *interest*

| | Urban scene evaluated | | | | | |
| | Scene 1 | | Scene 2 | | Scene 3 | |
| Monotony | Brazilian | Russian | Brazilian | Russian | Brazilian | Russian |
|---|---|---|---|---|---|---|
| Strongly agree and agree | 9 (12.3%) | 0 (0.0%) | 45 (60.8%) | 20 (62.4%) | 9 (12.2%) | 2 (6.2%) |
| Neutral | 5 (6.8%) | 1 (3.1%) | 13 (17.6%) | 3 (9.4%) | 5 (6.8%) | 2 (6.2%) |
| Desagree and strongly desagree | 59 (80.8%) | 31 (96.8%) | 16 (21.6%) | 9 (28.1%) | 60 (81%) | 28 (87.4%) |
| Total participants | 73 (100%) | 32 (100%) | 74 (100%) | 32 (100%) | 74 (100%) | 32 (100%) |
| Mann–Whitney mean rank* | 50.37 | 59 | 53.3 | 53.95 | 52.42 | 56 |
| Asymp. Sig. (2-tailed) | | 0.048 | | ns | | ns |

| | Urban scene evaluated | | | | | |
| | Scene 1 | | Scene 2 | | Scene 3 | |
| Interest | Brazilian | Russian | Brazilian | Russian | Brazilian | Russian |
|---|---|---|---|---|---|---|
| Strongly agree and agree | 41 (55.4%) | 20 (62.5%) | 11 (15%) | 10 (31.3%) | 49 (66.2%) | 24 (75.0%) |
| Neutral | 13 (17.6%) | 5 (15.6%) | 10 (13.7%) | 6 (18.8%) | 9 (12.2%) | 3 (9.4%) |
| Desagree and strongly desagree | 20 (27.1%) | 7 (21.9%) | 52 (71.2%) | 16 (49.3%) | 16 (21.6%) | 5 (15.6%) |
| Total participants | 74 (100%) | 32 (100%) | 73 (100%) | 32 (100%) | 74 (100%) | 32 (100%) |
| Mann–Whitney mean rank* | 54.7 | 50.73 | 56.63 | 44.72 | 54.93 | 50.2 |
| Asymp. Sig. (2-tailed) | | ns | | 0.029 | | ns |

*Notes.* Monotony = The scene is monotonous with respect to chromatic appearance of the buildings. Interest = The scene evokes interest, there is enough variation in the building colours. *The lower the mean rank value, the *more monotonous* is the scene and the *more interesting* is the evaluation of the scene. *ns* = not significant.

*calm nor exciting*), the Russians tended to classify this scene *as calm* and the Brazilians as *exciting*.

Thus, the differences in evaluating chromatic activity occurred predominantly in urban scene 2 with low complexity with the Russian cohort having more positive evaluations of this scene (as *calm*) than the Brazilian cohort. In the perception of the sense of security, the most colourful scenes, or those with higher chromatic complexity, when compared with the less colourful scenes, were assessed more positively (as *friendly*) by the Brazilian cohort. It seems that the presence of colours induced a greater sense of security than the absence of colour for this group of participants, and the scene with little colour seemed less safe for them. Refer to Table 4 for summary of results.

The results indicate a significant difference between the two cohort groups in relation to their appreciation of historical architectural design and colour.

In the opinion of the Brazilians, the pale neutral colours of scene 2, with little chromatic complexity, do not emphasize the historic character of the building (Mean Rank rus. = 41.31; Mean Rank bras. = 58.77; Mann–Whitney $U$, Asymp. Sig. = 0.003).

## Evaluation of the Chromatic Attributes

In evaluating the chromatic attributes of the urban scenes via two groups, the greatest similarities were found in terms of prevalence of positive indications of each attribute. The discrepancies could be noticed only in the intensity of indications, especially when scene 1 with higher complexity was evaluated. In the analysis of *colour saturation*, the Russian participants perceived the predominant colours of scene 1 as *more intense* than the Brazilian participants (93.7% and 87.8%, respectively). In the observation of the *amount of different colours,* in scene 1, the evaluation of the Russian cohort also was more intense. The majority of the participants in this group (90.7%) indicated the presence of a large amount of different colours, in opposition to 81% of the Brazilians. In the evaluation of the attribute *contrast among the predominant colours of the buildings* in the scene, the Russian cohort found the contrast in scene 1 as much stronger than the Brazilian participants (90.6% and 79.7%, respectively). With this data it is possible to infer that there exists an increased sensitivity of Russian participants regarding the saturated colours in scenes with high and medium complexity. Such scenes tend to be evaluated as more complex in terms of colour by this group of participants.

## Discussion and Conclusion

The findings of the study suggest that colour contributes to perception and evaluation of *coherence* and *complexity* of urban scenes by means of chromatic attributes (*saturation of colours, amount of different colours,* and *chromatic contrast among the buildings*).

**Table 4.** Perception of the symbolic features of urban scenes analysed using the two affective scales *calm – excited* and *friendly – aggressive*

| Scale calm – excited | Urban scene evaluated | | | | | |
| --- | --- | --- | --- | --- | --- | --- |
| | Scene 1 | | Scene 2 | | Scene 3 | |
| | Brazilian | Russian | Brazilian | Russian | Brazilian | Russian |
| Very calm and Calm | 8 (10.8%) | 1 (3.1%) | 36 (48.6%) | 26 (81.2%) | 13 (17.6%) | 12 (37.5%) |
| Neither calm nor excitement | 14 (18.9%) | 6 (18.8%) | 34 (45.9%) | 6 (18.8%) | 30 (40.5%) | 13 (40.6%) |
| Excited and very excited | 52 (70.3%) | 25 (78.2%) | 4 (5.4%) | 0 (0%) | 31 (41.9%) | 7 (21.9%) |
| Total | 74 (100%) | 32 (100%) | 74 (100%) | 32 (100%) | 74 (100%) | 32 (100%) |
| Mann–Whitney mean rank* | 52.01 | 56.94 | 58.88 | 41.06 | 57.99 | 43.11 |
| Asymp. Sig. (2-tailed) | ns | | 0.002 | | 0.014 | |

| Scale friendly – aggressive | Urban scene evaluated | | | | | |
| --- | --- | --- | --- | --- | --- | --- |
| | Scene 1 | | Scene 2 | | Scene 3 | |
| | Brazilian | Russian | Brazilian | Russian | Brazilian | Russian |
| Very friendly and Friendly | 28 (37.9%) | 16 (50%) | 21 (28.4%) | 13 (40.6%) | 36 (48.6%) | 20 (62.5%) |
| Neither friendly nor aggressive | 19 (25.7%) | 6 (18.8%) | 44 (59.5%) | 19 (59.4%) | 32 (43.2%) | 9 (28.1%) |
| Aggressive and very aggressive | 27 (36.5%) | 10 (31.2%) | 9 (12.2%) | 0 (0%) | 6 (8.1%) | 3 (9.4%) |
| Total | 74 (100%) | 32 (100%) | 74 (100%) | 32 (100%) | 74 (100%) | 32 (100%) |
| Mann–Whitney mean rank* | 55.26 | 49.44 | 56.61 | 46.3 | 55.43 | 49.03 |
| Asymp. Sig. (2-tailed) | ns | | ns | | ns | |

*The lower the mean rank value is, the *calmer and more friendly* is the assessment of the scene. ns = not significant.

Scenes with moderate complexity tend to be positively evaluated and preferred, while scenes with low and high complexity tend to be negatively evaluated and have fewer preferences. This result supports the existence of a curvilinear relationship between chromatic complexity of the scene and its aesthetic evaluation, in accordance with Berlynes' (1972) theory.

The scenes with medium chromatic variation (medium complexity) tend to transmit calm and provide a greater sense of security (seen as more friendly) than scenes with lots of saturated colours and also the scenes without colour (with little chromatic variety). In the scenes with high complexity, the sensation of excitement is directly correlated with the *amount of colours*, *intensity of colours*, and *contrasting combinations*. This means that the less intense and contrasting, used colours combinations are, the more positively evaluated the scene is, therefore transmitting more calm.

The study showed that urban scenes with old and new buildings can be considered coherent by the participants when they present similar colour, not so much for the hue, as for the general shade of the facades. This is linked with softness of the colour and contrast between the chromatic combinations used in the details.

The evaluation of urban scenes showed that despite having different reasons, the familiarity with the historic buildings did not significantly affect the responses about *pleasantness*, *coherence*, and *attractiveness* of the scenes. This revealed that possible symbolic associations related to the knowledge about the historic buildings and the specific urban context had no major impact on aesthetic evaluations of the participants of the two research cohorts.

At the same time the study reported there are perception peculiarities in the two groups based on cultural preferences and prolonged experience with the different urban environment, adding cognitive dimension in the evaluation. However, these peculiarities are perhaps not as strong as the interference of biological and emotional focus on formal aspects of observed urban scenes. The differences between groups often arise in the intensity of the evaluations, without changing the positive or negative significance of their answers.

These facts indicated that the increase of the general chromatic complexity of the urban environment modifies human ability to perceive colour. In particular, for the Brazilian group, the tolerance of the participants to the strong hues applied to the historic buildings in the urban environment increased significantly. The other observation is that the absence of colour does not convey calm, neither makes the scene friendlier (safer) in the opinion of this group of participants.

Many architectural practices argue that buildings are matched with their environment, primarily through its mass (Carlhian, 1980), as well as repetition of elements and details of the facade (Groat, 1992) The results of this study suggest that for the urban scenes to be considered more coherent and evaluated positively, by the subjects, the design strategies must incorporate chromatic organisation and some degree of replication of colours in terms of lightness and combinations). Further studies on the perception of the chromatic aspects in the urban environment are needed to clarify these issues.

The desire to promote and enhance local architectural designs and traditions is important in order to promote feelings of attachment and a sense of identity in a region.

Research in the role colour plays in this scenario is under researched at present, however, could provide a route to a more aesthetically pleasing and psychologically beneficial working and living environment. It is important to merge traditional aspects of design with new thinking in order to enhance existing architecture as well as providing a platform for modernisation, conducive to enhancing the environment for all users, whether local or tourist.

Interdisciplinary research is needed in order to advance our understanding of colour in the design process and provide guidelines for the development of planning policies and practices in historical and modern sectors of cities.

## Acknowledgements

This study was conducted with financial support from the Research Support Foundation of the State of Rio Grande do Sul (FAPERGS).

## References

Beach, L., Wise, B. K., & Wise, J. A. (1988). *The human factors of colour in design: A critical review.* Moffet Field, CA: National Aeronautics and Space Administration.

Berlyne, D. (1972). Ends and means of experimental aesthetics. *Canadian Journal of Psychology, 26,* 303–325.

Burchett, K. E. (2001). Colour harmony. *Colour Research and Application, 27*(1), 28–31.

Carlhian, J. P. (1980). Guides, guideposts and guidelines. In J. Biddle (Ed.), *Old and new architecture: Design relationship* (pp. 49–68). Washington, DC: Preservation Press.

Groat, L. N. (1992). Contextual compatibility in architecture: An issue of personal taste. In J. Nasar (Ed.), *Environmental aesthetics, theory, research, and applications* (pp. 228–253). Cambridge, UK: University Press.

Hope, A., & Walch, M. (1990). *The colour compendium.* New York, NY: Van Nostrand Reinhold.

Janssens, J. (2001). Facade colours not just a matter of personal taste. *Nordic Journal of Achitectural Research, 14*(2), 17–34.

Judd, D. B., & Wysezcki, G. (1975). *Colour in business, science and industry* (3rd ed.). New York, NY: Wiley.

Lenclos, J. P. (1999). *Colour of the world: The geography of colour.* New York, NY: Norton & Company.

Naoumova, N. (2009). *Qualidade estética e policromia de centros históricos* [Aesthetic quality and polychromy of the historical centers]. Porto Alegre, Brazil: Federal University of Rio Grande do Sul State, Architecture School Doctoral thesis in Urban and Regional Planning.

Nasar, J. L. (1997). New developments in aesthetics for urban design. In G. Moore & R. Marans (Eds.), *Advance in Environment Behavior and Design* (Vol. IV). New York, NY: Plenum Press, Toward the Integration of Theory, Methods, Research, and Utilization.

Nasar, J. L. (1998). *The evaluative image of the city.* London/New Delhi: Sage.

Ou, L.-C., & Luo, M. R. (2006). A colour harmony model for two-colour combinations. *Colour Research and Application, 31*(3), 191–204.

Purcell, A. T. (1984a). Aesthetics, measurement and control. *Architecture Australia, 73*(4), 29–38.

Purcell, A. T. (1984b). The organisation of the experience of the built environment. *Environment and Planning B: Planning and Design, 11*, 173–192.

Purcell, A. T., & Nasar, J. L. (1992). Experiencing other people's houses: A model of similarities and differences in environmental experience. *Environmental Psychology, 12*, 199–211.

Siegel, S., & Castellan, N. J. Jr. (1988). *Nonparametric statistics for the behavioral sciences* (2nd ed.). Singapore: McGraw-Hill.

Stamps, A. E. (2000). *Psychology and the aesthetics of the built environment.* San Francisco, CA: Kluwer.

Toska, T. F. (2002). Environmental colour design for the third millennium: An evolutionary standpoint. *Colour Research and Application, 27*(6), 441–454.

Ünver, R., & Öztuk, L. D. (2002). An example of facade colour design of mass housing. *Colour Research and Application, 27*(4), 291–299.

# Human Experience in Urban Sustainability

# Towards a Theoretical Basis for Anthropological People-Environment Studies

Ray Lucas

Manchester Architecture Research Centre (MARC), School of Environment, Education and Development, University of Manchester, UK

**Abstract**

This paper presents a review of theories that underpins the strong synergy between contemporary social anthropology and the field of people-environment studies. As anthropology is the study of people and their life-worlds, perhaps a carefully constructed, all be it contentious case, can be made to link the basic tenets of this discipline to the discipline of people-environment studies. However, rather than exploring a particular project or case study, this paper seeks to demonstrate the applicability of anthropological thought and ethnographic practices to both the understanding and design of the built environment. The formulation of an argument for the tenets of anthropological to be merged with people-environment studies to inform design of the built environment is a difficult one. There are natural consistencies between the two disciplines, such as they tend to be people centred and based in real-world research, but they also have some differences, such as methodological and analytical. Anthropology is conventionally understood as an observational practice; one which stresses engagement and participation, but methodologically atheist, apolitical, and philistine. The notion of taking these observations and making fundamental changes to the built environment is often anathema to anthropologists, where it is second nature to architects and urban designers. As an organisation, IAPS (International Association of People-environment Studies) has a clear cross-disciplinary approach, with a fundamental stated goal for a greater understanding of the relationship of people with their environment. Notable contributions to this have been made by anthropologists, of course, but there is a clear role for a deeper engagement with anthropological theory as a complementary focus to environmental psychology, architecture, and sociology. Anthropological theory, from conventional studies of: class, gender, alienation, embodiment, agency, and dwelling can inform and frame the multitude of different ways in which it is possible to engage with the environment – built or otherwise. In both disciplines there is a fundamental belief that each person has an individual perspective of the world, based on their education, genetics, personality traits, social, and cultural experiences. Indeed to some extent these concepts inform our perceptions and behaviours in different environments.

**Key words:** anthropology, architecture, cross-disciplinarity, people-environment studies, urban design

# Introduction

IAPS is the acronym for the *International Association of People-Environment Studies* which represents a wide range of disciplines and practices, each with contributions to knowledge founded on strong empirical methodologies and practices. It is interesting to note, that whilst some key members of the association, such as Peter Kellet, are anthropologists who actively contribute to the overall debate, there is an overwhelming focus on environmental psychology, urban design, planning, and architecture. The Social Sciences is a "broad church" which encompasses a diverse range of disciplines and methodologies. However, one of the basic questions of this paper is: Does anthropological studies have a valid role to play in anthropocentric research and environmental morphology? Are we potentially sketching out a discipline of *Contextual Studies* which addresses: how we engage with the world, our being-in-the-world, and the possibility of the multiple life-worlds which we inhabit?

I arrive at this from a cross-disciplinary context as an academic in architecture, but also as an anthropologist. My encounter with anthropology is unapologetically idiosyncratic, but theoretically and methodologically consistent, and grounded in the possibility of a *Graphic Anthropology* which parallels that of *Visual Anthropology*. One element of this paper shall address the cross-over between these disciplines in my pedagogical practices, but also as a fundamental challenge to the ways in which both of these disciplines operate. There is a value in the nature of anthropology, which stands both in terms of the personalised and individual nature of its engagement as well as the theoretical underpinnings of the discipline. Key to the synthesis of diverse empirical research disciplines is the practical elements and rigours of reliability and validity in data collection and analysis.

The immediacy of data gathered through anthropological inquiry removes some of the mediating issues of environmental psychology, for example. Drawing more on Gibson's (1966) school of thought, our perceptions, and other interactions with the environment are best studied whilst *in that environment*. The model of the sterile laboratory with large numbers of subjects being exposed to stimuli ignores the basic facts of our physical engagement with space, the excitement of several senses at once, and the feedback from even the most modest movements.

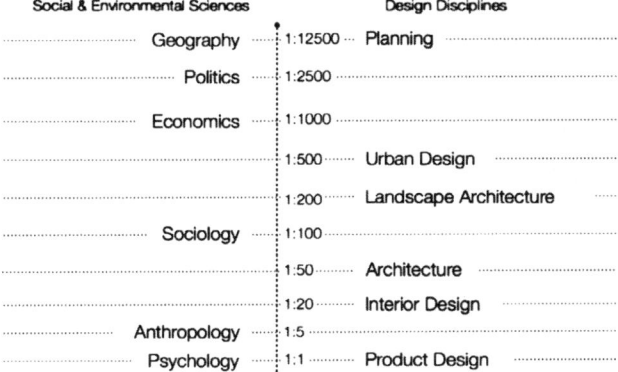

**Figure 1.** Scales of various built environment and social science disciplines.

None of this is designed to devalue the important and rigorous work carried out in other fields and by other means, but as a call for further methodologies to be used in order to explore the issues of our engagement within every day contexts. The position of this argument is that multiplicity is healthy, and each practice of knowledge production has something different to offer the understanding of real-world experiences. The theoretical lenses and filters offered by architecture and its graphic practices is variously complicated, augmented, detailed, and contradicted by the addition of anthropologies methods and theories.

This paper argues that these multiple "ways of knowing" help contextual exploration of the synthesis between anthropology and people-environment studies. In tackling this agenda several interesting questions are raised: How can we know a thing? What are the forms of engagement most appropriate to a given context? What do we learn through engagement with such practices? Perhaps more importantly: How do we then act on this? A number of issues are immediately raised. Defining disciplines is already a diverse and complex endeavour, however within the context of this paper we do need to understand the position of several disciplines and how they inform us. One of the key mechanisms for this shall be to consider the concept of scale, suggesting that each discipline has a focus on a scale (see Figure 1).

Whilst a great deal of this paper shall discuss practices as being important, it is not held that the practice of anthropology is to be found only in ethnographic field research. Such material does form an important foundation for the majority of anthropological works, but the production of knowledge in anthropology is also conducted through academic rigour. The theorisation, often resulting from ethnography, is often disregarded in our consideration of practices, but an idea or concept is a carefully crafted and considered construct. It is merely not some immediate flash of inspiration, made once the correct connections have been identified. It is from this point of view that I ask what might constitute

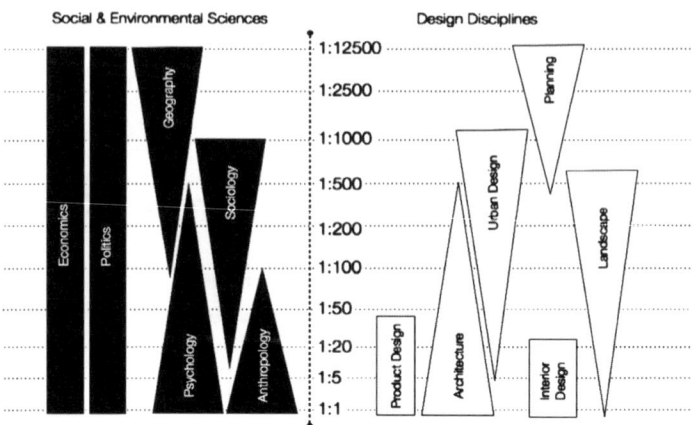

**Figure 2.** Extent of various built environment and social science disciplines.

a theoretical basis for anthropology (advisedly not ethnography) in People-Environment Studies.

The focus of the IAPS 22 conference encouraged the development of theoretical and applied areas of people-environment research. The anthropological stance this paper takes towards this process seems a natural endeavour as anthropology and its unique disciplinary characteristics can be matched to people and the environment from both a theoretical and applied view point. What anthropology offers is an understanding of alternative ways of being in the world and different practices of being human, that are fully enmeshed within the environment. For anthropology, all knowledge is produced *in* the environment with human *life-worlds* a key concept in contemporary anthropology research. These life-worlds are complex and rounded engagements with the natural and built environment and a recognition that we cannot think of our lives in the abstract. There is a need for this level of social and cultural understanding to be addressed at the level of design implementation as well as policy, and the first stage in this development is in design education and research (see Figure 2). The process of change in any discipline is complex and usually stems from the education of practitioners who work in a professional context such as planning, design, and architecture. The embryonic process of change can usually be found via the process of education. Educational pedagogical change is often slow and fraught with resistance.

## Graphic Anthropology

This lecture series is presented to second year architecture students, and confronts a number of theoretical issues in a manner consistent with the approach of Manchester School of

Architecture. It is shown here as a demonstration of the issues pertinent to anthropology and design, particularly architecture. This extends beyond the university context, and presents a broader approach as we shall see, towards truly *Multi-modal Representations of Urban Space*1 which can form the basis of a more holistic design discipline (see Lucas, Mair, & Romice, 2009).

The course content is pertinent to this paper as it has some resonance with work carried out between the writer and Tim Ingold on the delivery of the four A's project: Anthropology, Archeaology, Arts, and Architecture. The delivery of this course (detailed in Ingold & Lucas, 2007) was based on a frustration with the degree to which conventional anthropological education engaged with its own findings: that learning is a form of *understanding in practice*, and that one *learns by doing*. This suggests that *practice* is fundamental to teaching and learning.

> I have argued that it is wrong to think of learning as the *transmission* of a ready-made body of information, prior to its *application* in particular contexts of practice. On the contrary, we *learn by doing*, in the course of carrying out the tasks of life. In this the contribution of our teachers is not literally to pass on their knowledge but rather to establish the contexts or situations in which we can discover for ourselves much of what they already know, and also perhaps much that they do not. In short, we crow *into* knowledge rather than having it handed down to us. This is what Jean Lave (1990) means when she says that learning is a matter of *understanding in practice* rather than *acquiring culture*. (Ingold & Lucas, 2007, p. 288)

This is not the place to discuss the institutional frameworks of different Universities and Departments, but the circumstances of Graphic Anthropology were somewhat different, particularly the cohort size, which ranges from 160 to 190 students. This coupled with the prescribed nature of architectural education places some interesting constraints on the content and delivery of this lecture series 2. However, one basic structure remained: the field note exercise (Ingold & Lucas, 2007, p. 289).

The lecture series presents alternating practices of graphic representation and key anthropological theories in order to understand a site in the city of Manchester. Students are asked to: visit this place every week, observe, and interact with the place in a different manner each week, and directly relate the contextual experience to the content of the lectures. Each of these engagements is a practice, an exercise, and a model for understanding the site. Site selection reflects the course interests, and students are asked to pick a place which they can visit regularly and which falls into one of the following categories:

- Marketplace (such as a shopping mall, open-air market, car-boot sale),
- Transit space (e.g., a railway or bus station, or on the tram),
- Public square (any public open space where people can gather freely),
- Museum (a gallery, or other space of cultural display).

Lectures are grouped as follows:

*Sensory Perception*: Lectures on sensory perception approach the phenomenology of place with reference to particular methods of: sense-walking, sensory notation, soundscape studies, models of how movement through space can be conceptualised from Laban's approach to the body, to Augoyard's (2005) taxonomy of urban walking. Each sensory register demands different methodological ways of working, research combining sensory inputs requires synthesis of methodologies in order to gain valid data. What is interesting is so much of our experience of space is left out of the geometric bias of architecture and urban design.

*Representational Practices*: The section on representational practices presents students with the wide variety of inscriptions from: conventional architectural drawing, what it means to draw in plan, section, and elevation, the mental mapping of Gould and White (1986), urban graphics including Nolli, Gandelsonas (1987, 1998) and Bacon (1976) an appreciation of sketching, time-based media, and bearing witness through processes of drawing as understanding. These lectures address what it *means* to draw a perspective or an elevation, and how one edits and selects from reality in order to bring forth a particular understanding.

*Anthropology and Site*: Finally, key types of site are associated with fundamental forms of social exchange presenting marketplaces as sites of exchange such as, museums as centres of cultural display and the relation between home and identity. Other social issues and discussions of what it fundamentally means to live, occupy, pass through, and interact with a space. Why do we linger in some places but not others, how can the same space embody both wonder and colonialism?

Field note exercises include compiling a simple taxonomy, informed by: methods used by the essayist and author, Perec (1997, 2010); definitions and descriptions of the soundscape as explored by Schafer (1977), Augoyard and Torgue (2006), Chion (1994, 1999), and others, different forms of abstraction in drawing, exploring serial sketching as proposed by Cullen (1971), or movement notations inspired by Laban's work in modern dance and ballet (Laban, 1966; Laban & Lawrence, 1979; Laban & Ullman, 1971).

Whilst Humanities teaching has a great deal of ground to cover, what is offered by this course is the opportunity to build research methods. In addition to this, an openness to the idea that the means in which we engage with sites is more than a visual decision on what looks best, but is also instrumental to: the kinds of design produced, the understanding on which the architecture is based, and a set of concerns for how we dwell. As such, students are equipped with applied skills and the ability to develop these into an architectural agenda: much more than imparting a body of knowledge such as the details of a given architectural period.

Pedagogical practice and development has an impact upon the profession and policy, when taken over the long term. The impact of having large cohorts of design professionals schooled in anthropology is not to be underestimated. The RIBA validation process of UK schools of architecture ensures a strong humanities basis for both undergraduate and postgraduate study. It is significant that pedagogical development in architecture courses is understood as more than simply in terms of the history and theory of architecture. Built environment disciplines always look beyond their boundaries in order to understand the social role of building, and anthropology offers a nuanced approach to this social life.

This critique of urban design and architectural practice is not novel, of course. There are periodic moves towards a closer integration of social theory and design, such as tying anthropology to architecture (Amerlinck, 2001; Melhuish, 1996; Rappoport, 1969; Rykwert, 2010). These approaches all too often adopt an outdated form of anthropology. It is this papers aim to bring the disciplines together at the point of contemporary practice rather than with the benefit of critical historical distance. Cuthbert's research (2003, 2006, 2011) illustrates the use of historical anthropological models on contemporary research and therefore as an argument for exigency for the use of contemporary anthropological models. Cuthbert does identify the need for deeper understanding of social conditions in urban design, however, there remains a need to bring this into line with contemporary debates. The best way to do this is not to reflect on the outputs of alternative disciplines, but to collaborate directly with its practitioners. This reflects an attitude towards anthropology developed by this writer in ongoing research.

## Ethnographic Accounts as the Basis for Design

An interesting emerging approach can be identified in recent works by anthropologists such as Daniels' (2010) research, investigating the material culture of the Japanese Home. This book comprehensively explores the flow of objects and sentiment through family homes which highlights the role of storage as an important signifier in how people live. Other examples exist, such as Buchli's (2002) research focussing on the overt politics of the Soviet home or Bestor's (2004) research investigating the various spatial economies of the Tsukiji fish market in Tokyo. Sarah Pink's *Home Truths* (2004) discusses the minutiae of everyday domestic life and exemplifies this category of architecturally focussed anthropology, with a case-study approach focussing on concepts of cleanliness.

These approaches are strong examples of contemporary anthropology in architecture, which highlights an important distinction to be made. Whilst there is a great deal more to be learnt from such approaches, there is another, more substantial mode of cross-fertilisation between disciplines that does not subject one to the gaze of the other, but places them into a continuous dialogue in order to reconfigure the means by which spaces are specified, designed, and understood.

In using such understanding to construct better informed documents and briefs for buildings, might help to build a model for community engagement which affords a voice to the people in the concept build stage. This may avoid the inherent pitfalls of conservative tastes, replicating what has gone before, and the possibility of surpassing expectations or producing spaces which respond in novel and unexpected ways. In short, an alternative transdisciplinary approach may avoid the validation of conservative approaches, which respects and exploits the expertise of the professional designer.

## Multiple Inscriptive Practices

The crucial involvement of the inscriptive practice in all of this: more than simply an internal problem to architecture is a set of practices relevant to anthropologists. In this respect the suggestion from anthropological studies is that ethnographic fieldwork has a great deal to teach architects and urban designers.

The role of such representational techniques is important in discussions of architectural practice, where the prototype process available to product and industrial design is more difficult to achieve due to the scale and contextual nature of architecture. This tension between abstractions and context remains one of the most problematic in the practice of architecture, but also offers opportunities for creativity.

In order to further explore the nature of architecture, it is necessary to consider drawing and inscriptive practices, as well as understanding the flow of movement and temporality inherent to the practice. In many ways, a parallel practice can be found in the practice of improvisational dance described by Sheets-Johnstone (1999), p. 485. Sheets-Johnstone's concept of *thinking in movement* is helpful to the study of drawing and as a result, the design processes itself. The description of improvisational dance given above could easily reflect the close integration of drawing and the architectural design process. Thus, the process of creating is not the means of realising a design; it is the process of design itself: to draw is to design. In this way, thinking in movement is understood not as the transcription of a pre-formed mental image, but that "thinking is itself, by its nature, kinetic" (1999, p. 486). This idea has the potential of being an important new conceptualisation of design practices. As much as Sheets-Johnstone's focus on dance takes Bergson's critique of the homogenisation of time it also operationalises it as a means of understanding practices which have become embedded in disciplines without being understood fully.

The potential of such an understanding, in creative practice, as flows of movement is to understand the nature of thinking through drawing. Essayists such as Berger (2011) and architectural theorists including Pallasmaa (1996) and Merrill (2010) agree that there is a knowledge-seeking aspect to the drawing: that there is a desire (and ability) to understand and find things out by engaging in an inscriptive practice. Merrill's account (2010, pp. 12–14) is particularly useful, as it charts the development al drawings of Louis Kahn's practice (including those by Kahn himself as well as other architects and technicians) for an unrealised project: The Dominican Motherhouse inn. As such, it reflects the pure design process and reveals the fraught nature of architectural design by engagement with the wealth of archival material. This record or trace of the project is an important source for understanding the architectural project as it allowing access to presentation materials, designed for the consumption of a client, and also the sequence of drawings which lead to that point.

The preference expressed for the plan and other orthographic drawings by Merrill is, perhaps overstated, but is used to illustrate a shift in architectural practice with greater reliance on computer models, which serve as images more readily than the abstractions of plan, section, and elevation. This photorealistic representation is often held to be more direct or image-based, but I would argue that the same issues of abstraction and contextualisation remain at the heart of this way of thinking. Thus, the creative tension in terms of temporality and spatiality remains.

Discussions of improvisation lead to the work of Sudnow (2002) on learning to play jazz piano, as well as the strong linkage demonstrated by Hallam and Ingold in their editorial to the collection "Creativity and Cultural Improvisation" (2007, pp. 2–24). Fundamentally, each of these issues leads to better understanding of: flows, movements, intuition, and temporality. The work of Henri Bergson is particularly useful in describing this process, and how such practices occur temporally as heterogeneous and grounded activities. It is with Time and Free Will (2001 [1913], p. 97) that this description relating creative practices to a reappraisal of time offers an experiential alternative to the homogeneity of scientific time.

It is easy to fall into a trap where a preference is expressed for experiential time over mathematical time, but there is much greater potential in understanding and exploiting the differences between these two fundamentally different ways of understanding time or space. The homogeneous space is unique to human activity, an abstraction which offers a clarity that is sometimes dangerous and at other times crucial, to edit out that which is distracting or irrelevant. It is this operational inattention from specific context which allows the architect to act and provoke through intervention. It is much more useful to realise that there are abstracting and contextualising impulses at play in different aspects of the design process. It is sometimes absolutely necessary to work with measure (2001, p. 12) and to abstract generalisable principles before working again with the specific context. Measure is used interestingly by Bergson here to indicate not only a quantifiable, but an idea of anticipation, and the expectation of future movements.

We can trace both sides of temporality from an account which Bergson gives the simple mathematical procedure of counting. This can be understood as a temporal sequence of numbers, with the sequential process being key to the operation. What happens in mathematics, however, is that this sequence is abstracted from reality and experience (2001, p. 76).

This idea of neglecting the differences is important to the argument, and lies at the root of abstracting mechanism, in which attitudes towards temporality and spatiality alike are evened out into an undifferentiated homogeneous medium.

In defining the terms for his query, Bergson works with the categories of extensity and intensity. These two terms are understood to be possible conditions of the same thing:

> [...] we picture to ourselves, for example, a greater intensity of effort as a greater length of thread rolled up, or as a spring which, in unwinding, will occupy a greater space. In the idea of intensity, and even in the word which expresses it, we shall find the image of a present contraction and consequently a future expansion, the image of something virtually extended, and, if we may say so, of a compressed space. (Bergson, 2001 [1913], p. 4)

The conceptual "space" occupied, allows a categorical difference to be observed, More than merely compressing and internalising through the idea of intensity, we have a qualitatively different experience when sensations are so tightly coiled.

It is therefore more fruitful to think in terms of a cyclical process which flows from extensive to intensive and back again. The precise pattern of this being more descriptive of the creative process, than simply understanding the geometry, graphics, and eventual architecture produced. The return to measure in this description is important, as the denial of measure in the intensive phenomenon indicates a perpetual present which looks to memory but does not indicate a future position. There is a parallel to Bergson's concern for the temporal in Bollnow's significant work *Human Space* (2011). Bollnow himself is explicit in his description of this experiential space in drawing the connection to Bergson (2011, p. 18).

The recognition that the concept of experienced space and the intrinsic connection between spatiality and human life is difficult to grasp and must be done in contrast to the homogeneous mathematical space. The necessity of this contrast is interesting in itself, but it also reiterates the dichotomy between the abstract and the contextual. What we learn from the practice of architecture, however is that these two elements in time or space must be united: specifically that there is a flow and coexistence of these two concepts of space.

Bollnow details the "natural" co-ordinate system (2011, pp. 39–54) as being grounded in direct datum such as, things being *in front* or *behind of* our body, or related to the horizon in the distance which determines fundamental categories of up and down. This *centre* is conceptually similar to that expressed within dance theory and notation, particularly Laban's notation.

## Scales of Context

This paper confirms my interest in the inscriptive practices which lie at the heart of architecture. If we are to discuss the design disciplines involved in the production of our built environment, then we must consider the wide range of methods available to them. A commitment to working across scales and with different forms of editing, selection, and abstraction is crucial to the depth of understanding required. Additionally, by seeing the world through a range of theoretical frameworks, filters, and lenses, a designer can select the approach most appropriate to the site, people, and purpose at hand.

Understanding the underlying assumptions behind such inscriptions allows the designer to select the most appropriate tool for the job. Knowing that the elevation is equipped to discuss the proportions of a surface whilst the plan can articulate spatial relations and organisations seems like conventional wisdom, but this is not communicated in a sufficiently rigorous way within design pedagogy.

There are many ways of knowing, and the greater the number of methods used in solving a design issue, the more rounded and appropriate the result is likely to be. In suggesting that People-environment Studies can benefit from closer engagement with anthropology, I am suggesting a methodological and theoretical kinship between such studies. Anthropology deals in fine-grain information, which is difficult to quantify, but none the less important in the development of applied understanding of people-environment research. It reminds us of the wide variety of ways in which one can be human: rather than the defined populations of varying dimensions dealt with by other social, environmental sciences, and psychology sub-disciplines.

In concluding, I return to the scale diagram from the beginning of the paper (see Figure 3). This is perhaps an unrefined and deliberately provocative schema which does not map on to the reality of disciplinary engagement with context, people, and dwelling. It does, however, illustrate something of the ways in which the group of disciplines under the banner of IAPS might combine to address people-environment interactions (see Figure 4). The intent is not to reserve one scale for anthropology, another for sociology, and yet others for psychology and geography, but rather to see some of the potential corroborations and interactions between disciplines. However, there are interdisciplinary tensions that, although occupy a similar methodological stance there is still the potential to select an inappropriate anthropological scale for specific projects.

The purpose of developing the diagram is to inform discussion on where collaboration can and ought to take place. Like all good diagrams it should be: fluid, open to change and opportunities, map a set of conditions, and specifically in this case opportunities for improving the design of our built environment (see Figure 5). Exploiting these disciplinary intersections relies upon collaboration with contemporary practitioners, rather than on our reflections upon the outputs of anthropologists. Our alternative readings as designers, informs this collaboration significantly, as does the adoption of theories and practices. However, the way forward relies on the development of a parallel discipline, mirroring the development of Design Anthropology for industrial and product design but with the aims and needs of People-Environment Studies and the Built Environment kept in mind.

| Social & Environmental Sciences | | Design Disciplines |
|---|---|---|
| Census | 1:12500 | Regional Planning |
| Survey | 1:2500 | City Plan |
| Questionnaire | 1:1000 | Location Plan |
| | 1:500 | Site Plan |
| Experiment | 1:200 | Block Plan |
| | 1:100 | Office Plan |
| | 1:50 | House |
| | 1:20 | Interior Design |
| Interview | 1:5 | Technical Detailing |
| Ethnography | 1:1 | Furniture |

**Figure 3.** Scales of engagement and process.

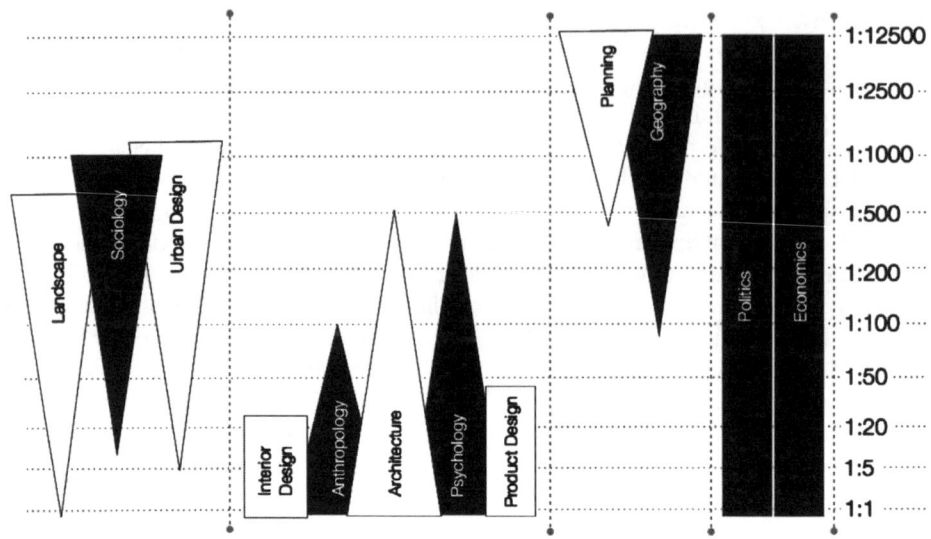

**Figure 4.** Mapping complementary disciplines.

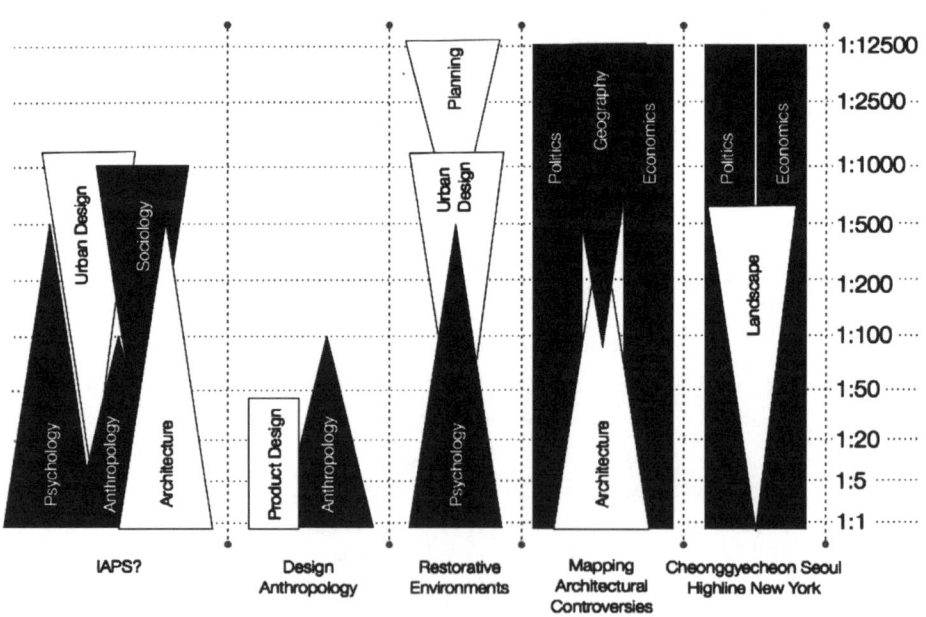

**Figure 5.** Mapping potential collaborations using the diagram.

# References

Amerlinck M. J. (Ed.). (2001). *Architectural anthropology*. Westport, CT: Greenwood Press.

Augoyard, J. F. (2005). *Step by step*. Minneapolis, MN: University of Minnesota Press.

Augoyard, J. F., & Torgue, H. (2006). *Sonic experience: A guide to everyday sounds*. Montreal, Canada: McGill-Queens University Press.

Bacon, E. N. (1976). *Design of cities: Revised edition*. London, UK: Penguin Books.

Berger, J. (2011). *Bento's sketchbook*. London, UK: Verso Books.

Bergson, H. (2001 [1913]). *Time and free will: An essay on the immediate data of consciousness*. New York, NY: Dover Books.

Bestor, T. C. (2004). *Tsukiji: The fish market at the center of the world*. Berkeley, CA: University of California Press.

Bollnow, O. F. (2011). *Human space* (C. Shuttleworth, Trans.). London, UK: Hyphen Press.

Buchli, V. (2002). Khruschev, modernism and the fight against petit-bourgeois consciousness in the Soviet Home. In V. Buchli (Ed.), *The material culture reader* (pp. 215–237). Oxford, UK: Berg.

Chion, M. (1994). *Audio-vision: Sound on screen*. New York, NY: Columbia University Press.

Chion, M. (1999). *The voice in cinema*. New York, NY: Columbia University Press.

Cullen, G. (1971). *The concise townscape*. Oxford, UK: Architectural Press.

Cuthbert A. R. (Ed.). (2003). *Designing cities: Critical readings in urban design*. Oxford, UK: Blackwell.

Cuthbert, A. R. (2006). *The form of cities: Political economy and urban design*. Oxford, UK: Blackwell.

Cuthbert, A. R. (2011). *Understanding cities: Method in urban design*. Oxford, UK: Blackwell.

Daniels, I., & Andrews, S. (2010). *The Japanese home: Material culture in the modern home*. Oxford, UK: Berg.

Gandelsonas, M. (1987). The order of the American city: Analytic drawings of boston. *Assemblage, 3*, 63–71.

Gandelsonas, M. (1998). The city as the object of architecture. *Assemblage, 37*, 128–144.

Gibson, J. J. (1966). *The senses considered as perceptual systems*. Westport, CT: Greenwood Press.

Gould, P., & White, R. (1986). *Mental maps*. London, UK: Routledge.

Hallam, E. & Ingold, T. (Eds.). (2007). *Creativity and cultural improvisation*. Oxford, UK: Berg.

Ingold, T., & Lucas, R. (2007). The 4 A's (Anthropology, Archaeology, Art and Architecture): Reflections on a teaching and learning experience. In M. Harris (Ed.), *Ways of knowing: New approaches in the anthropology of knowledge and learning* (pp. 287–305). Oxford, UK: Berghahn Books.

Laban R. (1966). *The language of movement: A guidebook to choreutics*. Boston, MA: Plays.

Laban, R., & Lawrence, F. C. (1979). *Effort*. London, UK: Macdonald & Evans.

Laban, R., & Ullman, L. (1971). *The mastery of movement*. London, UK: Macdonald & Evans.

Lave, J. (1990). The Culture of Acquisition and the Practice of Understanding. In J. W. Stigler, R. A. Shweder & G. Herdt (Eds.), *Cultural psychology: Essays on comparative human development* (pp. 309–27). Cambridge, UK: Cambridge University Press.

Lucas, R., Mair, G., & Romice, O. (2009). Making sense of the city: Representing the multimodality of urban space. In T. Inns (Ed.), *Designing for the 21st century: Interdisciplinary methods & findings* (pp. 190–207). Farnham, UK: Ashgate.

Melhuish C. (Ed.). (1996). *Architecture and anthropology*. London, UK: Academy Editions.

Merrill, M. (2010). *Louis Kahn, drawing to find out: The Dominican motherhouse and the patient search for architecture*. Baden, Germany: Lars Müller.

Pallasmaa, J. (1996). *The eyes of the skin: Architecture and the senses.* London, UK: Academy Editions.

Perec, G. (1997). *Species of spaces and other pieces.* London, UK: Penguin Books.

Perec, G. (2010). *An attempt at exhausting a place in Paris.* Cambridge, MA: Wakefield Press.

Pink, S. (2004). *Home truths: Gender, domestic objects and everyday life.* Oxford, UK: Berg.

Rappoport, A. (1969). *House form and culture.* Upper Saddle River, NJ: Prentice Hall.

Rykwert, J. (2010). *The idea of a town: The anthropology of urban form in Rome, Italy and the ancient world.* London, UK: Faber & Faber.

Schafer, R. M. (1977). *The soundscape: Our sonic environment and the tuning of the world.* Rochester, VT: Destiny Books.

Sheets-Johnstone, M. (1999). *The primacy of movement.* Amsterdam, The Netherlands: John Benjamins.

Sudnow, D. (2002). *Ways of the hand: A rewritten account.* Cambridge, MA: MIT Press.

# Participatory Public Policy, Public Housing, and Community Sustainability

## A Venezuelan Experience

Esther Wiesenfeld[1], Euclides Sánchez[1], and Fernando Giuliani[2]

[1] Institute of Psychology, Central University of Venezuela, Caracas, Venezuela
[2] School of Psychology, Central University of Venezuela, Caracas, Venezuela

**Abstract**

Environmental Community Psychology (ECP) has among its goals contributing to improved living conditions of residents in precarious settlements. Literature in ECP largely refers to projects that research the relationship between community and professionals. These professionals promote processes and actions in order to enhance communities' ability to empower themselves and participate, to improve their residential living conditions. Such endeavor is also expected to influence public policy. Nevertheless, little has been reported on communities' influence in public policies and on joint work with agencies in charge of devising and implementing them. This article focuses precisely on community guidelines for housing and habitat public policy, developed within a government agency. Guidelines were supported by: (a) ECP principles, (b) critical constructionist paradigm (Wiesenfeld, 2000), (c) an approach for public management based on community and agency members participation and co-responsibility, (d) sustainable development model, (e) information gathered in workshops, meetings, interviews and discussion groups, with the institution's personnel and community members in a Venezuelan State.

**Key words:** community sustainability, environmental community psychology, housing policy, participation, third agent

## Introduction

Since its inception in the Bruntland Report (1987), the Sustainable Development (SD) Model has to date become richer, more complex, and more widerspread worldwide. A contributing factor has been the realisation of the inadequacy and distortion that the emphasis on economic development imposes on the development of countries, at the expense of other inseparable dimensions. Among the limitations that have led to successive changes of the SD Model, the Commission on Sustainable Development (CSD) of the United Nations refers to the omission of conflicts, social inequalities, and cultural aspects specific to each country.

One of the model's most important changes has been to incorporate the social dimension and, more recently, the community dimension (Giuliani, 2006; Wiesenfeld & Giuliani, 2002). This recognised the difficulty of sustainability as a community goal, if the precarious conditions of the planet's numerous informal human settlements are not met. In 2005 it was reported that nearly one billion people in the world lived in precarious human settlements, and in Latin America the figure amounted to over 134 million, representing 30.8% of its urban population (United Nations – HABITAT, 2010).

In reality, the economic, environmental, social, community, and residential vulnerability in these settlements has put them on the public agenda as one of the priority challenges to be faced by multilateral, national, regional, and international agencies dedicated to solving the poverty problem. The Millennium Goal (UNDP, 2008), the Istanbul Habitat Declaration (United Nations – HABITAT, 1996) are examples of this.

In the case of Latin America, the magnitude of the poverty problem can be seen in recent ECLAC data indicating that 31.4% of its population are poor: 177 million people live in poverty, 70 million of which are destitute or living in extreme poverty (ECLAC, 2012). The concentration of poverty and the poor in the region, both in slums and in state constructed urban developments, shelters, or living in the streets, suggest that housing and habitat be made a priority for governmental agencies in their respective countries. It also assumes that public policies aimed at addressing this basic human right are dedicated to significantly reducing the housing deficit and improving living conditions of existing housing, for the sake of the inhabitants' quality of life.

## Public Policies, Housing, and Habitat in Latin America

Housing and habitat problems are often located in self-managed, high risk areas, without basic infrastructure and social services, highlighting the lack of effective public policy strategies (Gabaldón, 2006). These policies tend to be formulated from spaces and positions of power, alien to the needs, experiences, and perspectives of poor communities. In other words, public policy makers in housing and habitat understand little of the policy recipients' particular needs.

A repeated claim by poor communities and non-governmental agencies is that there is a lack of local community involvement in the formulation and management of public policies. One example is the Constitution of the Bolivarian Republic of Venezuela (1999) that confers community participation a central role. However, this prescription is not as closely followed as desired, which threatens the sustainability of and in these environments (Cilento, 2010; Rodríguez & Sugranyes, 2004).

Regarding this, Wiesenfeld and Sánchez (2010) consider community participation as an inescapable component for the application of the SD model. Similarly Ling, Dale, and Hanna (2007) formulated a long-term model to develop community sustainability, together with social and economic sustainability. The authors believe this plan represents a critical, integrating process that differentiates it from the conventional ones. The model differs because it incorporates community participation in its development and implementation, thereby facilitating local influence on planning policies. The plan, which integrates the quality of the place, the people, and the economy, hopes that community efforts, coordinated with input from specialists and other relevant actors, will actually affect public policies of planning. However, looking at context particularities, in our case precarious settlements or lower income urban developments in Latin America, these aspirations are incomplete, without interventions addressed to policy makers and implementers. In this sense, a strategy we suggest for bringing communities towards public policies and vice versa, is to include government agencies or third agents as necessary actors in managing actions aimed at community participation and influencing public policies. This proposal seeks to open processes with officials, so they re-signify a communities' conditions and rights, and themselves as public servants, with their demands, resources, and duties.

The proposal is grounded in contributions from Environmental Community Psychology (ECP), critical constructionist theoretical perspective, and qualitative methodology. ECP refers to an Environmental Psychology that aspires to understand and contribute to solving problems inherent in person-environment poverty settings, and to a Community Social Psychology that addresses community requirements, and environmental problems associated with those settings. Thus by promoting community and residential psychosocial processes in the communities, to help them overcome the adverse conditions, they endure (Wiesenfeld, 1994, 2001; Wiesenfeld & Sánchez, 2012). In this way, the Social Psychology community in Latin Americas' commitment to research and action to change conditions of economically and socially disadvantaged communities is combined with Environmental Psychology's efforts to understand and stimulate human-environmental transactions that promote welfare as well as social, community, and environmental sustainability (Wiesenfeld & Sánchez, 2010).

Critical constructionism (Wiesenfeld, 1998a, 1998b) is a theoretical approach that complements certain aspects of social constructionism and critical theory. Both perspectives share a subjective transactional approach to reality that highlight their historic nature, the influence of context and power relations in the social construction of human experience, and consider theory as a product of research, in which everyone involved is a co-participant (Guba & Lincoln, 1994). Though both perspectives emphasise the importance of discourse, the critical approach incorporates action, as a facilitator of change processes.

Thus, social constructionism maintains that reality is socially constructed from our experiences and communicative practices with groups and in particular contexts. Its transformation, therefore involves deconstructing the contextualised, temporal and spatial meanings of those experiences (Ibáñez, 1989, 1994). However, we believe that, as a social practice, this is not sufficient; such a deconstruction should involve other practices based on critical and reflective dialogues informed by situations and actions that have come to be considered natural or part of everyday life.

Relevant to this are some notions and methods of critical theory, or what Guba (1990) calls "ideologically oriented search," which see in false conscience the risk of maintaining the hegemony of dominant sectors and perpetuating the oppression of the excluded sectors. In agreement with Fals Borda (1959) and Freire (1974) some social psychologists (Lane, 1984; Martin-Baró, 1985; Wexler, 1983) and community psychologists with a critical orientation (Fryer, 2008; Prilleltensky, 1994) suggest problematisation and denaturalisation are strategies that conscienitise and re-signify oppressive conditions. The empowerment that this triggers in those involved stimulates them to actions that are reflected upon and transformers of such conditions. In this line of thought, critical perspectives contribute to the constructionist proposal that incorporation of change strategies go beyond discourse, on to reflected action.

Qualitative methodologies are appropriate to the presented theoretical approach because, like ECP, they assert forms of knowledge production and social practices committed to equity and social justice (Kendall & Michael, 1997). Despite their variety, qualitative approaches share the value of local narratives in the formulation of policies and actions to eradicate oppression, (Brydon-Miller, 1997; Gergen, 1996; Kendall & Michael, 1997; Potter & Wetherell, 1995, 1997; Sarbin, 1986; Spears, 1997).

Thus, ECP, critical constructionism, and qualitative methodology integrate the disciplinary, theoretical, and methodological foundations to address habitat unsustainability associated with poverty and community participation in public policies. These are relevant to our proposal to incorporate the third agent to this complex picture, through interventions that jointly involve him/her with ethical, political positions, in so far as they: (a) acknowledge the plural and diverse nature of communities and invite debate and confrontation of views on poverty, its places and its protagonists, (b) call for the bond with its members through mutual respect, that emerges from the problematisation and consciousness raising of their experiences and knowledge, (c) facilitate the familiarisation and appropriation by public officials of community and residential psychosocial processes that resonate cognitively and affectively for them, by being inherent to their own dwelling experiences.

## Community-Third Agent Rapprochement

Community psychosocial literature abounds with proposals and analysis on relationships between professionals in the field, other external agents and communities (Goncalves, 2005; Quintal de Freitas, 1998). Given the nature of community psychosocial research it is perhaps natural that the main thrust of dialogue in this area should be with deprived communities. On the other hand, there is little information about the link between communities and government agencies, which are often held accountable for the inequitable conditions suffered by poor communities. The transformation of those conditions is precisely one of ECP's goals, for which their representatives act, together with the communities.

On the other hand, there is little information about the link between communities and government agencies, which are often held accountable for the inequity conditions suffered by poor communities. The transformation of those conditions is precisely one of ECP's goals, for which their representatives act, together with the communities.

Given that: (a) improving population's quality of life is an unavoidable commitment of the third agent, and the public policies he/she is in charge of are key instruments in achieving this goal, (b) communities mistrust third agent's actions for the lack of success of public policies in improving poor communities' living conditions, (c) the third agent is reluctant to include communities as co-participants in the design and management of public policies that concern them, (d) ECP professionals possess knowledge and skills to facilitate processes that promote a rapprochement between the two stakeholders, there are fundamental questions that should be explored in order to overcome the problems posed. Such as: How to incorporate ECP professionals into government spheres, to advocate for community participation in public policies? How to build the trust of the third agent towards ECP professionals, a necessary condition for the job at hand, without losing the trust that the communities have placed on these professionals? How to encourage the third agent to problematise and be sensitive to the social, ethical, and political implications of their decisions, so he/she opens up to the influence of the communities on public policies? How to get the third agent to see him or herself as a subject of rights and duties, as a builder of a just society, from his/her own involvement in public policies?

Answering these questions demands a familiarisation and bonding with third agents, from their perspective, circumstances, problems, and needs in order to strengthen their skills and encourage psychosocially orientated processes (Giuliani & Wiesenfeld, 2011). Such an approach calls on the conceptualisation and promotion of community psychosocial processes and the development or adoption of procedures similar to those used by ECP in its work with communities. It also warrants stimulating the incorporation of governability models, such as participatory public management, that support the proposed objectives, and development models that harbour the technical, economic, social, environmental, and community imperatives of sustainability in a comprehensive manner (Natera, 2004). Both models converge with ECP on the importance of participation in claiming human rights and sustainability (Dryzek, 1999).

Thus, the methodology for psychosocial community work, context analysis, the participative public management model and the SD model, make up the guidelines that substantiate our research proposal that promotes the design of programmes and policies in housing and habitat, with community participation. The guidelines were developed through a series of activities carried out within the framework of a government institution in charge of the design and implementation of public policies in housing and habitat in a

Venezuelan state. They became the conceptual and methodological platform to train the officials of said institution and of the communities in guiding the proposal.

## Psychosocial Community Guidelines for Housing and Habitat Policies

Psychosocial community guidelines (PSCG) are based on ECP postulates that consider: (a) equity and justice possible, from acknowledgement, understanding and respect for diversity, and (b) reflective dialogue with and between the parties is a necessary mechanism to understand and negotiate affective and cognitive experiential plurality, within and between sectors, and trans-disciplines. In harmony with the ECP approach, these postulates, when transferred to the problem of precarious human settlements, involve: (1) assuming a comprehensive conception of housing and habitat, (2) re-signifying housing as a human right, (3) contextualising housing and habitat public policies. Additionally, the guideline assumptions are: (1) it is not possible to build habitat without considering the processes (community, psychosocial, residential, and cultural) that energize its occupants in different contexts; (2) efficient, effective and sustainable public management cannot be achieved without the active involvement of the communities in the formulation and implementation of the housing and habitat policies, programmes and projects suitable to their needs, (3) the co-managed construction of sustainable housing and habitat demand the sensitivity and training of those involved in the processes aimed at achieving it (Wiesenfeld & Giuliani, 2002). This means that institutions and communities should incorporate the psychosocial and community dimension as a central axis of management and development. The development of the guidelines, and the training involved, required work by ECP professionals throughout 2010 and was organised into the following stages and activities.

### Preliminary-Diagnostic Stage (Stage I)

This consists of identifying, collecting, and analysing information from different sources and procedures, namely conducting one discussion session with academics and specialists, and another with the communities. They were both structured around seven themes; each one dealt with at a discussion table where 6–8 participants sat according to their interests. The objectives of the discussions were: (a) to learn participants' perspectives on the agency's programmes and on issues relevant to housing and habitat, (b) to generate ideas in order to optimise, add others and/or implement programmes given criteria of efficiency, participation and sustainability. Activities in this stage included:

- Job analysis in the management offices of the agency, based on seven interviews with eight key participants.
- Analysis of the agencies policies and programmes on the subject of housing and habitat, based on existing documents.

- Identification of community psychosocial needs, explicit or implicit in the agency's programs. These were derived from information provided in the discussion sessions, review of the programmes, and interviews with key participants.
- Detection of staff training needs were obtained from our knowledge of the difficulties faced by members of different management offices in their work with communities, and the limitations of community participation in the management of housing and habitat projects. This was a dynamic process as some needs continued to show up throughout the PSCG training and implementation.

## Development of Psychosocial Community Guidelines for Housing and Habitat Policies (Stage II)

The PSCG drew on information produced at the preliminary stage, along with the experience in community work of the environmental community psychologists in charge of this project, and the contributions of specialised literature. They were organised into following modules:

1. Participative public management, which included some background on Venezuela's public management model, a historical review of how management alternatives emerged, ending with a descriptive analysis of the current context of public management, a characterisation of the Participative Public Management model and the challenges it involves for the housing organism.
2. The SD model and its implications for housing and habitat, which provides a presentation of the concept of development, its implications for public administration, and a description of the effects of the application of the prevailing models. It also describes the main features of the SD model and its implications for housing and habitat management. Finally, it presents factors associated with the habitat concept, its socio-community dimension and the sustainability criteria that are part of the guidelines.
3. Political-territorial, economic, geographic, cultural and institutional Characterisation of the agency's geographical setting, as a context for the implementation of Participative Public Management, Sustainable Development, and the psychosocial community perspective on habitat. This module includes the description of the region, its main characteristics, potentials and problems, and the characteristics of its public policies and housing and habitat criteria. Finally, we provide information about the agency and its programmes.
4. The methodology for psychosocial community work in housing and habitat, based on ECP postulates, principles and methods. Besides incorporating the participative public management model and promoting sustainable development, it adapts to

context particularities, calls for cross-sector work between communities with the third agent, vindicates diversity and articulates local and interdisciplinary knowledge. The module describes the main characteristics of the methodology proposed (participatory, dialogical, flexible, culturally relevant), the requirements for its application (holistic understanding of housing and habitat, knowledge diversity, intersectoriality), the guiding principles (organisation, participation, consciousness raising, co-management) and phases for conducting community work (preliminary contacts and encounters, diagnosis of resources and needs, design of action plans, implementation of action plans, continuous evaluation).

## Development of a Training Programme (Stage III)

This is a training programme for the personnel (managers, coordinators, and others) based on the modules. This programme aims to encourage, in the personnel, a shared vision of the goals, values, and means of the agency's policy on the development of housing and habitat. This is in order to foster their favourable relationships with the communities they are involved with and to promote satisfactory residential and community processes.

## Agency Personnel Training (Stage IV)

Training is provided, through workshops, discussion groups, practical exercises, and meetings with communities. Although training was based on the described training programme and guidelines, as it developed, other training demands emerged that required additional programmes, such as the following.

## Preparation of the Training Programme and Training in the Use of Methodological Tools to Evaluate Their Interventions in Housing and Habitat (Stage V)

## Development of a "Communication and Information Transmission Plan" for the Agency (Stage VI)

A need that appeared in the course of our work and that is an indispensable tool for the various activities that are carried out.

### Development of Community Psychosocial Guidelines for Attending Critical Situations in and With Communities (Stage VII)

### Development of a Training Programme for Communities (Stage VIII)

The purpose of this is to strengthen their organisation and participation in the management of their housing and habitat needs.

## Applying the Psychosocial Community Guidelines to a Pilot

In what follows we illustrate the application of the PSCG to the "I'm an owner" (IAO) programme, aimed at regularising ownership in urbanisms and housing. The programme arises from the large number of requests to the agency for home ownership, which reveals a concern for this topic. A concern, that was ratified in the discussions, conclusions and suggestions of the group discussions with specialists and communities, who made this requirement a priority. The following phrases, taken from the petitions collected by the agency and the transcripts of the discourses during the discussion groups, illustrate its importance:

> The land property deed generates and complements the communities' sense of belonging; The land deed is a necessary requisite to qualify for credits; The view of the communities must change "we are not invaders," "we are tenants"; It is a community need to know and manage the existing legal instruments; Land committees should be created and strengthened as active participants, to make the legal framework known; The communities should inventory usable land.

In addition, the following expectations were gathered regarding the agency's role in the co-management of ownership, which reinforce topics of co-management through community participation, sustainability, and training:

> It should guide, support, and promote; The Institute's priority could change from building to educating; The community should be trained to be self-sustainable; It should work with the communities, they are the ones who really know the problems; The support of various agencies is necessary to ensure the existence of the necessary infrastructure on site, to prevent this from becoming an obstacle when processing land ownership; Soil studies should be prior to granting land deeds and thus determine risk areas; Bring this type of experience to all the communities in the State.

According to the Committee on Economic, Social, and Cultural Rights of the United Nations, in General Comment number 4 (United Nations, 1991), ownership is precisely one condition that housing should undoubtedly be considered adequate or decent. However as demonstrated by Arébalo, Landaeta, and Solares (2003) and PROVEA (2008), consistent with what was requested and with the conception of housing as a right, the programme proposed a general objective:

> To promote and generate legal, urbanistic, construction, subsidiary and community conditions that ensure the completion of viable processes of regularisation of urbanism and housing tenure, so that the human right to housing is perfected in the full ownership of land and homes, and in urbanization conditions that ensure human development, quality of life, and healthy coexistence. (INVIHAMI, 2010, p. 23).

Likewise, the specific objectives included, amongst others: "Establishing types of legal, urbanistic, subsidiary and community intervention according to the legal status of each urban development and the state of its physical infrastructure." In addition to: "achieving sustainable conditions in the urban developments, by giving comprehensive technical advice to organized communities and encouraging conservation and maintenance."

In accordance with the PSCG, the listed objectives show a comprehensive view of housing and habitat, emphasising the psychosocial and environmental dimension, and the specific objectives point to community sustainability, through cross-sector, participative strategies, and the corresponding training. Furthermore, the programme implementation was facilitated by our familiarisation with and systematisation of the situations faced by the agency's officials and the communities that contributed to: (a) identify the legal, technical, psychosocial, community, administrative, political aspects, with implications for this and other Agency Programmes, revealing a comprehensive approach to the issues, (b) prepare the conditions for its implementation, from interdisciplinary and cross-sector standpoint, (c) develop the Operations Procedure (INVJHAMI, 2010), to make it easier to understand, (d) adapt the PSCG to the Programme and select the features, principles, and stages of the Socio-Community Methodology to guide the way for officials in charge of different areas to work with each other and with the communities in the implementation of the Programme.

The preceding contributions were integrated into a "Handbook on procedures and general plan for the implementation of the Programme," which was classified into five groups of materials. Each group representing a stage of the Programme and containing instructions and supportive documents, namely materials for the comprehensive diagnosis of the urbanisms pre-selected for the IAO programme strategy for the onset of the IAO programme with the communities, instruments for gathering information in urbanisms selected for the IAO programme, materials for the implementation of the IAO in cooperation with community organisations, training programme aimed at agency officials and representatives of community organisations, to familiarise them with its contents, train them to handle it and foster its appropriation.

Likewise, the stages of the Programme implementation procedure conform to those described in the Socio-Community Methodology and correspond to the PSCG (Participative Public Management, comprehensive concept of housing and habitat, Sustainable Development), promoting community processes (organisation, participation, coexistence, co-management) and community capacity for joint management of Sustainable Human Settlements.

It is worth pointing out that each stage incorporated cross-sector work, encouraged the exchange of knowledge and acknowledged perspective and context diversity. Also, encounters between actors were preceded by the development of strategies that included the contents or topics to be dealt with, as well as the community (organisation, participation, consciousness raising, co-management, sense of community, empowerment) and residential processes (sustainability, identity, rootedness, attachment) involved.

Let us consider the stages and their general activities.

*Preliminary stage*: Information gathering from different sources with various procedures.

*Preparatory stage*: Familiarisation of officials with IAO and the criteria for inclusion and prioritisation of the urbanisms selected for the first stage of IAO implementation.

*Stage 1*: Onset, including: contact with leaders and/or representatives of community organisations to present the programme, reach agreements for its implementation and provide material about the programme and the guide to implement it.

*Stage 2*: Comprehensive diagnosis of the programme components (legal, technical, architectural, socio-community). The activities of the socio-community diagnosis included:

- Conduction of a population census,
- Diagnosis of community organisation,
- Identification of community needs and resources through participative and dialogic processes,
- Information processing,
- Preparation of the Diagnostic Report,
- Coordinating the Dossier.

*Stage 3*: Design of action plans by component. On one hand, the Socio-Community Action Plan required the articulation between the community (s), the Agency, and other entities. It also considered population characteristics, community organisations, community needs and resources, land ownership, the Programme's objectives, the criteria for housing and habitat sustainability described in the Socio-Community Guidelines, the Government Plan for the development of the State.

Based on the aforementioned criteria, the action plan involved:

1. Meeting with local government teams,
2. Designing the strategy for joint action of the local Government Head Offices with the Agency,
3. Discussing the joint action strategy with community representatives,
4. Presenting and discussing the Action Plans with community representatives,
5. Presenting the dossier information and the Plans to a citizens' assembly in the community.

*Stage 4*: Implementation of action plans.

*Stage 5*: Granting of property deeds.

The preliminary diagnosis of the IAO Programme has identified physical assets of 10,371 homes, an equivalent number of families, and a population of approximately 51,855 people (INVIHAMI, 2010). The Programme was first implemented in 2010, and from that period to 2012 property deeds have been given to 3,000 families, which constitutes an important achievement in meeting the aspiration to ownership.

## Conclusions

The experience showed the relevance and potential of cross-sector, interdisciplinary collaboration, and training, in order to achieve a comprehensive approach to housing and habitat, its vindication as a right, and in promoting sustainable conditions in precarious settlements, starting from work with the third agent. It also shows the contributions of ECP in making this agent aware of the importance of the psychosocial community dimension in housing and habitat policies, positioning him/her as a subject of rights and eventual beneficiary of these policies. Thus providing conceptual tools that facilitate his/her understanding of community context and problems, and training in the use of methodological tools that support his/her work with the communities and other actors, in an atmosphere of mutual exchange and respect.

Programme implementation also revealed obstacles and critical situations. First, sustainable development and new Participatory Public Management require employee changes towards collaborative work with communities. Environmental community psychologists can contribute to this endeavour based on the discipline's corresponding concepts and methods.

It is also necessary to foster institutional articulation between and beyond their current stated principles. This a complex challenge that needs further research and undoubtedly fundamental change in attitudes by both professionals and institutional organisational in order to facilitate a paradigm shift in cultural structures. This is particularly relevant for implementing pubic policies at a local, regional, and national level. Although in principle the prevailing rhetoric claims to agree on tenet of collaboration and community involvement, in practice collaborative work is resisted. Unless this obstacle is urgently addressed, isolated and top-down programmes and policies will continue. In this respect we propose carrying out planned actions, oriented towards stakeholders' articulation.

Additionally, a systematic participatory evaluation, for programme improvement and accountability is required. Evaluation should also aim at strengthening both, the programme and its relation with the third agent and communities. Its reliance on mutual trust and co-responsibility opposes traditional, assitentialist, and hierarchical relations between public institutions and communities.

Finally, without denying the difficulties faced throughout the experience presented in this article, it is necessary to recognise the opportunities that this type of initiative opens up, for academia, for poor communities and for public policies, among others. We invite you to continue efforts in this line of work, as a contribution to the production of knowledge, the improvement of quality of life, and environmental, residential, and community sustainability.

# References

Arébalo, M., Landaeta, G., & Solares, H. (2003). *Suelo urbano y vivienda popular en América Latina* [Urban soil and popular housing in Latin America]. San José, Costa Rica: Centro Cooperativo Sueco.

Brundtland, G. H. (1987). *Our common future*. Oxford, UK: Oxford University Press (Report of the World Commission on Environment and Development WCED).

Brydon-Miller, M. (1997). Participatory action research: Psychology and social change. *Journal of Social Issues, 53*(4), 657–666.

Cilento, A. (2010). Sostenibilidad urbana: el caso de las ciudadades venezolanas [Urban sustainability, the case of Venezuelan cities]. *Portafolio, 21*(1), 28–37.

Dryzek, J. (1999). Transnational democracy. *The Journal of Political Philosophy, 7*(1), 30–51.

ECLAC (Economic Commission for Latin America and the Caribbean). (2012). *Panorama social de América Latina 2011* [Social Panorama of Latin America 2011]. New York, NY: United Nations. Retrieved from http://www.eclac.org/publicaciones/xml/1/45171/PSE2011-Panorama-Social-de-America-Latina.pdf

Fals Borda, O. (1959). *Acción comunal en una vereda colombiana* [Communal action in a colombian sidewalk]. Bogotá, Colombia: National University of Colombia.

Freire, P. (1974). *Educación para el cambio social* [Education for social change]. Buenos Aires, Argentina: Tierra Nueva.

Fryer, D. (2008). Some questions about "the history of community psychology". *Journal of Community Psychology, 36*(5), 572–586.

Gabaldón, A. (2006). *Desarrollo Sustentable. La salida de América Latina* [Sustainable Development. Latin America way out]. Caracas, Venezuela: Grijalbo.

Gergen, K. (1996). *Realidades y Relaciones* [Realities and Relations]. Barcelona, Spain: Paidós.

Giuliani, F. (2006). *Desarrollo Sostenible, Psicología Social Comunitaria y Articulación Barrio-Ciudad. El caso de la comunidad de Catuche* [Sustainable Development. Community Social Psychology and City-Slum Articulation]. Master's Thesis in Social Psychology, Central University of Venezuela, Caracas.

Giuliani, F., & Wiesenfeld, E. (2011). La intervención comunitaria en Venezuela. Nuevos tiempos, nuevos retos para la psicología social comunitaria [Community intervention in Venezuela. New times, new challenges for community social psychology]. *Investigación en Psicología, 16*(1), 15–28.

Goncalves, M. (2005). La relación investigador-comunidad en el trabajo psicosocial comunitario. Su lugar en la producción del conocimiento [The relationship researcher-community in psychosocial community work. Its place in knowledge production]. Master's Thesis in Social Psychology, Central University of Venezuela, Caracas.

Guba, E. (1990). *The paradigm dialog*. Newbury Park, CA: Sage.

Guba, E. G., & Lincoln, Y. S. (1994). Competing paradigms in qualitative research. In N. K. Denzin & Y. S. Lincoln (Eds.), *Handbook of qualitative research* (pp. 105–117). Thousand Oaks, CA: Sage.

Ibáñez, T. (1989). *La psicología social como dispositivo construccionista en el conocimiento de la realidad social* [Social psychology as a constructionist device for social reality knowledge]. Barcelona, Spain: Sendai.

Ibáñez, T. (1994). Construccionisno y Psicología [Constructionism and Psychology]. *Interamerican Journal of Psychology, 28*(1), 105–123.

INVIHAMI (Housing and Habitat Institute of Miranda State). (2010). *Lineamientos Psicosociales Comunitarios para la Política de Vivienda y Hábitat* [Community psychosocial guidelines for housing and habitat policy]. Caracas, Venezuela: Author.

Kendall, G., & Michael, M. (1997). Politicizing the politics of postmodern social psychology. *Theory and Psychology, 7*(2), 7–29.

Lane, S. T. M. (1984). A Psicologia uma nova concepcao de homem para a "Psicologia" [Psychology: A new conception of man for Psychology]. In S. T. M. Lane & W. Codo (Eds.), *Social Psychology: Man in movement* (pp. 10–19). Sao Paulo, Brazil: Brasiliense.

Ling, C., Dale, A., & Hanna, K. (2007). *Integrated Community Sustainability Planning Tool. Infrastructure/SSHRC Funded Project.* Royal Roads University. Retrieved from http://www.crcresearch.org/sites/default/files/icsp-planning-tool.pdf

Martin-Baró, I. (1985). *Acción e ideología. Psicología social desde Centroamérica* [Action and ideology. Social Pschology from Central America]. San Salvador, El Salvador: Central American University José Simeón Cañas.

Natera, A. (2004). La noción de gobernanza como gestión pública participativa y reticular [The notion of governance as participatiry and reticular public management]. *Politic and management.* Madrid: Department of Political Science and Sociology, University Carlos III. Retrieved from http://e-archivo.uc3m.es/bitstream/10016/590/1/cpa040202.pdf

Potter, J., & Wetherell, M. (1995). Discourse analysis. In J. A. Smith, R. Harré, & L. van Langenhove (Eds.), *Rethinking methods in psychology* (pp. 80–92). London, UK: Sage.

Potter, J., & Wetherell, M. (1997). Social representations, discourse analysis and racism. In S. Moscovici & U. Flick (Eds.), *The psychology of the social* (pp. 138–155). Berlin, Germany: Rowohlt.

Prilleltensky, I. (1994). *The morals and politics of psychology: Discourse and the status quo.* New York, NY: State University of New York Press.

PROVEA (Venezuelan Program for Education-Action in Human Rights). (2008). *Vivir con dignidad. El derecho humano a una vivienda y hábitat adecuados* [Living with dignity. Human Right to adequate housing and habitat]. Memoirs of the VI Seminar of formation in economic, social and cultural rights. Caracas, Venezuela: Author.

Quintal de Freitas, M. F. (1998). Inserção na comunidade e análise de necessidades: reflexões sobre a prática do psicólogo [Community insertion and needs analyss: Reflections about psychological practice]. *Psychology, reflection and critique, 11*(1), 175–189. Retrieved from http://www.scielo.br/scielo.php?script=sci_arttext&pid=S0102-79721998000100011&lng=en&nrm=iso

Rodríguez, A., & Sugranyes, A. (2004). El problema de vivienda de los "con techo" [Housing problem in those "with roof"]. *EURE (Santiago), 30*(91), 53–65. Retrieved from: http://www.scielo.cl/scielo.php?script=sci_arttext&pid=S0250-71612004009100004&lng=es&nrm=iso

Sarbin, T. (1986). *Narrative psychology. The storied nature of human conduct.* New York, NY: Praeger.

Spears, R. (1997). Introduction. In T. Ibañez & L. Iñiguez (Eds.), *Critical social psychology* (pp. 1–26). London, UK: Sage.

United Nations. (1991). *General Observation No. 4 the International Pact of economic, social and cultural human rights.* New York, NY: Secretary of the Publications board.

United Nations Development Programme [UNDP]. (2008). *End of poverty millennium development goals.* Retrieved from http://www.un.org/millenniumgoals/2008high level/sgstatement.shtml

E. Wiesenfeld et al.
Participatory Public Policy, Public Housing, and Community Sustainability

**155**

United Nations – HABITAT. (1996). *Istanbul decleration on human settlements*. Retrieved from http://www.unhabitat.org/content.asp?ID=407&catid=366&typeid=24

United Nations – HABITAT. (2010). *Estado de las ciudades de América Latina y el Caribe* [State of Latin American and Caribbean Cities]. United Nations Program for Human Settlements Retrieved from http://gaportal.org/resources/detail/el-estado-de-las-ciudades-de-america-latina-y-el-caribe-urbanizacion-desarrollo-humano-y-democracia

Wexler, P. (1983). *Critical social psychology*. University of Michigan, MI: Routledge & Kegan Paul.

Wiesenfeld, E. (1994). La psicología ambiental en el contexto de la comunidad: Hacia una Psicología Ambiental Comunitaria [Environmental Psychology in the context of community. Towards and environmental community psychology]. *Contemporary Psychology, 1*(2), 40–49.

Wiesenfeld, E. (1998a). El construccionismo crítico: su pertinencia en la psicología social comunitaria [Critical constructionism: Its pertinence for community social psychology]. *Psychology and Society, 10*(2), 137–157.

Wiesenfeld, E. (1998b). Desarrollo teórico en psicología ambiental: el enfoque construccionista-crítico [Theoretical development in environmental psychology: The critical constructionist approach]. *Journal of AVEPSO XXI, 2*, 33–61.

Wiesenfeld, E. (2000). La problemática ambiental desde la perspectiva psicosocial comunitaria. Hacia una psicología ambiental del cambio [Environmental problematic from the psychosocial community perspective. Towards an environmental psychology for change]. *Environment and Human Behavior, 1*(2), 1–19.

Wiesenfeld, E., & Giuliani, F. (2002). Promoting sustainable communities: Theory, research and action. *Journal of Community, Work and Family, 6*(2), 159–182.

Wiesenfeld, E., & Sánchez, E. (2010). Community sustainability: Orientations and implications from environmental community psychology. In V. Corral (Ed.), *Psychology and sustainability* (pp. 317–336). New York, NY: Nova Science.

Wiesenfeld, E., & Sánchez, E. (2012). Participación, pobreza y políticas públicas: 3P que desafían la psicología ambiental comunitaria [Participation, poverty and public policies: 3P that challenge environmental community psychology]. *Intervención Psicosocial/Psychosocial Intervention, 21*, 225–243.

# Programming for Behaviour in Educational Environments

Doris C. C. K. Kowaltowski, Daniel de Carvalho Moreira,
Marcella S. Deliberador, and Paula R. P. Pereira

School of Civil Engineering, Architecture and Urban Design, University of Campinas – UNICAMP,
Campinas-SP, Brazil

---

## Abstract

To attain a quality built environment the design process needs structure, rigour and rich, varied data on technical, functional, and behavioural issues of architectural design. Considering the complexities involved in architectural design the brief and design program are specific instruments of fundamental importance to the successful outcome of the overall design project. During the 1950s architects and engineers, aware of scientific theoretical developments, endeavoured to apply new methods to the building design process. During this period of development, the programming phase gained not only importance but specific methods such as "Problem Seeking" by Peña and Parshall, today in its 5th edition. This paper discusses the architectural program as part of the building design process. In most developed countries this design phase, especially for school buildings, is participatory and usually orchestrated by a well-informed design team who stimulate debates based on recent research findings. In countries like Brazil, public school building design still lacks a participatory programming debate. In addition important design data is rarely structured to produce effective documents for use in the pre-design phases of the design process. A study is presented where data on learning environments and especially behavioural issues are structured according to the "Problem Seeking" programming method. The public school environment found in the State of São Paulo, Brazil, form the backdrop to this study. The "Problem Seeking" material should enable participatory briefing to be introduced in a more productive way in the local public school building design process, in order to improve learning environments directly and education as a whole indirectly.

**Key words:** architectural design process, architectural program, behaviour and built environment, school architecture

---

## Introduction

Public education has been an essential instrument to promote social progress. In rapidly developing countries, like Brazil, the importance of education cannot be underestimated. This paper presents further developments of a continuing study, on the public school environment in the State of São Paulo, Brazil. Emphasis is given to the school building design process. For the design process to be successful, designers have to understand the end users needs and requirements. In the case of school environments designers need to have an appreciation of the functional aspects of the building that are needed to facilitate the pedagogy and educational systems adopted by the school to happen in a comfortable and positive environment, and to be able to adapt to changing needs over time.

Comfort includes, not only the typical environmental aspects of acoustic, thermal, and visual comfort, but also functional and psychological wellbeing. Spaces and their relation to each other must adequately accommodate the necessities of learning and social activities, as well as the emotions and stress felt by users. These feelings are related to environmental psychology and include a sense of belonging, security, and spatial orientation.

Discussion between designers and users should be supported by technical and quantitative research data, as well as subjective and qualitative elements specifically related to architectural designs of schools. Such data should not only contain the latest research results but should be placed in the context of the design debate.

An extensive study on the public school building design process found in Brazil, and specifically in the State of São Paulo, that the process lacks a participatory briefing phase, thus stunting necessary debates. An enriched design process, based on structured data to stimulate participatory debates, is seen as capable of producing improved educational spaces. These spaces can subsequently be evaluated according to key benchmarks set in the architectural program or brief phase (Deliberador, 2010).

## The Architectural Design Process With Emphasis on the Briefing Phase

A typical architectural design process model, shown in Figure 1, can be divided into five important phases: Programming (briefing), designing, constructing, occupying, and evaluating (Post-Occupancy Evaluation – POE) with adjustments or refitting. In most developed countries commissioning is added between the construction and occupation phases: To prepare the building for its users and their activities, adjust the infrastructure to optimum operational levels, train staff for best potential use and maintenance, and introduce minor retrofits of perceived problems.

To attain a quality built environment the design process needs structure, rigour, and rich varied data on technical and functional aspects of design and the relation of human behaviour to the physical environment. To this end, the architectural program is an important instrument. During the 1950s architects and engineers, aware of scientific theoretical developments, endeavoured to apply new methods to the building design process and the

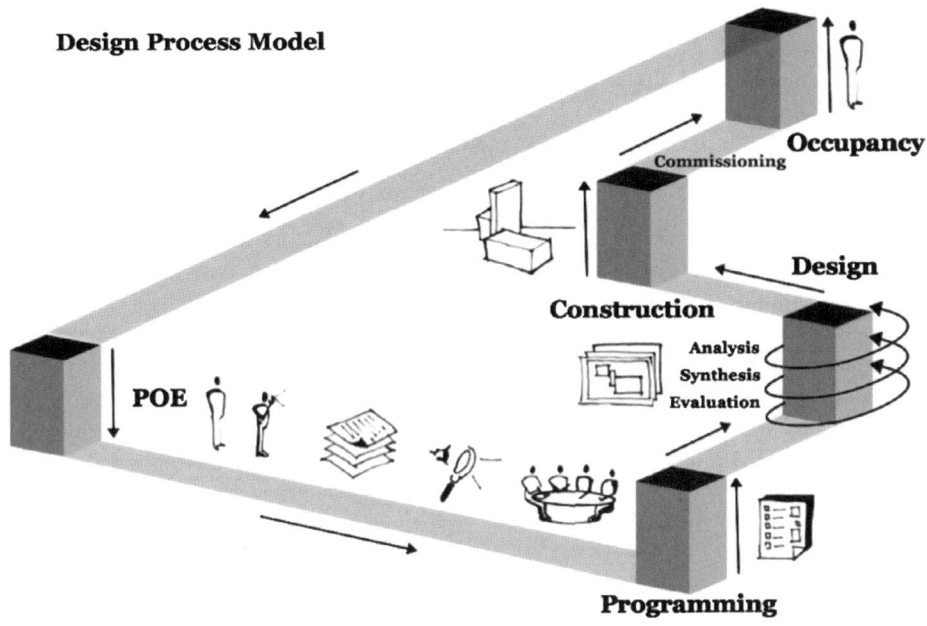

**Figure 1.** A model of the typical architectural design process.

programming phase gained specific methods such as Problem Seeking by Peña and Par-shall, today in its 5th edition (2012). A design process that supports the development of a quality school environment is first and foremost based on educational goals and values. The physical environment is considered an essential partner, or the third teacher, to achieve productive learning experiences. A multidisciplinary team should therefore conduct the process of defining the spaces for such experiences. Appropriate tools are introduced into the design process to simulate comfort levels and other important functions of a building. Decisions are made and evaluated along a loop, where knowledge is accumulated and passed on to new projects through feedback.

Users or potential users should be involved in the decision-making process, since participation can enrich design discussions. Ideas are generated, conflicts removed, misunderstanding avoided, and design intentions explained during the design dialogue (Woolner, 2009). In support the briefing activities, a specific analytical data collection phase is important. Post-Occupancy Evaluation and case study data are essential to enrich the programming discussions in the design process. It is also necessary to have access to regulations and recommendations for environmental comfort standards (Moreira & Kowaltowski, 2009). Data from research findings and technical standards should be structured and referenced to support and direct productive debates.

According to Peña and Parshall (2012), five steps are essential in the briefing phase. These are: setting goals, collect and analyse facts, uncover and test concepts, determine needs, and finally state the design problem adequately in the architectural program. To structure these steps, a detailed list of issues are organised in the "Problem Seeking" method according to four frameworks of: function (people, activities, relationships); form (site, environment, quality); economy (budget, operating costs, life cycle costs); and time (past, present, future).

Yu, Shen, Kelly, and Hunter (2006) establish success factors for briefing which are: a clear and agreed upon objective, carefully thought-out requirements (space standards, activity descriptions, equipment and furniture lists; performance standards), provision of essential information, flexible approach between a balance of quality/costs/deadlines, and finally trusting relationships. The same authors list another 37 points of critical success factors for design project briefing, which include advice on how to conduct a programming phase such as honesty, openness, and trust. It is important to reiterate, that the design process should have access to all relevant information in a clear and structured manner in order to ensure a frank and open dialogue between relevant actors, particularly the valuable skills of the architect.

## The Public Education Scenario in Brazil

For some time now the quality of public education has been under debate in Brazil, especially in light of recent unsatisfactory performance levels obtained by students. To evaluate education, as a whole, governments and independent agencies use several matrixes. In Brazil the Basic Index of Educational Development (IDEP) measures the performance of students through average scores that in 2013 at the high school level were 3.7 out of 10 (public) and 5.7 out of 10 (private), highlighting a need for improvement (IDEP, 2013).

This need can also be corroborated by results of POE studies of school buildings in Brazil. Such evaluations show that problems related to environmental comfort are frequent in schools, which also lack a satisfactory range of spaces to support the array of recommended educational activities (Kowaltowski et al., 2003; Ornstein & Moreira, 2008), suggesting an urgent need for review of design policies.

Many efforts have been made to improve the design of school buildings including the periodic engagement of well-known professionals, especially in the State of São Paulo, through the implementations of FDE (Deliberador, 2010; Fundação para o Desenvolvimento da Educação, 2013; Ornstein & Moreira, 2008). FDE has a long tradition in administrating school building construction and maintenance, with a responsibility in 2013 for over 5,200 schools, attended by approximately 5 million children in the State of São Paulo. FDE is also considered an important institution for advising other Brazilian States and Municipalities, due to its proven experience in school construction.

São Paulo has seen various different individual and design bodies control the development of its educational establishments. FDE was based on a legacy of previous

D. C. C. K. Kowaltowski et al.
Programming for Behaviour in Educational Environments

**161**

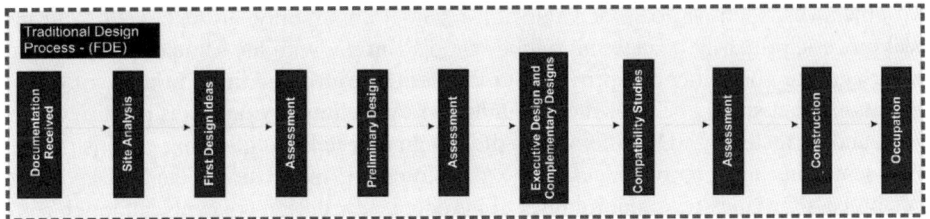

**Figure 2.** A model of the local school design process based on the process administered by FDE.

government agencies in charge of public schools and has produced varied types of school buildings over its 25-year history. There were also periods when renowned professionals were engaged in the development of school the design process. Then, for many years, ready-made plans were used with a view to provide continuity of standards for all localities which was seen as a more democratic process in public education. Recently, this process has changed again, via the Deliberador (2010) study; which resulted in a linear structure model, shown in Figure 2. An example of a recent school building as a result of this process is shown in Figure 3 (Deliberador, 2010), emphasising the importance that should be given to the programming phase.

At the present time the public school design process of the State of São Paulo, managed by FDE, is initiated by contracting local accredited architectural firms. The chosen professionals receive a predefined architectural program, formulated by the State Secretary of Education and construction detailing instructions, based on modular design and prefabricated reinforced concrete components. The brief consists of a list of spaces and their dimensions, with some recommendation on environmental comfort aspects. More subjec-

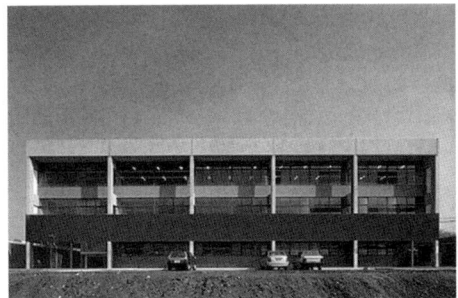 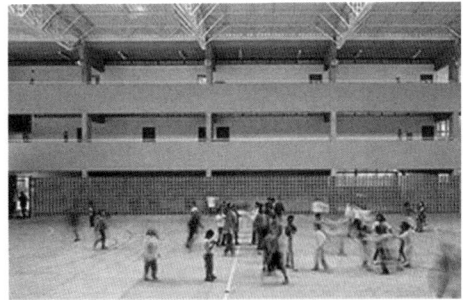

**Figure 3.** Example of a recent school building, administrated by FDE in the State of São Paulo, Brazil (E.E. Jose Roberto Magalhaes Teixeira Prefeito, Campinas, SP, Brazil). (Sources: Left image: http://file.fde.sp.gov.br/portalfde/images/Escolas/065473.jpg; right image: http://file.fde.sp.gov.br/portalfde/images/EscolasRede/065473_1.jpg)

tive objectives, such as goals or values of a school community, are excluded from this local process, primarily because all public schools comply with the same educational program. The site conditions are provided to the design team in addition to a list of design regulations, that should be consulted, is indicated. A preliminary design is produced, analysed, and corrected by FDE, after which the design proceeds, culminating in construction, documentation, and complementary designs (structural, installations, etc.; FDE, 2000). This process provides few opportunities to introduce new design concepts, although some change is under way with the recent adoption of the AQUA sustainable design process (FCAV, 2007).

From the characterisation of the school building design process it is evident that the process is essentially linear, lacking a feedback loop for positive or negative design solution revisions. Thus, a valuable learning mechanism is excluded from the process. Architectural decision-making deals with often conflicting parameters, which implies that design methods should display interferences and provide adequate information for the proper conduct in finding the best solution for specific problems. Research on local Brazilian professional practices shows, that designers use little reference material while developing their ideas, limiting them to codes and eventually some checklists (Graça, 2008a). Evaluations in the form of simulations and optimisations are rarely applied to designs and do not include the participation of users. POE studies are not a regular activity of school design teams, and therefore building performance assessment data is not readily available for application to new designs.

Despite advances in teaching methods and higher educational expectations there is still a reliance on traditional style class room designs. This seems to highlight a dichotomy between the two strands of professional inputs in the design and use of educational environments. Dynamics of education require the constant updating of architectural programmes, based on reflections of users and agents involved in planning and design of new schools or remodelling of old buildings. The wide diversity of users: students (of very different ages, with different backgrounds, and at different stages of development), parents, staff, teachers, and the community in general of surrounding urban areas need to be heard, to facilitate the complexity of contextual educational issues (Kowaltowski, 2011). Most Brazilian cities still have a large deficit of schools, demanding the construction of new schools. These new buildings must reflect the new demands coming from recommendations and the introduction of educational programs (FDE, 2013).

## Structured Information to Support Productive Briefing Debates

To improve the local school design process it is important to expand the programming phase to reflect on contemporary issues in education as well as traditional aspects. To do so it is crucial to incorporate the thoughts and beliefs of local educational authorities, teaching practitioners, and students, in any design dialogue that will eventually affect the daily working environment. This is contrary to the current prescriptive, standardised methods employed, which excludes local involvement and avoids a focus on the diverse needs,

D. C. C. K. Kowaltowski et al.
Programming for Behaviour in Educational Environments

**163**

wants, and aspirations of a wide range of local communities. This process perpetuates old models, without a learning loop based on previous experiences and evaluations.

Most discussions to improve public education in Brazil centre on the system of public education, curriculum, and pedagogy, but should also touch on the adequacy of the physical environment to support necessary educational changes that increase performance levels (Gomes da Silva, Kowaltowski, Pereira, Minette, & Deliberador, 2009). When a school design is started the technical and functional issues are usually given priority. During the analytical and briefing phase however, other types of data are important. Data from environmental psychology is essential to understand underlying issues relating to an individual's identity within school environments, where different age groups will be present and different social and cultural backgrounds can affect user and community characteristics. Privacy, security, segregation, the social/psychological environment, individuality, wayfinding, behavioural patterns, groupings and densities, functioning of the brain, emotions and stress are many of the issues with profound impacts on the decisions to be taken at the briefing stage (Rashid & Zimring, 2008).

Lackney (1998) has translated some of this research data into design recommendations, based on at least 12 principles of brain-compatible learning, suggesting that school environments should be stimulating places, facilitate positive social interaction, provide both passive and active zones, allow access to outside areas for sport and recreation, provide easy access to equipment and learning materials as well as allowing personalisation of the internal and external space. In addition to this, the environment should have: an appropriate colour scheme, allow colour and light to enhance the environment, and perhaps more importantly facilitate feelings of security.

The community around the school should play an active part in daily school activities, so that learning can be more practical and occur in the real world. However, data on behavioural issues are not usually readily available and often unrelated to physical elements of the built environment. For a productive design briefing, such data should be organised and referenced for analysis, reflection, questioning, and application. The structure of the data should also be easily accessible. Another important contribution comes from research by Lippman (2010), who gives an indication as to the most important activities that must be able to be performed in school environments. Eighteen experiences are listed, each demanding a specific space configuration and furniture layout for effective teaching and learning to take place.

To improve the local school design process this type of information has been structured according to the "Problem Seeking" architectural programming method. Figure 4 shows how this information was structured." This data should be made available to design teams and agents of change; a role FDE is capable of playing. Structured data should enrich briefing debates, direct a participatory process, and stimulate research on the productive school environments that facilitate a positive relationship between human behaviour and the physical environment.

The literature on school buildings is vast and diverse, and convincing data that architecture affects academic performance is available although dispersed. Especially poor

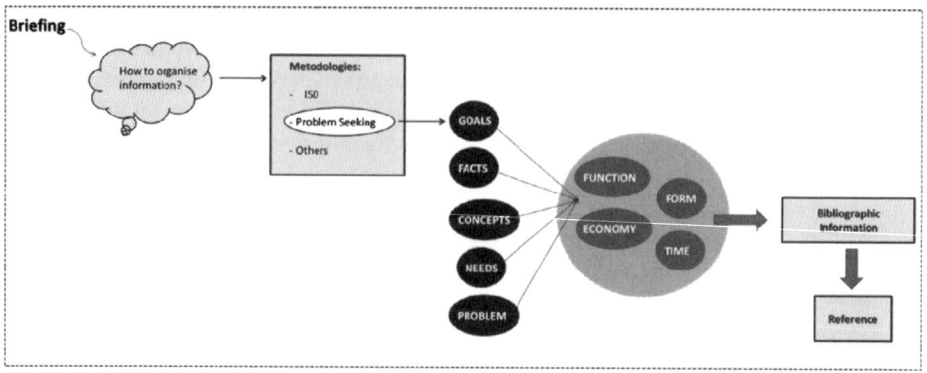

**Figure 4.** Organisation of behavioural data related to school buildings structured according to the "Problem Seeking" programming method.


conditions, with leaking roofs, broken windows, dark and sombre classrooms are related to lower achievement rates of students (Upitis, 2004).

Information should be readily available to a briefing team, with access to original studies focusing on design issues (references), through hyperlinks. For example, discussions on learning groups should dwell on space configurations that give groups autonomy (territoriality and privacy) and at the same time encourage interaction with other groups for social contact. The issue of crowding (positive and negative) and space requirements that define densities need clarification. The functional area of educational productive spaces can then be calculated on the basis of research data. For instance, recommendations on the maximum number of students for a productive school, state that this should be kept within 500 (Moore & Lackney, 1993). Such data however, should be tested in different cultural and economic conditions.

Schools should serve a student population with its specific characteristics, according to age groups, socio-economic conditions of family and risk situations that should be mitigated by the school environment (Argilaga, Velasco, & Arámburu, 2003; Bencostta, 2005). Different pedagogies have different goals, reflected in the educational activities, student grouping and their spatial arrangements. In Brazil, "Constructivism" based on the views of Jean Piaget, Lev Vygotsky, and John Dewey have had an important impact on public education, through the teachings of Paulo Freire and Darcy Ribeiro, who emphasise the importance of the learners' background and culture (Compayre, 1909; Salvatori, 2003). Established educational standards must be adapted to local conditions and the school environment must be adequately prepared for specific and varied activities, that teach not only the basics of education, but most importantly life skills and the environment needs to give signals as to appropriate uses (Lippman, 2010; van der Voordt & van Wegen, 2005).

The preparation of future generations for the challenges that lie ahead is an issue to be included in a quality school program, where the concept of sustainability should be incorporated into the building design. It is also prudent that teachers, who are often not aware of the potential of the educational spaces available, should be drawn into the briefing debate (Horne, 1998, 1999; Martin, 2006). Finally, programming debates should touch on antisocial behaviour in schools: drugs, bullying, gangs, vandalism, and extreme behaviours from timid to aggressive students (National Crime Prevention Council, 2003). Studies have found that vandalism in schools demands more robust design solutions to prevent damage as a result of boisterous, youthful playfulness. Good quality materials must be specified with the building having a pleasant, non-prison-like feel to it. Vandalism is also more common in public areas of schools, mainly in the more hidden parts of buildings. Thus, designs should avoid dead-end corridors without views to the exterior. Sanitary facilities and locker rooms must also be placed where supervision occurs naturally, through user movement. These, suggestions, based on user needs and educational outcomes, are similar to research by Freedman (2011) on avoiding antisocial behaviours and highlight the need for design principles to encompass a balanced approach to a wide range of user needs.

To structure this type of data an outline is presented in the Appendix, which shows data relating to "form" giving aspects of a programming discussion, and organised according to the "Problem Seeking" method. The method, once structured with a rich array of research findings, can support a participatory programming phase. Additional tools should also be applied. Evaluation tools such as DQI and CFA (Gann et al., 2003; van der Voordt, Vrielink, & van Wegen, 1997) for instance, must be made available (translated for local conditions), since they are directly applicable to preliminary design stages. They provide the design team: visual returns on the design development, appropriateness of building shape, size, and organisation in relation to vital issues of pedagogy, function, environmental comfort, universal design, and sustainability to mention just a few important aspects.

To stimulate the briefing debates several areas of research can be drawn upon. Sanoff (2001a, 2001b) for instance, has developed several design process activities, which can be applied directly to local needs. Others must be adapted to specific situations encountered in the public school realm in Brazil. Pattern languages, such as those of Alexander, Ishikawa, and Silverstein (1977) and Nair and Fielding (2009), can also be developed for the local public school design process. Some of the more urgent local Brazilian school architecture issues are: the question of security and control over schools sites, the importance of cross ventilation for the mostly tropical climates, found in the country, the proper connections between isolated buildings when the school complex is the result of an evolutionary building process, and the choice of architectural language or image a school portrays in urban areas of shanty towns or poor neighbourhoods where a local signature is difficult to define.

## Conclusions

This paper is part of a continuing study on the public school environment as found in the State of São Paulo, Brazil. The local school building design process was previously characterised and shown to lack a participatory briefing phase (Deliberador, 2010). In most developed countries this design phase, especially for school buildings, is participatory and a well-informed design team conducts the process, stimulating debates based on recent research findings. A discussion on the importance of this phase and specific methods, to be employed during the design process, could improve the local school environment. In countries like Brazil important design data is rarely structured to produce documents for effective use in the pre-design phases of school design. The structuring of the rich literature on environmental psychology and school building design according to the "Problem Seeking" architectural programming method is outlined in this paper. The focus of the research is to demonstrate that access to literature can enable change in the local school design process through the stimulation of productive participatory briefing debates. Finally, better buildings can support increased learning and productivity in schools and improved educational spaces can be evaluated according to benchmarks set in the architectural program itself.

# References

Alexander, C., Ishikawa, S., & Silverstein, M. (1977). *A pattern language: Towns, buildings, construction*. Oxford, UK: Oxford University Press.

Argilaga, M. T. A., Velasco, C. S., & Arámburu, M. C. E. (2003). Evaluating links intensity in social networks in a school context through observational designs. In R. García Mira, J. M. S. Sabucedo Cameselle, & J. R. Martínez (Eds.), *Culture, environmental action and sustainability* (pp. 287–298). Cambridge, MA: Hogrefe & Huber.

Balzani, M., & Borgogni, A. (2003). The body goes to the city project: Research on safe routes to school and playgrounds in Ferrara. In R. G. Mira, J. M. S. Cameselle, & J. R. Martinez (Eds.), *Culture, environmental action and sustainability* (pp. 313–324). Cambridge, MA: Hogrefe & Huber.

Barker, R., & Gump, P. V. (1964). *Big school, small school, high school size and student, behavior*. Stanford, CA: Stanford University Press.

Bencostta, M. L. (2005). *História da educação, arquitetura e espaço escolar*. [History of education, architecture and the school environment]. São Paulo, Brazil: Cortez Editora.

Bittencourt, L. S., & Batista, J. O. O efeito de dutos de luz verticais na iluminação natural de ambientes escolares [The effect of vertical light ducts on natural lighting in school environments]. In *Proceedings of III Conferência Latino-Americana sobre Conforto e Desempenho Energético de Edificações* (p. 559–566). Curitiba, Brazil: ANTAC.

Brubaker, C. W. (1998). *Planning and designing schools*. New York, NY: McGraw-Hill.

Buffa, E., & Almeida Pinto, G. de (2002). *Arquitetura e Educação: organização e propostaspe-dagógicas dos grupos escolares paulistas 1893/1971*. São Paulo, Brazil: EdUFSCar.

Building Futures. (2004). *21st Century Schools – learning environments of the future*. Retrieved from http://www.buildingfutures.org.br

Commission for Architecture and the Built Environment (CABE). (2003). *Achieving well designed schools thought PFI*. London, UK: Author.

Commission for Architecture and the Built Environment (CABE). (2004). *Being involved in school design*. London, UK: Author.

Commission for Architecture and the Built Environment (CABE). (2005). *Picturing school design*. London, UK: Author.

D. C. C. K. Kowaltowski et al.
Programming for Behaviour in Educational Environments

**167**

Commission for Architecture and the Built Environment (CABE). (2006). *Assessing secondary schools design quality*. London, UK: Author.

CHPS. (2008). *The collaborative for high performance schools best practices manual*. Retrieved from http://www.chps.net/manual/index.htm

CHPS. (2009). *The collaborative for high performance schools best practices manual*. Retrieved from http://www.chps.net/manual/index.htm#score

Clark, C., & Uzzell, D. L. (2006). The socio-environmental affordances of adolescents' environments. In C. Spencer & M. Blades (Eds.), *Children and their environments: Learning, using and designing spaces*. (pp. 176–198). Cambridge, UK: Cambridge University Press.

Compayre, G. (1909). *History of Pedagogy*. Boston, MA: Swan Sonnenschein & Co.

Deliberador, M. S. (2010). *O processo de projeto de arquitetura escolar no Estado de São Paulo: caracterização e possibilidades de intervenção* (Masters Dissertation). Universidade Estadual de Campinas – UNICAMP, Campinas, Brazil.

Dudek, M. (2000). *Architecture of schools: The new learning environments*. Oxford: Architectural Press.

Dudek, M. (2007). *Schools and Kindergartens – A design manual*. Berlin, Germany: Birkäuser.

FCAV. (2007). *Referencial técnico de certificação, Edifícios do setor de serviços – Processo AQUA, Escritórios – Edifícios escolares*. São Paulo, SP: FCAV.

FDE (Fundação para o Desenvolvimento da Educação). (2013). Retrieved from http://www.fde.sp. gov.br/pagespublic/Home.aspx

FDE. (2000). *Normas-de-Apresentação-Projetos-FDE (Norma)*. Retrieved from http://www.scribd. com/doc/62920581/NORMAS-DE-APRESENTACAO-PROJETOSFDE

Figueiredo, F. G. (2009). *Processo de Projeto Integrado para melhoria de desempenho ambiental de edificações: dois estudos de caso*, (Masters Dissertation). Universidade Estadual de Campinas – UNICAMP, Campinas SP.

Freedman, T. (2011). *7 ways to prevent vandalism to educational technology equipment*. Retrieved from http://www.ictineducation.org/home-page/2011/2/6/7-ways-to-prevent-vandalism-to-educational-technology-equipm.html

Gann, D., Salter, A., & Whyte, J. (2003). Design Quality Indicator as a tool for thinking. *Building Research & Information, 31*(5), 318–333.

Gifford, R. (1997). *Environmental psychology: Principles and practice*. Boston, MA: Allyn and Bacon.

Gomes da Silva, V., Kowaltowski, D. C. C. K., Pereira, P. P. R., Minette, L., & Deliberador, M. S. (2009, November). *Analysis of the building process and of energy efficiency of public schools in the State of São Paulo, Brazil*. Paper presented at the CSAAR, Tripoli, Libya.

Graça, V. A. C. (2008a). *A união de aspectos de conforto ambiental no projeto de escolas: viabilidade do uso da metodologia axiomática e de exemplos simplificados* (PhD Thesis). Universidade Estadual de Campinas – UNICAMP, Campinas, Brazil.

Graça, V. A. C. (2008b). *A integração dos aspectos de conforto ambiental no projeto de escolas: uso da metodologia axiomática e de exemplos simplificados* (Doctoral Thesis). Universidade Estadual de Campinas – UNICAMP, Campinas SP.

Graça, V. A. C., Scarazzato, P. S., & Kowaltowski, D. C. C. K. (2001). *Método Simplificado para a Avaliação de Iluminação Natural em Anteprojetos de Escolas de Ensino Estadual de São Paulo*. ANAIS do VI Encontro Nacional sobre Conforto no Ambiente Construído e III Encontro Latino Americano sobre Conforto no Ambiente Construído, São Pedro.

Hershberger, R. G. (1999). *Architectural programming and predesign manager*. New York, NY: McGraw-Hill Professional.

Heschong Mahone Group. (2003). *Daylighting in schools: Investigation into relationship between daylighting and human performance*. Sacramento, CA: CA Board for Energy Efficiency.

Horne, S. C. (1998). *Shared visions? Architects and teachers perceptions on the design of classroom environments.* Paper presented at the IDATER Conference, Loughborough University, UK.

Horne, S. C. (1999). *The classroom environment and its effects on the practice of teachers.* London, UK: University of London.

IDEP – Índice de Desenvolvimento da Educação Básica. (2013). Retrieved from http://ideb.inep. gov.br/resultado/resultado/resultadoBrasil.seam?cid=28870

Kowaltowski, D. C. C. K. (1980). *Humanization of architecture* (PhD Thesis). University of California Berkeley, Berkeley, USA.

Kowaltowski, D. C. C. K. (2011). *Arquitetura escolar: o projeto do ambiente de ensino* [School architecture: The design of the learning environment]. São Paulo, Brazil: Oficina de Textos.

Kowaltowski, D. C. C. K., Celani, M. G. C., Moreira, D. C., & Pina, S. A. M. G. (2006). Reflexão sobre Metodologias de projeto Arquitetônico. In *Revista online da ANTAC – AMBIENTE CONSTRUÍDO.* Porto Alegre, V6 no. 2, 7–19. Retrieved from http://www.antac.org.br/ambiente-construido/pdf/revista/artigos/Doc124154.pdf

Kowaltowski, D. C. C. K., Graça, V. A. C. da., & Petreche, J. R. D. (2007). An evaluation method for school building design at the preliminary phase with optimisation of aspects of environmental comfort for the school system of the State São Paulo in Brazil. *Building and Environment, 42*(2), 984–999.

Kowaltowski, D. C. C. K., Labaki, L. C., Pina, S. A. M. G., Ruschel, R. C., Borges, F. E., & Bertolli, S. R. (2001). *Melhoria do conforto ambiental em edificações escolares de Campinas.* [Environmental comfort improvements for school buildings in Campinas]. Campinas, Brazil: FEC/UNICAMP.

Kowaltowski, D. C. C. K., Pina, S. A. M. G., Ruschel, R. C., Labaki, L. C., Bertolli, S. R., & Filho, F. B. (2003). Environmental comfort and school buildings: The case of Campinas, SP, Brazil. In R. García Mira, J. M. Sabucedo Cameselle, & J. R. Martínez (Eds.), *Culture, environmental action and sustainability* (pp. 325–333). Cambridge, MA: Hogrefe & Huber.

Lackney, J. A. (1998), *12 design principles based on brain-based learning research.* Retrieved from http://www.designshare.com/Research/BrainBased Learn98.htm

Lawson, B. (2001). *How designers think: The design process demystified.* Burlington, MA: Architectural Press.

Lepper, M. R., & Greene, D. (1975). Turning play into work: Effects of adult surveillance and extrinsic rewards on children's intrinsic motivation. *Journal of Personality and Social Psychology, 31*(3), 479–486.

Lippman, P. C. (2010). *Can the physical environment have an impact on the learning environment?* Paris, France: OECD Publishing. Retrieved from http://www.oecd.org/education/innovation-education/centreforeffectivelearningenvironmentscele/46413458.pdf

Loughlin, C. E., & Suina, J. H. (1982). *The learning environment: An instructional strategy.* New York, NY: Teachers College Press, Columbia University.

Lynch, K. (2011). *A imagem da cidade* [In the image of the city]. (3rd ed.). São Paulo, Brazil: Martins Fontes.

Martin, S. H. (2006). The classroom environment and children's performance: Is there a relationship? In C. Spencer & M. Blades (Eds.), *Children and their environments: Learning, using and designing spaces,* (pp. 91–107). Cambridge, UK: Cambridge University Press.

Mimbacas, A., Leitão, E., Reis da, A. T. L., & Lay, M. C. D. (1998). Avaliação de desempenho térmico, lumínico e acústico – escola padrão de alvenaria (EPA) e projeto nova escola (PNE) [Evaluation of thermal, acoustic and lighting performances – standard school in masonry (EPA) and the New School Design (PNE)]. In *Proceedings of the ANAIS do VII Encontro Nacional de Tecnologia no Ambiente Construído* (pp. 339–346). Florianópolis: Antac e Universidade Federal De Santa Catarina.

Moore, G. T., & Lackney, J. A. (1993). *Design patterns for American schools: Responding to the reform movement.* US Department of Education, Educational Resources Information Center, EDRS.

Moore, G. T., & Lackney, J. A. (1995). *Design patterns for American schools: Responding to the reform movement.* US Department of Education, Educational Resources Information Center, EDRS.

Moreira, D. de. C., & Kowaltowski, D. C. C. K. (2009). Discussão sobre a Importância do Programa de Necessidades para a Qualidade no Processo de Projeto em Arquitetura [Discussion on the importance of the architectural program to ensure the quality in the architectural design process]. *Revista ANTAC, Ambiente Construído, 9*(2), 31–45.

Müeller, C. M. (2007). *Espaços de ensino-aprendizagem com qualidade ambiental: o processo metodológico para elaboração de um anteprojeto* (Masters Dissertation). Universidade de SãoPaulo (USP), São Paulo, Brazil.

Nair, P., & Fielding, R. (2005). *The language of school design: Design patterns for 21$^{st}$ century schools.* Designshare.

Nair, P., & Fielding, R. (2009). *The language of school design: Design patterns for 21$^{st}$ century schools.* Designshare.

Nasar, J. L., Preiser, W. F. E., & Fisher, T. (2007). *Designing for designers: Lessons from schools of architecture.* New York, NY: Fairchild.

National Crime Prevention Council. (2003). *Crime prevention through environmental design: Guidebook.* Singapore: Author.

Ornstein, S. W., & Moreira, N. S. (2008). *Evaluating school facilities in Brazil.* Paris, France: OECD. Retrieved from http://www.oecd.org/brazil/40051760.pdf

Ornstein, S. W., & Neto, J. B. (Coord.) (1996). *O desempenho dos edifícios da rede estadual de ensino: o caso da grande São Paulo* [The performance of state public school buildings: the case of Greater São Paulo]. São Paulo, Brazil FAU/USP.

Peña, W. M., & Parshall, S. A. (2012). *Problem seeking: An architectural programming primer.* New York, NY: Wiley.

Rashid, M., & Zimring, C. (2008). A review of the empirical literature on the relationships between indoor environment and stress in health care and office settings – Problems and prospects of sharing evidence. *Environment and Behavior, 40*(2), 151–190.

Salvatori M. R. (Ed.). (2003). *Pedagogy: Disturbing History, 1820–1930.* Pittsburgh, PA: University of Pittsburgh Press.

San Juan, G. A., & Rosenfeld, E. (1995). El diseño bioclimático de edificio de uso discontinuo en educacion. In *Proceedings of ANAIS do III Encontro Latino Americano de Conforto no ambiente Construído* (pp. 339–346). Gramado, Brazil: Antac and UFRGS.

Sanoff, H. (1994). *School design.* New York, NY: Willey.

Sanoff, H. (2001a). *A visioning process for designing responsive schools.* Washington, DC: National Clearinghouse for Educational Facilities.

Sanoff, H. (2001b). *School building assessment methods.* Washington, DC: National Clearinghouse for Educational Facilities.

Steele, F. I. (1973). *Physical settings and organizational development.* Boston, MA: Addison Wesley Longman Publishing Co.

Taralli, C. H. (2004), Espaços De Leitura Na Escola: Salas De Leitura/Bibliotecas Escolares. Boletim Salto Para o Futuro MEC, Rio de Janeiro, Brazil, pp. 31–39.

Trancik, A. M., & Evans, G. W. (1995). Spaces fit for children: Competency in the design of daycare center environments. *Children's Environments, 12*, pp. 311–319.

Upitis, R. (2004). School architecture and complexity. *Complicity: An International Journal of Complexity and Education, 1*(1), 19–38.

Ura, A. M., & Bertoli, S. (1998). A acústica das salas de aula das escolas da rede estadual de Campinas [Acoustics of classrooms of the state school in Campinas, SP]. In *Proceedings of ANAIS do VII Encontro Nacional de Tecnologia do Ambiente Construído* (pp. 333–337). Florianópolis: Antac e Universidade Federal De Santa Catarina.

van der Voordt, D. J. M., & van Wegen, H. B. R. (2005). *Architecture in use: An introduction to the programming, design and evaluation of buildings.* Oxford, UK: Architectural Press.

van der Voordt, D. J. M., Vrielink, D., & van Wegen, H. B. R. (1997). Comparative floor plan analysis in programming and architectural design. *Design Studies, 18*(1), 67–88.

Woolner, P. (2009, September). *Building schools for the future through a participatory design process: Exploring the issues and investigating ways forward.* Paper presented at the The British Education Association Conference, Manchester, UK.

Yu, A. T. W., Shen, Q., Kelly, J., & Hunter, K. (2006). Investigation of critical success factors in construction project briefing by way of content analysis. *Journal of Construction Engineering and Management, 132,* 1178–1186.

D. C. C. K. Kowaltowski et al.
Programming for Behaviour in Educational Environments

171

**Appendix.** School Design Data structured according to the "Problem Seeking" programming method by Peña and Parshall (2012)

| Code | Summary | Description | Bibliographic Information | Bibliographic Reference |
|---|---|---|---|---|
| **Goals Relating to FORM** | | | | |
| 14 | Bias on site elements | Identify any clients attitudes toward existing elements on the site (trees, water, open space, facilities and utilities) | Identification of reference points. Better orientation, wayfinding, feelings of belonging and security. | Gifford, 1997; Loughlin & Suina, 1982; Lynch, 2011 |
| 15 | Environmental response | Identify client attitudes toward the facility response to its environment | Sustainability behaviour, (recycling, efficient use of water and energy), care for the environment, community spirit. Promote environmental awareness to increase user participation. Teachers need environmental competence. | CHPS, 2008; Nair & Fielding, 2005; Steele, 1973 |
| 16 | Efficient land use | Investigate the land use policy for efficiency and environmental character | Incorporate sustainable elements to give visual cues towards sustainable behaviour. | CHPS, 2008 |
| 17 | Community relations | Identify policies concerning coincident planning and relations with the neighboring community | Identify the role of school in its community, improve community relations, create sense of belonging, increase the sense of value given to educational activities. Create feelings of security. Pride of school which increases productivity and educational outcomes. | CABE, 2004 |
| | | | Relation of the school with its surrounding. Avoid vandalism through community acceptance and use of school facilities by the community. | Sanoff, 2001a |
| 18 | Community improvements | Identify policies concerning the investment in, or improvement of, the neighboring community | Acceptance of community of school design. In line with community image of what a school should express. Better acceptance of school policies, better relations, better possibility of community involvement with school activities. | Sanoff, 2001a |
| 19 | Physical comfort | Identify the level of physical comfort required | Importance of environmental comfort and learning productivity. Avoid aggressive behaviour and apathy. | Kowaltowski et al, 2001; Nair & Fielding, 2005; Ornstein & Neto, 1996 |

(continued on next page)

**Appendix.** Continued

| Code | Summary | Description | Bibliographic Information | Bibliographic Reference |
|---|---|---|---|---|
| | | | Importance of verbal communication to avoid lack of understanding, feelings of confusion, lack of involvement. | Bittencourt & Batista, 2003; Mimbacas, Leitão, Reis, & Lay, 1998; San Juan & Rosenfeld, 1995; Ura et al., 1998 |
| | | | Acoustic conditions adjusted to activities to avoid interference between incompatible activities. Avoid failures in verbal communications. | Dudek, 2007 |
| | | | Give priority to natural lighting, to enhance the circadian cycle, avoid glare on tables and blackboard to avoid failure in visual communication. Correct lighting levels and mixture of light to increase the feeling of comfort and security. | Dudek, 2007; Graça, Scarazzato, & Kowaltowski, 2001; Nair & Fielding, 2005 |
| | | | In many schools there is a tendency for less space to play. Revise this. Children can no longer perceive the city as a place to live and play since so many limitations are imposed due to safety and security issues. Give opportunities to play in front of the school. Functional space requirements must be at ideal levels to perform desired activities with ease. Avoid disorder, crowding. Sense of order is an important feeling affecting positive behaviour towards learning. Reserve enough space for deposits of teaching equipment and material, cleaning products and tools. Scale and size of spaces affect density and crowding which can lead to aggression and less social interconnections. Teachers tend to overlook certain areas of a typical classroom. Teachers need training in environmental competence. The concept of affordance (what does the space show to be capable of supporting?). Legibility of space, presence of comprehensible patterns. Environmental awareness increases students autonomy and feeling of security. Importance of perception and experimentation. Awareness of introducing changes. Questioning the setting by new layouts. | Clark & Uzzell, 2006; Graça, 2008b; Kowaltowski et al., 2001; Lepper & Greene, 1975; Ornstein & Neto, 1996; Trancik & Evans, 1995; van der Voordt & van Wegen, 2005 |
| | | | Optimize environmental comfort indicators to provide for a comfortable learning environment. Comfort affects productivity and aggressiveness. | CABE, 2006; CHPS, 2008; Kowaltowski, Celani, Moreira, & Pina, 2006; Sanoff, 2001b |

(continued on next page)

D. C. C. K. Kowaltowski et al.
Programming for Behaviour in Educational Environments

173

**Appendix.** Continued

| Code | Summary | Description | Bibliographic Information | Bibliographic Reference |
|---|---|---|---|---|
| 20 | Life safety | Identify critical life safety considerations | Safe routes to school and playgrounds. Feeling secure affects learning attitudes and social behaviour. | Balzani & Borgogni, 2003 |
| 21 | Social/Psychological environment | Identify clients attitudes toward the social/psychological environment to be provided | High performance schools affect learning positively. Functions of space are: security, shelter, social interaction possibilities, expression of symbolic meaning, appropriate for tasks at hand, give pleasure, promote user involvement, give cues towards appropriate behaviour. Strange reactions should be checked against layout. | Brubaker, 1998; Dudek, 2000, 2007; Sanoff, 1994 |
| | | | Explore the relationship of spaces and buildings to cultural and social values of the community. Social interactions enhance learning. | Taralli, 2004; Mueller, 2007 |
| | | | Think of educational spaces as being learning facilitators or the third teacher. This will improve psychological feelings of comfort. Things children like in playgrounds: trees, fountains, sports grounds, sand, water, benches, cycle lanes, tunnels, caves, play structures, slide etc. | Deliberador, 2010 |
| | | | Give importance to the relation of teaching methods and the pedagogical concepts applied when making design decisions. Each type of pedagogy asks for specific spatial solutions. | Buffa et al, 2002; CABE, 2005; Building Futures, 2004; Upitis, 2004 |
| 22 | Individuality | Identify goals concerning the promotion of the personal individuality of the user | Give more importance to individual studies, through spaces where children can isolate themselves from the group. This will enhance self-esteem, autonomy and independence and increase learning. Personal space feeling. Need for quiet spaces to relax, concentrate and gain control over moods. Give opportunities for isolating aggressive behaviour. | Nair & Fielding, 2005 |
| | | | Children need their personal space to keep their belongings. Preserve self-esteem, increase feelings of security. Avoid bullying. | Nair & Fielding, 2005 |
| 23 | Wayfinding | Identify goals dealing with the flow of people and vehicles to provide wayfinding with a sense of orientation (knowing where you are) or a sense of entry (knowing where to enter) | Make school facilities fully accessible, improve wayfinding to increase feelings of security and self-esteem. Improve the way children go to school. Better parking facilities, better bike routes, bus stop near school. | CABE, 2005 |

(continued on next page)

**Appendix.** Continued

| Code | Summary | Description | Bibliographic Information | Bibliographic Reference |
|---|---|---|---|---|
| 24 | Projected image | Identify the image that must be projected | Choose an architectural language that expresses the local image of what a school should be. Increase feeling of belonging and pride in education. Avoid vandalism. Impact perception of space and place. Going from sensation to perception to cognition (recording the place in memory). These concepts are related to size and distance (proxemics) scale and movement in space, as well as social order. Evaluate what is perceived in foreground, background, verticality, symmetry, color, number of elements, their meaning their context. Is there a sense of territory? Think about space and time (Classroom activity intervals. Importance of space identity. If students have a lack of access to variety of art forms, schools need to address this issue.). | Lawson, 2001; Moore & Lackney, 1995; Sanoff, 2001a |
|  |  |  | Local signature is important to set the school apart from other schools, to increase pride in the school, feeling of belonging and caring. Territorial expression increases user involvement in school activities and caretaking. A school should be a point of reference. Less prison like design language. | CABE, 2005; Deliberador, 2010; Lynch, 2011; Nair & Fielding, 2005 |
| 25 | Client expectations | Identify clients attitudes toward the quality of the physical environment and the balance of space and quality | Quality designs express that public money is well invested. Community feels gratified and will get more easily involved in school activities. Lack of play space is often related to cost per area issues. Reflect on this. | CABE, 2003 |
| 53 | Site analysis | Analyse the existing site conditions to include: contours, views, natural features, buildable areas, access and egress, utilities, size and capacity | Elements which impact levels of sustainability, influence user attitudes towards the environment and sustainability behaviour (recycling, energy and water use efficiency). | Nair & Fielding, 2005 |
| 54 | Soil analysis | Evaluate the soil test report and determine its implication on cost and design | Not applicable to behaviour relations. | Hershberger, 1999 |
| 55 | FAR and GAC | Evaluate the floor area ratio, the ground area coverage, people per acre, and other comparative measures of density | Spatial densities affect feeling of belonging, crowding, aggressive and reclusive behaviour. | Gifford, 1997 |
|  |  |  | Provide a minimum of 1.5 sq. m per student in academic areas, avoid crowding. | Kowaltowski et al., 2001 |
| 56 | Climate analysis | Analyse the climate to include climatological data on seasonal temperatures, precipitation, snow, sun angles and wind direction | Thermal comfort affects productivity, alertness and excludes aggressive behaviour. | Hershberger, 1999 |

(continued on next page)

D. C. C. K. Kowaltowski et al.
Programming for Behaviour in Educational Environments

**175**

**Appendix.** Continued

| Code | Summary | Description | Bibliographic Information | Bibliographic Reference |
|------|---------|-------------|---------------------------|-------------------------|
| 57 | Code survey | Evaluate the form-giving significance of code and zoning requirements | School setting in relation to architectural values of the urban setting. Similar architectural language or contrast to impact the community. Feelings of creating a special place within the community. | CHPS, 2008 |
| 58 | Surroundings | Analyse local materials and the immediate surroundings of the site for possible influences | Environmental questions in relation to urban or rural context. Regard for and preservation of natural forms and elements. Humanization elements impact school maintenance and productivity through place attachment. | Hershberger, 1999 |
| | | | Choose good materials which impact a feeling of quality and values towards educational goals. Avoids vandalism. | CHPS, 2008 |
| 59 | Psychological implications | Understand the psychological implications of form on territoriality and movement of people and vehicles | Possibilities of: territorial feelings and ownership, sensory stimulation, social interactions, feelings of security and safety. | Kowaltowski et al., 2001; Gifford, 1997 |
| 60 | Point of reference/ entry | Define points of reference and entry | Create a sense of entry to impact a feeling of belonging and exploration of the school complex as a whole. | Nair & Fielding, 2005 |
| 61 | Cost/SF | Establish a mutual understanding of building quality on quantitative basis (cost per square meter) | | |
| 62 | Building or layout efficiency | Understand the effect of building layout efficiency (commonly referred to as net to gross ratio) on quality | Functional questions should provide possibility to change layouts to include educationally important activities with ease. Smooth running of a classroom increases productivity, individualization of attention, avoids monotony. Include generosity of space, surface areas, infrastructure (equipment availability, plugs, Wi-Fi, etc.). | Hershberger, 1999 |

(continued on next page)

**Appendix.** Continued

| Code | Summary | Description | Bibliographic Information | Bibliographic Reference |
|---|---|---|---|---|
| 63 | Equipment costs | Understand the effect of equipment cost on quality | | Hershberger, 1999 |
| 64 | Area per unit | Establish the functional adequacy (area/unit) of spaces as an indication of quality | Functional aspects go beyond mere space adequacy for each activity. They include dynamic possibilities, group involvement in space usage, rich and diverse activities, less monotony, more productivity. Impact on personal involvements. Feeling of belonging. Dependent on: space adequacy, spatial relations, flexibility, generosity of available space, equipment, surface areas, plugs etc.). | Hershberger, 1999 |
| **Facts Relating to FORM** | | | | |
| 90 | Enhancements | Evaluate the natural features of the site, and identify those to be preserved or enhanced | Identifiable objects that serve as reference points. In schools: special entrance elements, fountains, totems, amphitheater. | Lynch, 2011 |
| 91 | Special foundations | Evaluate the climate analysis and determine the implication on climate controls | Climate (hot and humid) may cause fatigue, apathetic behaviour, reduced productivity, reduced attention span, aggressive behaviour. | Heschong Mahone Group, 2003 |
| 92 | Density | Evaluate the for-giving implications of the code survey, and identify the salient safety precautions | Spatial densities. | Gifford, 1997 |
| 93 | Environmental controls | Evaluate the soil analysis report and determine the possibility of special foundations and their costs | Not related to behaviour of users. | |
| 94 | Safety | Evaluate climate, demographic data, site conditions and land value to establish general density standards | Environmental values. | Hershberger, 1999 |
| 95 | Neighbours | Evaluate the policy concerning the neighbouring community to uncover the concept of sharing or interdependence | Give importance to community expectancy in relation to the artistic value of the new school. | Hershberger, 1999 |
| | | | Determine the total population size to enhance community use of the school. Maximum recommended = 500 students | Barker & Gump, 1964 |
| 96 | Home base/Officing concepts | Uncover the need for an individual's home base or territoriality | Campfire-spaces and individual study and relaxation nooks. Impact of distance learning on social behaviour of students. | Nair & Fielding, 2005 |
| | | | Personal space for keeping personal items, value of the individual. | Nair & Fielding, 2005 |
| | | | Importance of individual study places distributed within the school compound. Increase concentration behaviour of students. | Nair & Fielding, 2005 |

(continued on next page)

D. C. C. K. Kowaltowski et al.
Programming for Behaviour in Educational Environments

177

**Appendix.** Continued

| Code | Summary | Description | Bibliographic Information | Bibliographic Reference |
|---|---|---|---|---|
| 97 | Orientation | Uncover the need for good orientation, maintaining a sense of direction through a building or campus | Importance of evaluating wayfinding issues in POE studies. Spatial orientation problems may cause apathy and learning dysfunctions. | Nasar, Preiser, & Fisher, 2007 |
| 98 | Accessibility | Uncover the need for the concept of accessibility, which promotes a sense of entrance and of arrival, providing directly access to public-oriented facilities | Promote the sense of entrance through architectural elements. Improve access and check accessibility in POE studies. Comparative floor plan evaluations are recommended. | Nasar et al., 2007; van der Voordt et al., 1997 |
| 99 | Character | Uncover the general character of the architectural form that the client intends to project as an image | Building should express the community spirit and have a special signature to distinguish one from another school. Feeling of belonging: ownership, territoriality, interventions by group users, sense of caring. The image of the school affects a sense of attachment, impacts care and a feeling of belonging and ultimately productivity and a liking of school. | CABE, 2005; Deliberador, 2010; Nair & Fielding, 2005 Sanoff, 2001a |
| 100 | Quality control | Understand that quality control is an operation concept used to provide the highest quality level feasible after the balance of quality/cost factors | Importance of commissioning phase. Relation of construction cost, running and maintenance cost. Quality is measured through intrinsic attributes: accessibility, adaptability, crowding, spaciousness, legibility wayfinding, meaning, possibility to personalize, feeling of ownership, physical comfort, privacy, safety and security. | CHPS, 2009; Deliberador, 2010 CHPS, 2008 |
| **Concepts Relating to FORM** | | | | |
| 118 | Site development costs | Identify the components of site development costs | | |
| 119 | Environmental influences on costs | Consider the factors of the physical and psychological environment, as well as site conditions as influences on the construction budget | Impact on vandalism | Kowaltowski, 1980 |

(continued on next page)

**Appendix.** Continued

| Code | Summary | Description | Bibliographic Information | Bibliographic Reference |
|---|---|---|---|---|
| 120 | Building costs/SM | Establish mutual agreement with the client on the construction quality expressed for each activity by organization, location, space type and time | Positive impact of a quality environment on users: feelings of belonging, better care and use of buildings and grounds, impact on reduction of vandalism. | Nair & Fielding, 2009 |
| 121 | Building overall efficiency factor | Evaluate the efficiency factor that was used to determine the useable, rentable or gross area requirements | Schools may rent out spaces to generate income for school installation, maintenance and upgrading | Nair & Fielding, 2009 |
| **Needs Relating to FORM** | | | | |
| 135 | Major form considerations that will affect building design | Identify and abstract the major form-giving influences of the site on the building design | It is important to evaluate the design at various stages of its design process. Include the school community in this. | Deliberador, 2010 |
| 136 | | Identify the salient environmental influences on the building design | Apply an integrated design process to evaluate the design from different perspectives, including environmental impacts. | Figueiredo, 2009 |
| 137 | | Identify the quality of the project and its implication on the building design | Importance of including a commissioning phase into the design process for retrofits, training of staff and education of users on full usage of infrastructure. | CHPS, 2009; Deliberador, 2010 |

# Complexity and Order in Commercial Streetscapes

## How to Maintain User Satisfaction With Visual Quality in Contemporary Cities

Adriana Portella[1] and Sinval Xavier[2]

[1]Department of Architecture and Urbanism, Federal University of Pelotas, Brazil
[2]Department of Civil Engineering, Federal University of Rio Grande, Pelotas, Brazil

**Abstract**

The aim of this study is to provide a tool, for planning practice and policy making, in order to preserve the visual quality of historic streetscapes located on commercial areas. This tool involves the development and testing of a comparative method to calculate complexity levels of commercial streetscapes and to ascertain their correspondence with levels as perceived by users. The concept of complexity is understood as a variety of elements and relationships, in an aesthetic configuration, which are structured according to some overall principles of Gestalt Theory. The method, developed here, to calculate levels of complexity in street facades was tested utilising urban users from different cities and countries, including Brazil and England. It is the intention of the authors that this tool is used by urban designers, architects, and planners, before a new building intervention is added to an existing context, to ascertain whether it will increase or decrease people's evaluation of overall visual quality. As there is a relationship between the affective dimensions of user satisfaction, with street scenes and levels of complexity, the model has potential implications for urban design professionals.

**Key words:** complexity, Gestalt, order, visual quality

## Introduction

The focus of the study is to provide a tool for planning practice and policy making, in order to preserve the visual quality of historic streetscapes located on commercial areas. This investigation attempts to calculate the level of complexity of a set of street facades and compare these results with user evaluation of these places. If it is confirmed, this method can become a useful tool to help the aesthetic design of the built environment. The theoretical background applied to define this methodological approach is discussed below, followed by the methodology, results, and further discussion.

## Theoretical Background: Visual Quality of Built Environment and Gestalt Theory

The concept of visual quality is related to the level and order among the physical elements of built space. Weber (1995) mentions the following relationship: "the more orderly a configuration, the higher its aesthetic value." According to Gestalt psychology principles, high visual quality of public places exists in the "good form" or "pragnanz" of the city. "Good" in this case concerns how elements in an aesthetic composition are related to each other through regularity, orderliness, simplicity, symmetry, and so on, which refer to specific Gestalt laws (Boeree, 2000; Landry, 2006). Streetscapes, where there are no aesthetic conflicts between physical elements of building and commercial signs are recognised as having high visual quality or high order. Following this approach, low visual quality is linked to disordered places and other characteristics (Arnheim, 1977).

Weber (1995) and Arnheim (1977) argue that order is an indispensable aspect in all kinds of configuration (physical and mental). According to these authors, ordered compositions cause positive reactions on user perception and evaluation. Although user evaluation can be influenced by particular experiences, preferences, and feelings, the perception of order is evaluated as positive by almost all people. Nasar (1998) suggests that ordered streetscapes are evaluated positively by people who live in different cultures and physical environments. On the other hand, disordered public spaces are evaluated negatively because observers are exposed to a series of disconnected aesthetic elements (such as commercial signs, buildings, and urban furniture) which provoke user saturation. This saturation experience means that people lose the enjoyment of variety, and their senses become insensitive to the succession of visual stimulus without order (Lozano, quoted in Nasar, 1988).

The process of user evaluation in the visual quality of public spaces involves two principles: perception and cognition. Perception is generally related to processing inputs via sensory stimuli. In city centres, these stimuli are physical elements of built form, open space, and infrastructure, in its widest sense such as: commercial signs, shapes and colours of buildings, street furniture, and so on. The cognitive process does not necessarily require visual stimuli linked to physical environmental characteristics to function as part of the evaluative process. The cognitive process concerns symbolic meanings associated with places, and can be influenced by the user, urban context, values, culture, and individual experiences. This definition agrees with Meader, Uzzell and Gatersleben (2006, p. 61) who suggest: "people do not perceive the environment through clear eyes, but through perceptual lenses coloured by their world view." The result of the combined processes of perception and cognition constitutes the mental representation of a public space. According to Golledge and Stimsom (1996), this representation is what people evaluate as positive or negative when the streetscape is analysed. In this regard the mental representation produced for evaluation is the focus of analysis in this paper. The study specifically analyses how commercial street facades are perceived and evaluated by users from different urban contexts.

## Gestalt and Order

The segregation and unification of visual stimuli from public spaces, which result in the perception of order, are determined by the principles of Gestalt Theory and related to the psychological organisation of visual compositions (Ellis, 1969; Kanizsa, 1979; Murray, 1995; Smith, 1980). The principles of Gestalt explain why a determined space is perceived as orderly, pleasant and interesting by users from different backgrounds, despite the complexity of stimulation this place presents. These principles suggest how human beings tend to organise their perceptions to give preference to more regular configurations (Weber, 1995). One of the most sustained analyses of architecture content, based on the Gestalt theory of perception, was conducted by Arnheim (1977). The approach adopted in his work can be summarized by the following: "Shapes can be analysed in detail by describing their forms in terms of geometry, size, quantity and location, also there are visual forces which expand and contract, push and pull, rise and fall, advance and recede – which determine meaning and expression in art" (Arnheim, 1977, p. 10).

According to Weber (1995) and Lang (1987), the principle of "good Gestalt" or "law of pragnanz" is defined as a tendency of users to take on as much regularity as possible which is focused on pattern perception. Seven Gestalt laws form the factors that influence user perception of form: proximity, similarity, closure, good continuance, closeness, area, and symmetry. Studies by Reis (2002), Stamps (2000), Nasar and Hong (1999), Nasar (1988), and Lang (1987) indicated that the principle of complexity, related to the Gestalt laws, has high influence user perception and evaluation of the built environment. The relevance of complexity has also been highlighted by early studies related to the built environment. Eighty years ago Birkhoff's (1933) research successfully linked aesthetic quality with two factors: order and complexity.

In the context of this study, commercial street facades are perceived as ordered, when physical characteristics of commercial signs and buildings are structured according to some overall gestalt principle. Although this study recognises that all laws of Gestalt and principles related to the visual composition of forms influence user perception and evaluation of public spaces, this investigation attempts to analyse the level of complexity of a set of street facades and compare these results with user perceptions and evaluations of these places.

## Complexity vs. Disorder

Complexity refers to a variety of elements and relationships in an aesthetic configuration, which is structured according to some overall principle based on Gestalt Theory. This concept is related to the level of order of elements that form an aesthetic composition. Places where order does not exist, are perceived and evaluated as chaotic and irregular, and not as complex (Prak, 1985; Von Meiss, 1993; Weber, 1995). In this regard, Salingaros (2000, pp. 292–293) argues that: "In a general complex system (...) certain rules of assembly are followed so that the parts cooperate and the whole functions well." According to Moudon and Ryan (quoted in Neary, Symes, & Brown, 1994), most commercial streetscapes lie between disorder and order in which the ones in this last group reflect different levels of complexity. In this regard, this study assumes that complex urban scenes are characterised by an ordered aesthetic composition formed by many visual points of attention and different aesthetic relationships between them. Here, the concept of complexity is related to the variation of physical characteristics of commercial signs and buildings. The present study assumes that order is a pre-requisite for complexity. If a street facade has a high variation of physical elements, but its aesthetic configuration is not governed by an overall principle, this is just a chaotic street with high variation. The principle of complexity is approached in this way by many other researchers that analyse the visual quality of street facades (Berlyne, 1972; Nasar, 1988; Nasar & Hong, 1999).

There is an agreement in the literature that complexity is a necessary condition for aesthetic satisfaction (Berlyne, 1960; Kaplan, 1976a; Lang, 1987; Nasar, 1988; Rapport, 1977; Venturi, 1977; Weber, 1995). Venturi's (1977) and Berlyne's (1960) studies were the first to explore the principle of complexity in urban streetscapes. Venturi confronted ideas related to modernist architecture which promoted places with low complexity. Alternatively, Berlyne addressed the same propositions as Venturi, but in an approach which attempted to identify variables that may result in places being perceived positively. Kaplan (1976b) further identified negative implications of environments perceived as too complex or too monotonous on user behaviour, such as difficult wayfinding due to too high or too low visual stimulations and lack of interest. In addition, other studies suggest that complex streetscapes are evaluated more positively than simple streetscapes because they provide more information (Elsheshtawy, 1997; Weber, 1995; Lang, 1987). At the same time, studies show that user preferences are associated with moderate levels of complexity and extreme low and high complexities are not evaluated positively by observers (Berlyne, 1960; Bexton, Heron, & Scott, 1954; Day, 1992; Nasar, 1988, 1998; Nasar & Hong, 1999; Widmar, 1984).

Weber (1995), Lang (1987), and Rapoport (1977 quoted in Lang, 1987) suggest that, according to user perception and evaluation, there is a relationship between the affective dimensions of "pleasure" and "interest" with complexity. In terms of the "pleasure" dimension, the relationship is directly proportional until an optimum is reached and when this limit is exceeded, the relationship becomes inversely proportional. Nasar (1988, 1998) and Lang (1987) suggest that there have been several attempts to define this optimum level, but the number of factors that influence user perception and evaluation of the physical environment is so high that no clear definition can be made. On the other hand, in terms of the dimension of "interest," the relationship with complexity is always directly proportional.

Taking into account the context described in the previous paragraphs, the present paper analyses a set of physical characteristics of commercial signs and buildings in order to define the complexity of commercial streetscapes. Studies have already demonstrated that specific characteristics of commercial signs and buildings can influence user perception and evaluation of complexity (Elsheshtawy, 1997; Nasar & Hong, 1999; Stamps, 2000). The method developed and presented here to calculate complexity of street facades was based on issues discussed by Stamps (2000), Elsheshtawy (1997), and Nasar (1988). This demonstrates it is possible to define levels of complexity in commercial streetscapes, through the analysis of the variation in a range of physical characteristics of commercial signs and buildings. These characteristics are presented below.

## Physical Characteristics of Commercial Signs and Buildings That Increase Complexity

According to Nasar (1988) and an early study of Hardin (1968), there is a significant relationship between user perception and evaluation of complexity and variation of commercial signs. As stated by Nasar and Hong (1999), Nasar (1988), and guidelines applied in some European and American city centres (Duerksen & Goebel, 1999; Scenic America, 1993, 2000), variation of the following physical characteristics of commercial signs can influence user perception and evaluation of complexity: size, shape, proportion, arrangement on facades, type of sign, location on facade, presence of images, lettering style, predominant lettering style, letter size (height), number of chromatic groups, chromatic contrast between letters and sign background, segregation between figure (letters or images) and sign background by size proportion. Moreover, the number of commercial signs, percentage of street facade covered by these media, and square metres of signs per linear street metre are factors that can increase complexity (Ashihara, 1983). In recent studies, Mollerup (2005) and Stamps (2004) analyse variation of commercial signs in terms of the following features and indicate that they influence user perception of complexity: sign shape, orientation (perpendicular or parallel to the building facade), and height. All the physical characteristics of commercial signs that were mentioned above are considered in this paper.

Considering buildings, according to Stamps (2000), three formal aspects of facades can influence user perception and evaluation of complexity in streetscapes: silhouette, facade details, and facade articulation (see also studies of Burden, 1995; Ching, 1996; Groat, 1982; Quilan, 1991). Visual character and colour variation are also two other important attributes related to user perception and evaluation of complexity in commercial street-scapes (Moughtin, OC, & Tiesdell, 1999; Naoumova, 1997; Portella, 2003). In this paper, a range of physical features of buildings related to these formal aspects are considered to calculate the level of complexity of commercial street facades.

# Methodology

## Selecting Countries and Cities

The study presented in this paper is part of a wider project encompassing different countries to specifically compare two divergent cohorts:

- User evaluation of commercial streetscapes where there is a national approach to control commercial signage in historic city centres.
- User evaluation of local authorities that are not involved in any nationally controlled approach to signage in historic city centres.

In comparing these differing strategies it is important to evaluate whether this level of control is necessary or not. The choice for the sample of countries was also based on the researchers' previous knowledge of commercial signage approaches applied in South America countries (Portella, 2003). In addition the researchers had already carried previous research related to the visual pollution caused by commercial signs in historic cities in Brazil, and have an understanding of the problem. Moreover, the choice for the sample was based on the fact that England, where the bigger research project was based, is an example where a national commercial signage approach is applied to help local authorities guide and control commercial signage in historic city centres. These facts contributed to the selection of England and Brazil. With regard to Brazil, this investigation concentrated the analysis in the southern most Federal State, Rio Grande do Sul, as part of the theoretical background of this study is based on the findings produced by an earlier Masters dissertation and PhD thesis (Portella, 2003, 2007) on historic cities in the south of Brazil. The territorial dimension of this country ($8,514,876.599$ km$^2$) was also taken into account in the selection of only one State; the concentration of this study in one Brazilian Federal State avoided data collection becoming exhausting and impractical in terms of financial resources and time spent travelling.

Having chosen the countries for the analysis, historic city centres were selected as case studies. The limited financial resources and time available suggested that in total no more than three case studies could be chosen.

A diagnostic exploration was conducted in terms of the size of population (i) in the thirty five major historic cities and towns of England, according to English Heritage (English Heritage, 2006), and (ii) in the main cities, colonies and villages, which marked the history of colonisation and urbanisation of the southernmost Federal State of Brazil (Barroso, 1992; Daros & Barroso, 2000). This analysis demonstrated that the majority of these places, in England and in the State of Rio Grande do Sul, can be classified as small or medium sized (population $\leq$ 400,000 inhabitants). Therefore, this became the first main criterion in the selection of the cities. Only small or medium cities, towns, colonies, or villages were considered as potential case studies. Taking this main criterion into account, the following aspects were also applied in the choice of the case studies:

1) They need to be small/medium cities because commercial activities are more intense in these places than in towns, colonies, or villages.
2) They need to have a historic city centre with intense commercial activity.
3) They need to be different in terms of how commercial signage controls are approached in relation to the preservation of historic heritage, in order to explore fully the effects that distinct commercial signage controls can have on the appearance of historic city centres.
4) They need to include streets that have similar relationships between commercial signs and building form to other historic cities in each country, in order to explore the effects of commercial signage controls on typical commercial streetscapes as opposed to individual cases.

With regard to the final item above, three analyses were carried out to select the most representative case studies: (i) photographic analysis of commercial streets of historic city centres in England and Brazil, (ii) fieldtrips to historic cities in England and in the Brazilian Federal State of Rio Grande do Sul, and (iii) analysis of legislation related to commercial signage controls in English and Brazilian historic city centres. While the impressions obtained from these explorative analyses cannot be taken to have more than superficial validity, as a measure of recognition of the physical characteristics of historic city centres and the commercial signage controls applied in these places, they did allow the identification of common features across commercial streetscapes in different settings.

The results from these analyses show that in England there is one common scenario that represents the majority of historic city centres: commercial signage controls are currently applied in order to preserve the historic character of these places so that the streetscape is ordered and characterised by preserved historic buildings.

In Brazil, two typical cases illustrate the majority of historic city centres: (i) commercial signage controls are designed and applied by the local authority in order to reinforce a manufactured image of the place, resulting in an ordered streetscape characterised by contemporary buildings; (ii) commercial signage controls are not applied, resulting in a disordered streetscape characterised by historic buildings harmed by shopfronts and window displays.

The following historic cities were selected as case studies because they conform to all of the criteria above: Oxford, in England, and Gramado and Pelotas in Brazil. In Oxford, commercial signage controls had been designed and applied to preserve the historic heritage of the city. In Gramado, commercial signage controls had been designed and applied to reinforce a manufactured image of the city promoted by the local authority. In Pelotas, commercial signage controls had not been applied. The study area in each of these case studies was limited according to the following criteria: it needs to be (i) in the city centre, (ii) in the historic core, and (iii) in zones of intense commercial activity.

## Criteria for Selection of Commercial Street Facades

Probability sampling was applied to select a set of street facades in each case study. Two street facades in each case study were selected because this number was considered to be representative of the historic core of each city, and it met the time constraints of the study (see Figure 1). The following stratification factors were adopted in their selection:

1) The street facade should reflect the general characteristics of the study area in terms of the relationship between commercial signs and buildings.
2) The street facade should be formed by (i) ordinary buildings and (ii) either lawfully recognised historic buildings or, in the Brazilian context, exemplars from the first period of the city which may not be currently recognised by law.
3) The street facade should have historic buildings with commercial signs displayed on their facades.
4) The street facade should have 80% or more buildings related to commercial activities. This is because this study analyses the relationship between commercial signs and buildings, and street facades where commercial activities are predominant and this relationship is conspicuous are preferred.
5) The street facade should not have empty plots, buildings in the process of construction or buildings in the process of restoration or renovation. As found by Portella (2003), these variables effect user perception and evaluation of commercial streets.
6) The width of the street needs to be 3 meters or more in order to allow photographs to be taken. A previous study suggested that road widths of less than 3 meters makes it difficult to produce the media representation of street facades (Portella, 2003).
7) The street facade should not have buildings with more than five floors. High buildings tend to be difficult to photograph, and usually, when photos can be taken, the level of parallax distortion is extremely high.

In order to analyse the influence of different physical characteristics of commercial signs and buildings on user perception and evaluation, the commercial street facades in the sample should vary in terms of (i) number of commercial signs and percentage of street facades covered by these media, (ii) square metres of commercial signs per linear street metre, (iii) number of buildings harmed by commercial signs, (iv) visual character, and (v) colour.

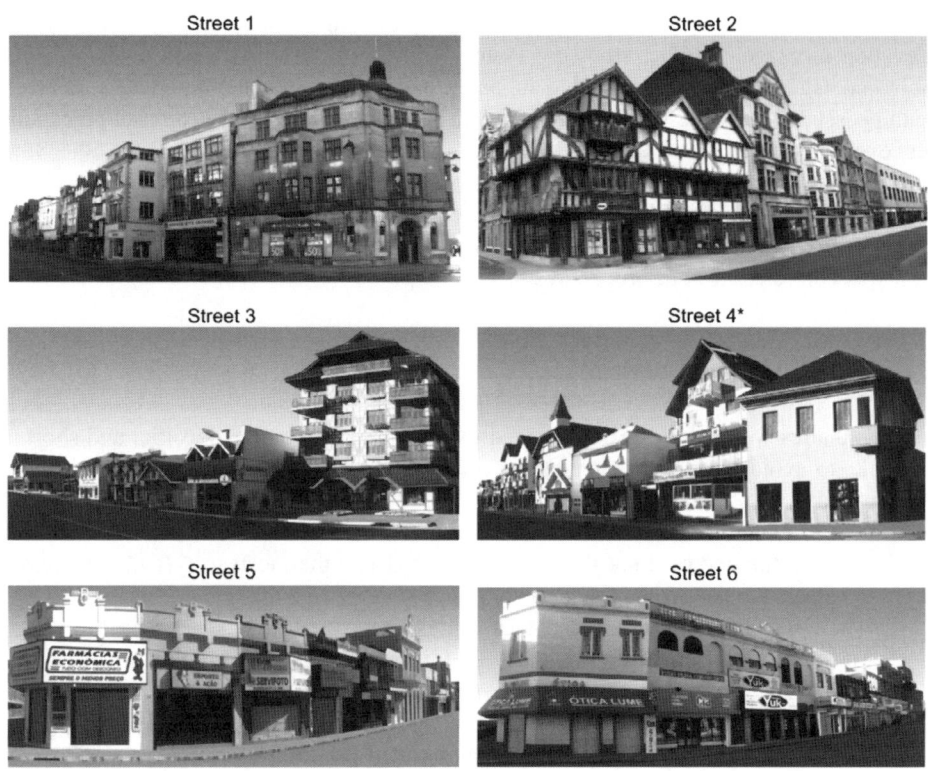

**Figure 1.** Commercial street facades investigated. (Source: author).
*Note.* Street numbered as 4 is not analysed in this article, as here it presented just the findings related with the streets pointed out as the best and the worst in terms of visual quality by users, street 4 did not appear in this classification.

## Media Representation of the Commercial Street Facades in the Sample

Ideally, to ensure maximum realism, users from England and Brazil should observe the sample of commercial street facades on-site. However, because of the impracticality of bringing users from England to Brazil and vice versa, the experiment was based on colour photomontages attached to a questionnaire.

The media representations adopted here were based on the method developed by Stamps (1993). Each commercial street facade was represented by two kinds of photomontage. In the first one, the entire row of buildings was photographed from one station point generating a two-point perceptive image, while for the second one, each building was photographed separately and the photographs pasted together to form an elevation montage. Another study by Stamps (1997) suggests that users tend to dislike photomontages of streetscapes with cars, poles, and wires, while photomontages of streets with pedestrians and trees tend to be preferred. As this research focuses on user perception and evaluation of the relationship between commercial signs and building form, other variables which may interfere with users' answers (such as trees, cars, poles, wires, pedestrians, scaffolding, and street furniture) were deleted from the photomontage. These deletions were done to avoid misinterpretation of the findings. In addition, parallax distortion was corrected in both procedures.

## Data Collection: Questionnaires

Questionnaires were applied and designed to be as simple, precise, specific, and short as possible, to avoid respondents getting bored, confused, or tired. The following questions were asked:

1. Look at the photos; rank the streets from 1 (I like the most) to 6 (I like the least):
   ( ) street 1   ( ) street 2   ( ) street 3   ( ) street 4   ( ) street 5   ( ) street 6
2. The BEST street in terms of appearance is:
   ( ) street 1   ( ) street 2   ( ) street 3   ( ) street 4   ( ) street 5   ( ) street 6
3. The WORST street in terms of appearance is:
   ( ) street 1   ( ) street 2   ( ) street 3   ( ) street 4   ( ) street 5   ( ) street 6
4–5. Rate the BEST/WORST street along each of the following scales:
   ( ) Very ordered ( ) Ordered  ( ) Neither ordered nor chaotic ( ) Chaotic ( ) Very chaotic
   ( ) Very complex ( ) Complex ( ) Neither complex nor simple ( ) Simple ( ) Very simple
6–7. Look at the poster attached to this questionnaire, mark the alternative that best describes the BEST/WORST street:

| | Very high | High | Moderate | Low | Very low |
|---|---|---|---|---|---|
| The variation of commercial signs is: | ( ) | ( ) | ( ) | ( ) | ( ) |
| The variation of buildings is: | ( ) | ( ) | ( ) | ( ) | ( ) |

To select respondents, a random volunteer sample, comprising people who were willing to participate in the survey were considered. As the nature of this study assumes that people cannot be forced to be part of the survey, users decided whether they would like to answer the questionnaire or not. The only pre-requisites to be part of the sample were to be resident in one of the case studies, and to be 18 years old or more.

Posters were displayed in universities, cafes, public places, and City Council halls and were given to pedestrians in Oxford, Gramado, and Pelotas as pamphlets to search for volunteers. These media explained the purposes of the questionnaire and invited people to participate. Invitation letters were also sent by post to professionals and lay people, selected randomly from phone lists. In addition, a snowballing approach was adopted with volunteers allowed to invite friends to participate. As a result of these techniques, several people contacted the researcher by e-mail or phone (contact information was included on posters, invitation letters, and cover pages of questionnaires, which most volunteers kept) and asked to take part in this study. Articles in local newspapers of the Brazilian case studies were published in order to encourage people to become involved in the survey. The other techniques mentioned above (such as posters and invitation letters) were not effective in the Brazilian case studies.

The sample size was not pre-fixed, as a result of a self-selection process; the sample sizes in the three case studies were different: 114 respondents in Oxford, 120 respondents in Gramado, and 127 respondents in Pelotas. The total sample was 361 respondents.

The questionnaire was delivered in person, and the researchers explained to the respondent what was expected to be done and made an appointment to collect it. Usually questionnaires were collected on the following day. Clear instructions were presented in an introductory statement to avoid possible misinterpretation, as the respondents completed the questionnaire on their own. The researchers also mentioned that participants could contact them at any time if they had any doubts about how to answer or interpret the questions. Direct contact between the researchers and the participants was an important factor in committing them to complete the questionnaire. In addition, the sample criteria adopted, to select users was a contributing factor to engage people with interest in participation in the survey coming from the respondents who contacted the researcher. Therefore, this was interpreted as a sign that they were committed to completing the task.

In terms of the questionnaire format, as suggested by Sommer and Sommer (2002), appeal to the eye was an important issue. A cover letter introducing the researcher, the purpose of the survey, general information, such as how long the questionnaire takes to be completed, confidentiality of users' responses and so on, was printed in colour on official University paper. This gave credibility to the research in the eyes of the respondents. The media representation of the commercial street facades attached to questionnaire was printed on A1 (84.10 cm × 59.40 cm) gloss (photo) paper, using the best quality of resolution.

The results of the questionnaire were analysed through Kruskal-Wallis and Mann-Whitney statistical tests, Mean and crosstabs.

## Analysis of the Commercial Street Facades in the Sample

By making field visits to the study areas, a systematic observation of the commercial street facades was carried out to identify the level of order among commercial signs and buildings. At this stage, the following criterion was applied to identify the street facades which are ordered and disordered: the percentage of street facade related to buildings harmed by commercial signs. If more than 40% of the street facade is harmed by signage, it is classified as a disordered street. According to this criterion, the sample of street facades is classified as follows: street 1 (most ordered), 2, 3, and 4 (least ordered). Streets 6 and 5 are classified as disordered; this initial classification converged with user perception and evaluation of these streets (see Table 1). As this study assumes that order is a pre-requisite to complexity, the term "complexity" is not applied to streets 5 and 6. These streets are identified as having just higher or lower variation of commercial signs and buildings.

Record cards were designed and applied to aid observation of the physical characteristics of the commercial street facades in the sample on-site and to allow the same characteristics observed in one street for comparison in another. These characteristics are presented in Table 2.

## The Complexity Method

The method developed and tested here to calculate the level of complexity in commercial street facades is called "the complexity method". This method is used to determine the level of complexity of commercial street facades by analysing the variation of a range of physical features of commercial signs and buildings (see Table 2). The application of this method consists of numbering the street facades in the sample according to the level of variation of physical characteristics of commercial signs and buildings, where the higher the variation, the lower the number allocated to each street. For example, when analysing the variation in the size of commercial signs, the street facade with the highest variation was numbered one and the street facade with the lowest variation was numbered six. After all of the physical features had been analysed, the numbers allocated to each street for every single feature were summed to provide a total figure indicating the final level of complexity of each street. The street with the lowest final sum was classified as having the highest complexity, while the street with the highest final sum was classified as having the lowest complexity. Table 3 shows the final level of complexity of each street facade in the sample, as a result of this method. In this study, the method took into account, that all the physical characteristics of the street facades related to signage and buildings have the same height value, consequently the numerical values of variation of each characteristic where sum as equal. However, it is recognised that it can create discrepancies which is intended to be identified when comparing the results from this method with users' responses to the appearance of street facades.

Looking at Table 2, it is necessary to define what is meant by the expression "lettering style" as a physical feature of commercial signs to avoid vagueness and ambiguity of terms. This expression means a group of letters that has the same structure. According to Williams' study (1994), there are several lettering styles grouped into six categories: (i) old style, (ii) modern, (iii) slab serif, (vi) sans serif, (v) script, and (vi) decorative. These categories were adopted to classify the level of variation of "lettering style". In addition, it is important to note that when symmetry of shape perimeter (street as a whole) was analysed to calculate building silhouette, three levels of variation were considered: (i) level 1 – silhouette of street facade has high variation (main turns on shape perimeter $\geq$ 6); (ii) level 2 – silhouette of street facade has variation but some similarity can be noted

**Table 1.** Comparison between the initial categorisation of the streets according to the criterion adopted to define order and user evaluation of order

| Street facades | Percentage of street facade related to buildings harmed by commercial signs* | Level of order |
|---|---|---|
| Street 1 | 0 | Most ordered |
| Street 2 | 0 | |
| Street 3 | 4% | |
| Street 4 | 35% | |
| Street 6 | 46% | Disordered |
| Street 5 | 56% | |

| Users responses to: Rate the street >x< along the following scale: | Street facades chosen as the BEST by users in terms of appearance: | | | Street facades chosen as the WORST by users in terms of appearance: | |
|---|---|---|---|---|---|
| | Street 1 | Street 2 | Street 3 | Street 5 | Street 6 |
| Very ordered + ordered | 123 (80.39%) | 66 (89.19%) | 82 (77.36%) | 18 (12.08%) | 20 (11.83%) |
| Neither ordered nor disordered | 20 (13.34%) | 7 (9.46%) | 20 (18.87%) | 23 (15.44%) | 29 (17.16%) |
| Chaotic + very chaotic | 10 (6.53%) | 1 (1.35%) | 4 (3.78%) | 108 (72.48%) | 120 (71.01%) |
| Total | 153 (100%) | 74 (100%) | 106 (100%) | 149 (100%) | 169 (100%) |
| Mean* | 2 | 1.45 | 1.83 | 3.98 | 4.02 |

*The lower this value, the more ordered the commercial street facade. In mathematics and statistics, the mean is another name for the average. The mean is calculated by adding all of the values together, then dividing by the number of original values. Street 4 is not indicated by a significant number of users as the best or the worst street in terms of appearance; so in this case this street is not analysed in this report.

**Table 2.** Physical features of commercial signs and buildings analysed to calculate complexity

| Physical features of commercial signs | | Size; shape; number of chromatic groups; chromatic contrast between letters and sign background; proportion; arrangement on facades; type of sign; location on facade; presence of images; lettering style; predominant letter style; size of letters in relation to sign background; size of images in relation to sign background; letter size (height). |
|---|---|---|
| Physical features of buildings | Silhouettes | Symmetry of shape perimeter (street as a whole); number of vertexes; number of turns in shape perimeter (street as a whole); symmetry of building perimeter; height of buildings; width of buildings; type of coronation. |
| | Facade details | Type of details; number of buildings with details; architectural styles; texture of revetments. |
| | Articulation | Size of facades; fenestration; percentage of street facade fenestration; shape of windows and doors; overall proportion of windows and doors; number of building with broken mass; percentage of street facade cover by buildings with broken mass; proportion of buildings; presence of horizontal and vertical partition on building facades; presence of vertical features on building facades; thickness of vertical features on building facades; localisation of buildings on plots; presence of vegetation. |
| | Visual character | Architectural styles; number of storeys; roof line; building symmetry. |
| | Colour variation | Colour of building facades; colour of body facades. |

(main turns on shape perimeter $\leq 5$); and (iii) level 3 – silhouette of street facade has few variation and looks almost symmetric (main turns on shape perimeter $< 4$).

In relation to colour variation, a colour palette was defined to each street facade in the sample which was based on the colours of buildings and commercial signs. The colours were grouped into three main categories: hue, colour-temperature, and colour-saturation. The following groups of hues were identified: (i) blue to purple; (ii) green to yellow green, (iii) yellow to orange, and (iv) brown to red. In terms of colour-saturation, colours were divided into dark, medium, and light; and in terms of colour-temperature, colours were classified as cold and hot. The relationships between colours were also classified as harmonious or not and they were linked with the position of colours in the chromatic disc.

**Table 3.** Final level of complexity of each street as a result of the application of the method

| Commercial street facades | Commercial signs | Variation of physical features related to: | | | | | Final level of complexity (sum of the numeric classifications of each street facade) | |
|---|---|---|---|---|---|---|---|---|
| | | Building facades | | | | | | |
| | | Silhouette | Details | Articulation | Visual character | Colour variation | | |
| Street 4 | 38 | 10 | 15 | 37 | 9 | 5 | 114 | Highest variation |
| Street 1 | 43 | 22 | 6 | 35 | 11 | 5 | 122 | |
| Street 3 | 44 | 23 | 12 | 29 | 12 | 5 | 125 | |
| Street 6* | 39 | 25 | 20 | 35 | 15 | 8 | 142 | |
| Street 2 | 48 | 28 | 9 | 41 | 16 | 12 | 154 | |
| Street 5* | 49 | 29 | 16 | 45 | 18 | 7 | 164 | Lowest variation |

*The term complexity is not applied to Streets 5 and 6 because they are disordered. These streets are understood as having just higher or lower variation.

Colours of body facades were delimited to this analysis, because they usually correspond to the biggest part of a building facade, and seven harmonic groups were identified in this study: (i) achromatic harmony, (ii) monochromatic harmony, (iii) harmony by proximity, (iv) harmony by dominance, (v) harmony by contrast, (vi) harmony by complementary colours, and (vii) harmony by light-dark contrast.

## Comparing the Levels of Complexity Defined Through the Method With Users Evaluation

The results relating to user perception and evaluation of street complexity are presented in terms of best and worst appearance. The findings are related to streets 1, 2, and 3 chosen as the best streets by 92.3% of users, and streets 5 and 6 chosen as the worst streets by 88.1% of users. Street 4 is out of the analysis as only 6.9% of users pointed this one as the best street, and 8.9% of users as the worst street (see Table 1).

The results from the analysis of user perception and evaluation regarding the semantic scales of "complex-simple" (questions 4 and 5 of the questionnaire) indicate that there are significant differences between streets 1, 2, and 3 (KW = 20.009, DF = 2, $p$ = .001) in terms of complexity. Street 2 is evaluated by users as less complex than street 1 (U = 3,723.0, N1 = 153, N2 = 74, two-tailed $p$ = .001). According to user evaluation, street 1 is evaluated as "very complex" or "complex" (49.02% of users), while street 2 is evaluated as "very simple" or "simple" (48.65% of users) (Table 4). These results converge with the findings obtained from the application of the method adopted to calculate complexity, which show that street 1 has the second highest level of complexity and street 2 has the second lowest level of complexity when compared to the other streets in the sample.

**Table 4.** User evaluation of complexity when the appearance of streets chosen as the best and worst in terms of appearance were analysed

Users responses to: Rate the street >x< along the following scale

| | Street facades chosen as the BEST by users in terms of appearance: | | | Street facades chosen as the WORST by users in terms of appearance: | |
|---|---|---|---|---|---|
| | Street 1 | Street 2 | Street 3 | Street 5 | Street 6 |
| **The whole sample (361 respondents)** | | | | | |
| Very complex + complex | 75 (49.02%) | 14 (18.96%) | 32 (30.19%) | 55 (36.91%) | 50 (29.58%) |
| Neither complex nor simple | 37 (24.18%) | 24 (32.43%) | 36 (33.96%) | 57 (38.26%) | 66 (39.05%) |
| Simple + very simple | 41 (26.80%) | 36 (48.65%) | 38 (35.85%) | 37 (25.83%) | 53 (31.36%) |
| Total | 153 (100%) | 74 (100%) | 106 (100%) | 149 (100%) | 169 (100%) |
| Mean* | 2.71 | 3.43 | 3.14 | 2.88 | 3.08 |

*The lower this value, the more complex the commercial street facades. The mean is calculated by adding all of the values together, then dividing by the number of original values.

Users responses to: Mark the alternative that best describes the street:

| | Street facades chosen as the BEST by users in terms of appearance: | | | Street facades chosen as the WORST by users in terms of appearance: | |
|---|---|---|---|---|---|
| | Street 1 | Street 2 | Street 3 | Street 5 | Street 6 |
| **The variation of commercial signage is:** | | | | | |
| Very high + high | 22 (14.38%) | 0 | 39 (36.79%) | 127 (85.24%) | 156 (92.30%) |
| Moderate | 47 (30.72%) | 31 (41.89%) | 46 (43.40%) | 15 (10.07%) | 10 (5.92%) |
| Low + very low | 84 (54.90%) | 43 (58.1%) | 21 (19.81%) | 7 (4.7%) | 3 (1.78%) |
| Total | 153 (100%) | 74 (100%) | 106 (100%) | 149 (100%) | 169 (100%) |
| Mean score* | 3.56 | 3.73 | 2.80 | 1.74 | 1.70 |
| **The variation of buildings is:** | | | | | |
| Very high + high | 75 (49.02%) | 21 (28.38%) | 44 (41.5%) | 72 (48.32%) | 64 (37.87%) |
| Moderate | 65 (42.48%) | 37 (50%) | 51 (48.11%) | 55 (36.91%) | 89 (52.66%) |
| Low + very low | 13 (8.50%) | 16 (21.62%) | 11 (10.37%) | 22 (14.76%) | 16 (9.46%) |
| Total | 153 (100%) | 74 (100%) | 106 (100%) | 149 (100%) | 169 (100%) |
| Mean* | 2.44 | 2.89 | 2.63 | 2.54 | 2.62 |

*The lower this value, the higher the commercial signage and building variation. The mean is calculated by adding all of the values together, then dividing by the number of original values. The total sample (100%) is related with the number of users who chose each street as the best or the worst in terms of appearance.

When comparing the findings obtained from the method applied to calculate complexity and user evaluation of complexity, a difference is found in relation to the appearance of street 3. According to the method, street 3 has the third highest level of complexity, when compared to the other streets. However, respondents evaluate this street as "very complex" or "complex" (30.19% of users), "neither complex nor simple" (33.96% of users), and "very simple" or "simple" (35.85% of users). In this regard, taking into account the physical characteristics of this street, this study indicates that when a street facade is comprised of buildings similar in visual character and architectural style, some users will perceive this similarity[1] as simplicity. Therefore, street 3 was not evaluated as "complex" or "very complex" by the majority of users.

There are no statistical differences between streets 5 and 6 in terms of user evaluation of variation.[2] A significant number of respondents classify both these streets as "very complex" or "complex" (street 5: 36.91%; street 6: 29.58%), "neither complex nor complex" (street 5: 38.26%; street 6: 39.05%), and "simple" or "very simple" (street 5: 25.83%; street 6: 31.36%). The findings from the method applied to calculate complexity show that street 5 have a lower final level of commercial signage and buildings variation than street 6. In this regard, the results from user evaluation indicate that a set of physical characteristics of commercial signs and buildings in streets 5 and 6 may balance this difference and have different height of importance to users' perceptions. Therefore, users classify the level of variation of commercial signs and buildings in both these streets as the same. This study indicates that user evaluation of variation in street 5 is increased because, when compared to street 6, this street has (i) higher commercial signage variation in terms of size, number of chromatic groups, position in relation to facades, size of images, and size of letters, and (ii) higher building variation in terms of fenestration, presence of horizontal and vertical partitions, and colour. On the other hand, user evaluation of variation in street 6 is decreased because, when compared to street 5, this street has (i) lower commercial signage variation in terms of chromatic contrast between letters and sign background, and size of images, and (ii) lower building variation in terms of turns of shape perimeter, overall proportion of windows and doors, articulation, roof line, colour, and facade details.

Taking into consideration the responses of users regarding the semantic scale of "high variation-low variation" (questions 6 and 7 of the questionnaire), there are significant differences between streets 1, 2, and 3 in terms of commercial signage variation (KW = 47.467, DF = 2, $p$ = .001). These differences are placed between streets 2 and 3 (U = 1,829.0, N1 = 74, N2 = 106, two-tailed $p$ = .001), and streets 1 and 3

---

[1]   The concept of similarity rests either on exact or approximate repetitions of physical features of buildings.
[2]   The term "complexity" is not applied to interpret the findings related to streets 5 and 6 as both these streets are disordered, and order is a pre-requisite to complexity. Therefore, user responses to streets 5 and 6 are interpreted as variation of physical characteristics of commercial signs and buildings. However, in the questionnaire the semantic scale of "complex-simple" was applied to investigate all streets to not confuse the respondents.

(U = 4,854.5, N1 = 153, N2 = 106, two-tailed $p$ = .001). According to users, street 3 has the highest commercial signage variation, followed by streets 1 and 2.

The majority of users evaluate street 1 (54.90% of users) and street 2 (58.10% of users) as having "very low" or "low" commercial signage variation, while 43.40% of respondents classify street 3 as having "moderate" commercial signage variation (Table 4). Reviewing the results from the method applied to calculate complexity, streets 1 and 3 have almost the same level of commercial signage variation, while street 2 has the second lowest level of commercial signage variation when compared to the other streets. Although the level of commercial signage variation, defined by this method, of streets 1 and 3 is similar, some differences are found between the physical characteristics of these streets. Street 3 has higher commercial signage variation in size, arrangement in relation to facades, location on facades, presence of images, and size of letters and images in relation to sign background. In this regard, this study indicates that these factors may have a major impact on user perception than the other physical aspects analysed.

There is no statistical difference between streets 5 and 6 in terms of commercial signage variation regarding users' responses. According to the results from the method, street 5 has lower commercial signage variation than street 6. However, the majority of respondents agree that both these streets have "very high" or "high" commercial signage variation (street 5: 85.25%; street 6: 92.30%). In this regard, this study indicates that the following characteristics of street 5 are having stronger impact on user perception and evaluation of commercial signage variation: in comparison to street 6, street 5 has higher commercial signage variation in size, number of chromatic groups, arrangement in relation to facades, size of images in relation to sign background, and size of letters.

User evaluation of building variation (Table 4) suggest there are significant differences between streets 1, 2, and 3 (KW = 13.409, DF = 2, $p$ = .001) regarding users responses. These differences are placed between streets 1 and 2 (U = 4,097.0, N1 = 153, N2 = 74, two-tailed $p$ = .001), and streets 2 and 3 (U = 3212.0, N1 = 74, N2 = 106, two-tailed $p$ = .02). According to users, street 1 has higher building variation than street 2, and street 3 has higher building variation than street 2.

These results confirm the findings obtained from the method applied to calculate complexity in commercial streetscapes. Findings from this method show that street 2 has the lowest building variation, when compared to streets 1 and 3. The majority of users from the whole sample (50% of users) agree that street 2 has moderate variation, while, in relation to streets 1 and 3, respondents are divided between those who mention a "very high" or "high" (street 1: 49.02% of users; street 3: 41.51% of users) and a "moderate" (street 1: 42.48% of users; street 3: 48.11% of users) variation.

Analysing street facades chosen as the worst, there is no statistical difference between streets 5 and 6 in terms of building variation when the responses of users were analysed. In both these streets, users are divided between those who mention a "very high" or "high" (street 5: 48.32% of users; street 6: 37.87% of users), and a "moderate" building variation (street 5: 36.91% of users; street 6: 52.66% of users). Taking into account the results from the method applied to calculate complexity; street 5 has lower building variation than street 6. However, some differences can be seen between the physical characteristics of buildings in both these streets. In this regard, this study indicates that higher building variation in number of turns of facade shape perimeter, facade width, facade details, percentage of fenestration on building facade, overall proportion of windows and doors, presence of horizontal or vertical partition on building facade, and colour are increasing user evaluation of building variation in street 5.

## Discussion

The main contribution of this study is not so much in the specific finding, but in the method applied to discuss the level of complexity of streetscapes in commercial and historical areas and the potential repercussions it could have on practice and policy making. The method applied in this study to calculate complexity produces results which, in general, converge with the perception and evaluation of users. In this sense, this method can be integrated into a general commercial signage approaches in order to help local authorities monitor levels of complexity in commercial and historic streetscapes. This method can also be adopted to predict whether the level of complexity of a street facade, in terms of commercial signage and building variation, will increase too much with the insertion of a new commercial sign or building. For example, the application of this method could identify whether a new commercial sign would increase the complexity of a street facade too much, before the sign was displayed in the city centre. If these results indicated that the complexity would be increased too much with the insertion of this new sign, the local authority could ask the shop owner to re-design the media based on objective measures of evaluation to request this. This study recognises the method as a potential tool to help planning practice in the preservation of historic heritage and visual quality, avoiding the decrease of user satisfaction with the appearance of our cities.

Evidence presented in this study suggests that some users can perceive similarity as simplicity in terms of street facade when the street is comprised of buildings similar in visual character and architectural style. In addition, the findings indicate a set of combinations of physical aspects have different influences on user evaluation of complexity. Variation of commercial signs in terms of: size, number of chromatic groups, arrangement in relation to facades, size of images and size of letters; variation of buildings in terms of fenestration, presence of horizontal and vertical partitions, turns of shape perimeter, proportion of windows and doors, articulation, roof line, facade details and colour seem to have a major impact on user evaluation of complexity than other physical aspects.

Results from the analysis of user evaluation show that the commercial street facades chosen as the best streets in terms of appearance are evaluated as having moderate commercial signage and building variation; and the commercial street facades chosen as the worst streets in terms of appearance are evaluated as having high commercial signage and building variation. Findings also show that the ordered streetscapes are classified by a significant number of users as having "very low/low or moderate" commercial signage variation, and "very high/high or moderate" building variation, and disordered streetscapes are classified as having "very high/high" commercial signage variation, and "very high/high or moderate" building variation. The outcomes reinforce the idea that is essential to control commercial signage variation; however it is positive to allow high variation of buildings. This corroborates the literature review, which argues people will prefer places with more information within a degree of order.

In addition, a further stage of the research methodology could be the non-selection of residents in the cities where the street samples are located. This could allow the exploration of user perception of complexity whilst excluding the possible influence of resident familiarity with particular streetscapes and symbolic meanings attributed to buildings. It was not supported that the findings of this report were influenced by this variable, but it could be interesting to replicate the study with a sample of users not familiar with the streets investigated. Moreover, the small sample of street facades can be a limitation to generalising the results across a wider population. Therefore the findings in this report act as hypotheses to be tested on other case studies with a higher range of streetscapes.

Further investigation into the subject of visual quality and complexity in the built environment could also be conducted in order to explore how commercial signage controls might be developed in city centres where the historic component is not a dominant issue. Application of the same methodology used here, in places where the visual character of commercial streetscapes is mainly carried or deliberately constructed through commercial signage, such as in Las Vegas, Times Square, and Hong Kong, might produce different results from those verified here when compared to user perception. In these cases, the signage itself constitutes the architecture, and therefore very different issues related to the control of the complexity might be taken into account in such places.

# References

Arnheim, R. (1977). *Dynamic of architectural form*. Berkeley, CA: University of California Press.
Ashihara, Y. (1983). *The aesthetic townscape*. Cambridge, MA: MIT Press.
Barroso, V. L. M. (1992) Povoamento e Urbanizacao do Rio Grande do Sul [Colonization and Urbanization of Rio Grande do Sul]. In G. Weimer (Ed.), *Urbanismo no Rio Grande do Sul* (pp. 35–55). Porto Alegre, Brazil: Editora da Universidade.
Berlyne, D. E. (1960). *Conflict, arousal and curiosity*. New York, NY: MacGraw-Hill.
Berlyne, D. E. (1972). Ends and means of experimental aesthetics. *Canadian Journal of Psychology, 26*(4), 303–325.
Bexton, W. H., Heron, W., & Scott, T. H. (1954). Effects of decreased variation in the sensory environment. *Canadian Journal of Psychology, 8*(2), 70–76.
Birkhoff, G. D. (1933). *Aesthetic measure*. Cambridge, MA: Harvard University Press.
Boeree, G. (2000). *Gestalt psychology*. Retrieved from http://www.ship.edu/~cgboeree/gestalt.html
Burden, E. (1995). *Elements of architecture*. New York, NY: Van Nostrand Reinhold.
Ching, F. D. (1996). *Form, space and order*. New York, NY: Van Nostrand Reinhold.
Daros, M., & Barroso, V. L. M. (2000). *Raizes de Gramado – V Encontro dos Municipios Originarios de Santo Antonio da Patrulha* [Roots of Gramado – V Meeting of the Cities Originary from "Santo Antonio da Patrulha"] (2nd ed.). Porto Alegre, Brazil: Edicoes Estacoes.

Day, L. L. (1992). Placemaking by design: Fitting a large new building into a historic district. *Environment and Behavior, 24*(3), 326–346.

Duerksen, C. J., & Goebel, R. M. (1999, December). *Aesthetic, community character and law* (pp. 489–490). Chicago, IL: Scenic America.

Ellis, W. D. (1969). *A source book of Gestalt psychology*. London, UK: Routledge & Kegan Paul.

Elsheshtawy, Y. (1997). Urban complexity: Toward the measurement of the physical complexity of streetscapes. *Journal of Architecture and Planning Research, 14*(4), 301–328.

English Heritage. (2006). *Historic towns & city surveys*. Retrieved from http://www.english-heritage.org.uk/server/show/conwebDoc3963

Golledge, R. G., & Stimsom, R. J. (1996). *Spatial behavior: A geographic perspective*. New York, NY: Guilford Press.

Groat, L. (1982). Meaning in post-modern architecture. An examination using the multiple sorting task. *Journal of Environmental Psychology, 2*(1), 3–22.

Hardin, G. (1968). The tragedy of the commons. *Science, 162*(3859), pp. 1243–1248.

Kanizsa, C. (1979). *Organization in vision, essays on gestalt perception*. NewYork, NY: Praeger.

Kaplan, S. (1976a). Adaptation, structure and knowledge. In G. T. Moore & R. G. Golledge (Eds.), *Environmental knowing: Theories, perspectives and methods* (pp. 32–45). Stroudsburg, PA: Dowden, Hutchinson and Ross.

Kaplan, S. (1976b). Wayfinding in the natural environment. In G. T. Moore & R. G. Golledge (Eds.), *Environmental knowing: Theories, perspectives and methods* (pp. 3–24). Stroudsburg, PA: Dowden, Hutchinson and Ross.

Landry, C. (2006). *The art of the city making*. London, UK: Earthscan.

Lang, J. (1987). *Creating architectural theory, The role of the behavioral sciences in environmental design*. New York, NY: Van Nostrand Reinhold.

Meader, N., Uzzell, D., & Gatersleben, B. (2006). Cultural theory and quality of life. *European Review of Applied Psychology, 56*(1), 61–69.

Mollerup, P. (2005). *Wayshowing: A guide to environmental signage, principles & practices*. Vicenza, Italy: Graphicom srl.

Moughtin, J. C., OC, T., & Tiesdell, S. (1999). *Urban design: Ornament and decoration*. Oxford, UK: Architectural Press.

Murray, D. J. (1995). *Gestalt psychology and the cognitive revolution*. London, UK: Harvester Wheatsheaf.

Naoumova, N. (1997). *A Policromia da Cidade: Aspectos Culturais, Simbolicos e Estruturais - Teoria e Pratica* [The policromy of the City: Cultural, Symbolic and Structural Aspects – Theory and Practice]. Supplement Material for the Technical Course "Colours of the City." Pelotas, Brazil: Federal University of Pelotas.

Neary, S. J., Symes, M. S., & Brown, F. E. (Eds.). (1994). *The urban experience: A people-environment perspective*. London, UK: E & FN Spon.

Nasar, J., & Hong, X. (1999). Visual preferences in urban signscapes. *Environment and Behavior, 31*(5), 671–691.

Nasar, J. L. (1988). *Environmental Aesthetics: Theory, Research and Applications*. Cambridge, MA: University Press.

Nasar, J. L. (1998). *The evaluative image of the city*. London, UK: Sage.

Portella, A. A. (2003). *A Qualidade Visual dos Centros de Comércio e a Legibilidade dos Anúncios Comerciais* [Visual quality of commercial city centres and legibility of commercial signs] (Unpublished dissertation). Federal University of Rio Grande do Sul, Porto Alegre, Brazil.

Portella, A. A. (2007). *Evaluating commercial signs in historic streetscapes: The effects of the control of advertising and signage on user's sense of environmental quality* (Unpublished dissertation). Oxford Brookes University, Joint Centre for Urban Design, Oxford, UK.

Prak, N. (1985). *The visual perception of the built environment.* Delft, The Netherlands: Delft University Press.

Quilan, P. T. (1991). Differing approaches to two-dimensional shape recognition. *Psychological Bulletin, 109*(2), 224–241.

Rapport, A. (1977). *Human aspects of urban form: Towards a man-environment approach to urban form and design.* New York, NY: Pergamon Press.

Reis, A. T. da. L. (2002). *Repertorio, Analise e Sintese: uma Introducao ao Projeto Arquitetonico* [Repertory, analysis and synthesis: An introduction to the architectural design]. Porto Alegre, Brazil: UFRGS.

Salingaros, N. A. (2000). Complexity and urban coherence. *Journal of Urban Design, 5*(3), 291–316.

Smith, P. F. (1980). Urban aesthetics. In B. Mikellides (Ed.), *Architecture for people: Explorations in a new humane environment* (pp.74–85). London, UK: Studio Vista.

Scenic America. (1993). Aesthetics and commercial districts. *Technical Information Series, 1*(6), Washington, DC: Scenic America.

Scenic America. (2000). Scenic beauty benefits business: Design guidelines for business and historic districts. In *Facts for action.* Washington, DC: Scenic America.

Sommer, R., & Sommer, B. (2002). *A practical guide to behavioral research* (5th ed.). Oxford, UK: Oxford University Press.

Stamps, A.E. (1993). Simulation effects on environmental preferences. *Journal of Environmental Management, 38*(2), 693–707.

Stamps, A. E. (2000). *Psychology and the aesthetics of the built environment.* San Francisco, CA: Kluwe Academic.

Stamps, A. E. (2004). Entropy and visual diversity in the environment. *Journal of Architectural and Planning Research, 21*(3), 239–256.

Venturi, R. (1977). *Complexity and contradiction in architecture.* London, UK: Architectural Press.

Von Meiss, P. (1993). *Elements of architecture – from form to place.* London, UK: E & FN Spon.

Weber, R. (1995). *On the aesthetic of architecture, a psychological approach to the structure and the order of perceived architectural space.* San Francisco, CA: Ashgate.

Widmar, R. (1984). Preferences for multiple-family housing: Some implications for public participation. *Journal of Architectural and Planning Research, 1*, 245–260.

Williams, R. (1994). *The non-designer's design book: Design and typographic principles for the visual novice.* Berkeley, CA: Peachpit Press.

# Global Environment Challenges

# The Local Impact of Encountering Global Environmental Problems

## Rural Residents' Appraisal of Changes as to the Better or the Worse

Eja Pedersen and Maria Johansson

Environmental Psychology, Department of Architecture and Built Environment, Lund University, Sweden

**Abstract**

It is important to ensure that changes made to counteract global environmental problems do not undermine local sustainability by causing stress amongst local residents that could reduce well-being and affect health. Rural residents' appraisals of local environmental changes, for example, through the construction of renewable energy plants and infrastructure for more sustainable travel, were analysed in three empirical studies in Sweden and the Netherlands. Residents' appraisals were affected by their perceptions of the physical environment (whether or not this was conducive for economic growth and closeness to nature), the social climate (providing opportunities for participation or not being receptive), together with individual resources (sensitivity to environmental stressors, reduced well-being, and coping strategies). It is proposed that rural residents' opportunities for restoration and place attachment are particularly vulnerable to local changes. Planners must employ participatory approaches and treat local views seriously in order to advance local sustainability and not interfere with rural residents' need for a healthy environment.

**Key words:** cognitive stress theory, environmental changes, place attachment, restorative environments, rural areas

## Introduction

One of the most important ways to achieve a sustainable society is to reduce human emissions of carbon dioxide to the atmosphere. Various initiatives to this end, such as the construction of wind turbines and biogas plants, more frequent freight trains, and the creation of bike lanes to reduce road traffic, though not fundamental, may change the local living environment and residential conditions. Reactions could expectedly be greater amongst residents of non-urban environments where such changes are more visually and aurally prominent than they are in urban or industrial areas (Devine-Wright & Howe, 2010). Moreover, people choosing to live in non-urban environments may value certain local environmental qualities, such as natural beauty and tranquillity, which are important for restorative experiences (Herzog, Maguire, & Nebel, 2003; Laumann, Gärling, & Stormark, 2001; van den Berg, Koole, & van der Wulp, 2003). Given these findings, it could be argued that perceptions of local environmental changes should be studied separately for urban and rural settings (Sell & Zube, 1986). From a sustainability perspective, it is important to ensure that changes made to counter global environmental problems do not cause adverse stress reactions amongst local residents, as this could reduce well-being and negatively affect health. A change in the environment becomes a stressor if a person's appraisal of the proposed or implemented change leads to reactions that are unfavourable to the individual (Kudielka & Kirschbaum, 2001). It may also be the case that minor environmental changes that in comparison appear to be relatively mild stressors, could be negative, if repeated or if combined with the presence of other stressors (Folkow, 1987).

The strength of the psychological and physiological effects is largely determined by situational and individual factors (Cox, 1988). A broader understanding of what determines an individual's appraisal of a local environmental change, can contribute to improved management leading to less distress amongst local residents. This paper addresses local residents' perceptions specifically related to the impact of environmental changes that occurred in a rural and semi-rural area in Sweden and the Netherlands. The areas investigated in the two countries are dominated by agricultural land and small towns and although some people earn their living locally, a large proportion commutes to work in nearby cities.

Individual reactions to a proposed change, or evaluations of a change that has already occurred, can be understood in light of Lazarus and Folkman's (1984) cognitive stress theory. According to this theory, an individual who experiences a change initially assesses what the change means (appraisal). Depending on whether the change is considered trivial, intimidating, or even harmful, the individual considers whether its effects must be mitigated and, if so, whether he or she has the resources to do so and what it would cost (reappraisal). This is an ongoing process influenced by internal and external factors. Devine-Wright (2009) proposed a theoretical framework in which *knowledge* of a planned environmental change leads to an appraisal process where the individual *interprets* and

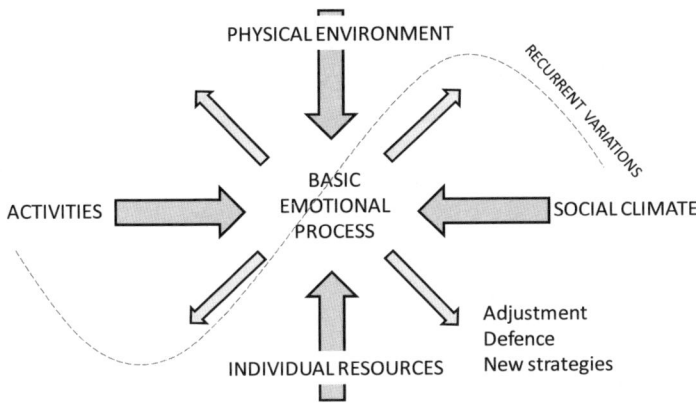

PHYSICAL ENVIRONMENT

RECURRENT VARIATIONS

ACTIVITIES

BASIC
EMOTIONAL
PROCESS

SOCIAL CLIMATE

INDIVIDUAL RESOURCES

Adjustment
Defence
New strategies

**Figure 1.** The Human-Environment Interaction (HEI) model. (Based on Küller, 1991)

*evaluates* the significance of the change. The outcome of the process will depend on whether the change is perceived as threatening the individual's pre-existing emotional attachment to the place and his or her place-related identity processes.

The Human-Environment Interaction (HEI) model posits a similar appraisal process accounting for awareness/activation (comparable to *knowledge*), orientation (comparable to *interpretation*), evaluation (comparable to *evaluation*), and control (Küller, 1991). This notion is central to all HEI, short-term and long-term, and should thus be applicable not only to individual expectations but also to reactions to an actual change in the local environment. The outcome of this emotional process in a given situation is thought to be governed by the individual's perception of the *physical environment* and *social climate*, in light of the *person's individual resources* and of the *activity* that takes place, in this case, living in the countryside (Figure 1). A model of the process extending from the experience of the change to the perception of it should therefore also explicitly take into account these factors. The overarching aim of this paper is to contribute to a wider understanding of the factors that may contribute to an individual's appraisal of a local environmental change. The more specific objective is to analyse the following three factors that may influence local residents' appraisals of recent changes (positive or negative) in rural and semi-rural areas:

- environmental, that is, perception of values and qualities in the local environment;
- social, that is, perception of local authorities' openness for dialogue;
- individual, that is, socio-demographics, sensitivity to environmental stressors, well-being, and coping strategies.

**Table 1.** Characteristics of respondents in the three datasets and the frequencies of respondents perceiving changes for the better and for the worse

|                             | Study A | Study B | Study C         |
| --------------------------- | ------- | ------- | --------------- |
|                             | Sweden  | Sweden  | The Netherlands |
| Year                        | 2000    | 2005    | 2007            |
| Response rate               | 68%     | 58%     | 37%             |
| n                           | 351     | 750     | 725             |
| Mean age, years             | 48      | 51      | 54              |
| Gender, % male/female       | 42/58   | 44/56   | 51/49           |
| Mean residence time, years  | 15      | 15      | 18              |
| Changes for the better      | 24%     | 21%     | 23%             |
| Changes for the worse       | 40%     | 26%     | 35%             |

## Method

Data from three empirical studies conducted in Sweden in 2000 (Study A) and 2005 (Study B) and in the Netherlands in 2007 (Study C) were used for the analyses. In the three studies, questionnaires entitled "Living in the Countryside" were sent to residents of rural and semi-rural areas, resulting in response rates of 68%, 58%, and 37%, respectively (Table 1). The studies were originally initiated to measure the response to wind turbine noise. However, the studies were designed as general studies on perception of living conditions in the countryside. This was partly to mask the focus on wind turbines, in addition to gaining a general picture of how changes in a rural environment influence individual residents. Results concerning the response to wind turbine noise have previously been published elsewhere (Pedersen & Persson Waye, 2004, 2007; Pedersen, van den Berg, Bakker, & Bouma, 2009), but results from the more general part have not been systematically analysed before. This is a longitudinal study spanning 7 years, over different rural and semi-rural location in two countries. Three independent locations were selected for analysis in this article. The results of these analyses are also presented separately, although they are organised thematically. The findings are then jointly depicted in a conceptual model and the results discussed.

The main part of the questionnaire was the same in all three studies. The questionnaire was originally written in Swedish and translated into Dutch for the study in the Netherlands. The research focus has changed somewhat over the years and some supplementary questions were added as described below. In all three studies, the questionnaires opened with the same two questions: "Have there been any changes for the better in your living environment in recent years?" and "Have there been any changes for the worse in your living environment in recent years?" (response alternatives were: "no/yes: if 'yes,' what changes?"). In the analyses, these variables were used as dependent outcome variables.

Perceptions of the *physical environment* were measured in Study A by an item focussing on the main reasons for choosing to live in the surveyed area followed by five response alternatives:

- closeness to the sea,
- closeness to nature,
- appreciate the peace and tranquillity,
- my or my partner's job,
- closeness to relatives or friends.

In Studies B and C, valued qualities in the current living environment were measured by three items:

- I live in a place where I can restore myself and regain energy.
- My area is suitable for economic development.
- I feel a sense of community with people living in this area.

Perceptions of the *social climate* were measured in Study A via the question *"How do you rate your community as regards the following?"* followed by four response alternatives:

- transparency/information on municipal issues,
- opportunities to influence municipal issues,
- opportunities to make contact with officials,
- office hours/telephone access hours.

Confirmatory factor analyses showed that one factor could account for 68% of the variance (Cronbach's $\alpha = .84$) with factor loadings of $.79–.84$. A median value of the four items was calculated for each respondent (Svensson, 2001), measuring the perception of whether the *social climate* provides opportunities for participation. The receptiveness of the *social climate* was also measured in Study A by the question "Would you consider making a complaint to the municipality to have a disturbance remedied?" with the response alternatives: "yes," "no, it would be no use," "no, it would be better to talk with the person causing the disturbance," and "do not know."

In all three studies, *individual resources* were measured as sensitivity to environmental stressors (i.e., air pollution, noise, and odour). A sensitivity score was calculated as the median value of these three items; all values of Cronbach's $\alpha = .85$ and 77%–78% of the items' variances captured. In all three studies, the frequencies of possible reduced well-being were measured using four-point scales ranging from $1 =$ "never or almost never" to $4 =$ "daily or almost daily" for the following four items:

- headache,
- undue tiredness,

- being tense or stressed,
- being easily irritated.

The four variables formed one factor that explained 66% of the variance in the variables in Study A (Cronbach's $\alpha = .82$), 57% in Study B (Cronbach's $\alpha = .75$), and 56% in Study C (Cronbach's $\alpha = .73$); a median of the four variables was calculated for each respondent. In Study B, coping strategies were measured by the question "How do you react in general when confronted with a problem or a difficult situation?" Two coping styles were identified using explorative principal component analyses with orthogonal rotation (varimax). The Kaiser-Meyer-Olkin (KMO) measure verified the adequacy of the sampling for the analysis (i.e., KMO = .64), and Barlett's test of sphericity indicated that correlations between items were sufficiently large (i.e., $\chi^2(15) = 751.7$, $p < .001$). The existence of an active coping strategy (Cronbach's $\alpha = .69$) was measured by three items (here presented with rotated factor loadings): "I act in a targeted way to solve the problem" (.79), "The first thing I do is analyse the problem" (.79), and "I find several options for solutions to the problem" (.76). The existence of a passive coping strategy (Cronbach's $\alpha = .65$) was also measured by three items (here presented with rotated factor loadings): "I occupy myself to distract myself from my thoughts" (.82), "I try to think of other things" (.82), and "I assume that the problems will disappear by themselves" (.64). Median scores were calculated as described above.

In the case of perceived environmental changes for both the better and worse, the analyses were conducted separately for each study. Variables of interest for this study, as presented above, together with gender and age, were tested using binary logistic regression as predictors of whether a resident would report recent changes in the area as being for the better ("no/yes"). The variables were simultaneously entered into the regression and a forward conditional approach was used to find the best model, for as many independent variables as possible, having a significant impact on the dependent variable. The procedure was repeated for changes for the worse. The results are presented as odds ratios (ORs), which indicate the change in odds resulting from a unit change in the predictor. Two values of $R^2$ (i.e., Cox and Snell's and Nagelkerke's) describe the variance of the dependent variable explained. Hosmer and Lemeshow's $\chi^2$ test is a test of differences between data and the model, and the $p$-values for this test should therefore be >.05 (no significant difference).

## Results

Changes for the better were reported by 21–24% of the respondents (Table 1). Many of the respondents reported several such changes, the most common of which were improvements such as bike lanes, green areas, playgrounds, and schools (stated in 52%, 34%, and 46% of the comments included in this category for studies A, B, and C, respectively). Improvements to infrastructure for public transport, broadband provision, sewage handling, and road traffic (both better roads and slowed traffic were mentioned) were also perceived as positive (stated by 26%, 43%, and 22% of the comments in this category). Respondents also reported personal changes (stated by 6%, 25%, and 23% of the comments in this category) such as improvements they had made in their dwellings. In Study B, the average residential time of those who reported changes for the better was 12 years versus 17 years for those *not* reporting changes for the better ($F = 5.2, p < .001$); no such differences were found in Study A or C.

Changes for the worse were reported by 26%–40% of the respondents (Table 1); the specified changes in the area included cuts in public services, thefts, fewer shops, and reduced outdoor lighting (mentioned in 27%, 45%, and 31% of the comments included in this category for Studies A, B, and C, respectively). The respondents also stated changes connected with industrialisation, including construction of wind turbines, industrial facilities, and biogas plants (mentioned in 44%, 19%, and 34% of the comments in this category) as well as busier infrastructure, mainly caused by road traffic (mentioned in 24%, 25%, and 28% of the comments in this category). Only a few respondents reported personal changes for the worse (mentioned in 3%, 9%, and 7% of the comments in this category). No associations were found between residential time and the likelihood of reporting changes for the worse.

Changes for the better were, as seen in Table 2, predicted by perceiving the physical environment as conducive for economic growth (Studies B and C) and included restorative values (Studies B and C). Residents were also more likely to report changes for the better if they experienced their social environment as providing opportunities for participation, even in the sense that complaining to the municipality about a nuisance was seen as a viable alternative (Study A). Changes for the better were more often reported by younger than older residents (Studies A and B). Individuals with passive coping strategies were less likely to report changes for the better than those with other coping strategies (Study B).

Changes for the worse were associated with perceiving the physical environment as *not* conducive for economic growth (Study C) and with greatly valuing closeness to nature (Study A). The likelihood of reporting changes for the worse increased if the social environment was such that complaining about a nuisance was perceived as useless (Study A). In addition, respondents who claimed they would complain were more likely to perceive changes for the worse. Individual factors that predicted reports of changes for the worse were sensitivity to environmental stressors (Studies A and C) and impaired well-being (Study C). People with passive coping strategies were also less likely to report changes for the worse, just as they were less likely to report changes for the better (Study B).

## Discussion

The present study suggests that the consequences of large-scale environmental changes also generate local changes that could be appraised as improving or degrading

**Table 2.** Models predicting perceived changes in the living environment tested with binary logistic regression using a forward conditional approach

| | OR[a] (95% CI)[b] | p |
|---|---|---|
| **Study A** | | |
| Model A1 – Changes for the better. $R^2$ = .06–.09, H-L $\chi^2(8)$ = 11.9, $p$ = .155 | | |
| Perceived participation opportunities (from bad to good) | 1.51 (1.06–2.16) | < .05 |
| Yes, I would complain to the municipality (do not agree/agree) | 1.87 (1.09–3.18) | < .05 |
| Age (from young to old) | 0.97 (0.95–0.99) | < .01 |
| Model A2 – Changes for the worse. $R^2$ = .14–.17. H-L $\chi^2(8)$ = 2.8, $p$ = .149 | | |
| Closeness to nature (from low to high) | 2.02 (1.23–3.33) | < .01 |
| Yes, I would complain to the municipality (do not agree/agree) | 3.12 (1.77–5.51) | < .001 |
| No use complaining to the municipality (do not agree/agree) | 4.55 (2.24–9.23) | < .001 |
| Sensitivity (from not sensitive to very sensitive) | 1.55 (1.16–2.08) | < .01 |
| **Study B** | | |
| Model B1 – Changes for the better. $R^2$ = .04–.07. H-L $\chi^2(8)$ = 8.5, $p$ = .391 | | |
| Restorative values (from low to high) | 1.72 (1.25–2.38) | < .001 |
| Economic growth (from low to high) | 1.23 (1.03–1.46) | < .05 |
| Age | 0.99 (0.97–0.99) | < .05 |
| Passive coping (from low to high) | 0.83 (0.69–0.99) | < .05 |
| Model B2 – Changes for the worse. $R^2$ = .01–.02. H-L $\chi^2(3)$ = 2.6, $p$ = .451 | | |
| Passive coping (from low to high) | 0.83 (0.70–0.98) | < .05 |
| **Study C** | | |
| Model C1 – Changes for the better. $R^2$ = .02–.04. H-L $\chi^2(7)$ = 12.3, $p$ = .090 | | |
| Restorative values (from low to high) | 1.45 (1.12–1.87) | < .05 |
| Economic growth (from low to high) | 1.21 (1.02–1.43) | < .05 |
| Model C2 – Changes for the worse. $R^2$ = .05–.07. H-L $\chi^2(8)$ = 8.9, $p$ = .355 | | |
| Economic growth (from low to high) | 0.83 (0.72–0.97) | < .05 |
| Sensitivity (from low to high) | 1.21 (1.04–1.41) | < .05 |
| Impaired well-being (from seldom to often) | 1.46 (1.18–1.81) | < .01 |

*Notes.* [a]OR = odds ratio. OR < 1 indicates that the independent variable reduces the likelihood of the dependent variable. OR > 1 indicates that the independent variable increases the likelihood of the dependent variable. [b]95% confidence intervals.

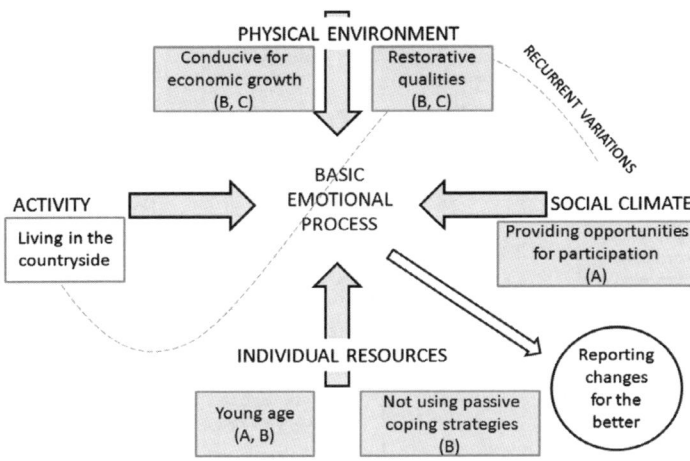

**Figure 2.** Conceptual model of variables influencing the basic emotional process that leads to reports of changes for the better, based on results from separate analyses of data from three empirical studies (A, B, and C).

the residential environment potentially influencing the local population's well-being and health. The appraisal of changes, either for the better or worse, seems partly determined by various factors linked to individual psychological resources and perceptions of the physical and social environment.

Passive coping strategies led to not reporting any changes, for either the better or worse. The chances of reporting changes for the better or worse were predicted by different factors. However, reviewing these factors (Figures 2 and 3) reveals that they can be traced to the need for personal restoration in association with the living environment. Residents who reported changes for the better experienced the local environment as having restorative qualities, even after the changes. They also felt that the area was conducive for economic growth, indicating that the environment was perceived as able to tolerate the changes that had taken place while retaining, and perhaps even augmenting, its original beneficial qualities. Perceiving the social environment as facilitating those who want to participate in societal concerns and thus be able to influence the changes taking place also increased the likelihood of perceiving changes for the better, meaning that changes would not be seen as uncontrollable threats. No differences were found between men and women in this regard, though younger people tended to report more changes for the better than did older people. This could be because younger people assigned a higher value to certain reported changes that benefitted their families, such as playgrounds and bike lanes.

The connection with the need for personal restoration, or rather reduced opportunities for personal restoration, is even clearer in the case of changes for the worse. Residents who felt that closeness to nature was an essential quality of their living environment,

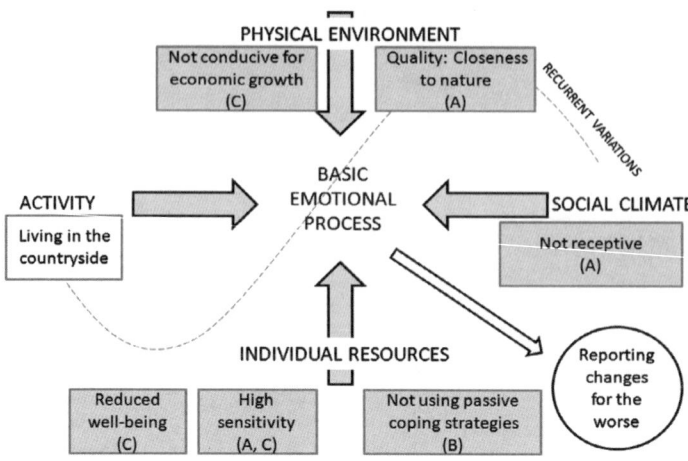

**Figure 3.** Conceptual model of variables influencing the basic emotional process that leads to reports of changes for the worse, based on results from separate analyses of data from three empirical studies (A, B, and C).

but who did not perceive their environment as conducive for economic growth, were more likely to report changes for the worse. Given that they were more sensitive to environmental stressors and reported lower well-being than others, and thus had a greater need for restorative peace and quiet, one can assume that they perceived the changes as reducing the potential to recover from stress. Perceiving the social climate as unreceptive to efforts to moderate the effects of these changes increased the risk of reporting changes for the worse. Most changes for the worse reported in this study would likely increase the exposure to "daily hassle" stressors, rather than to stressors having a major impact on people's lives. Kanner, Coyne, Schaefer, and Lazarus (1981) defined daily hassles as irritating, frustrating, and distressing demands originating from everyday transactions with the environment, including interaction with family members, work overload and underload, and exposure to environmental stressors such as noise and air pollution. A change in itself does not induce stress; it is only if the change involves a perceived loss of any kind that stress occurs (Hobfoll, 1989) – in this case, a loss of restorative qualities. However, the results could also be viewed as indicating a different type of loss, caused by disruption of the individual's pre-existing emotional attachments to the place and his or her place-related identity processes, leading to the appraisal of a change as for the worse (Devine-Wright, 2009).

In our study, several parallel but interrelated appraisal processes, for example, disrupted place attachment and reduced personal restoration opportunities, might have resulted in the appraisal of changes for the worse. The concepts of place identity and the restorative environment may be linked (Korpela & Hartig, 1996). Emotional and self-regulation processes are assumed to underlie the development of place identity, and environments perceived as supporting personal restoration (usually places with natural features) are used in such processes. However, the two processes may be differently weighted by different groups of residents, leading to different responses. People who have lived for a prolonged period in one place are usually strongly attached to the location (Hay, 1998; Knez, 2005), often via ties that emerge from childhood place experiences (Morgan, 2010), and may therefore perceive any change as disrupted place attachment. People who have moved to the countryside for its particular qualities may primarily perceive change in the environment as threatening suggesting that the restorative nature aspect of place attachment does not seem to depend on length of residence (Raymond, Brown, & Weber, 2010; Scannell & Gifford, 2010; Stedman, 2002). Soini, Vaarala, and Pouta (2012) identify two groups with a differing sense of place. One group are short and medium term residents "committed to the place" with strong emotional but weak social ties who value its natural landscape features. Alternatively, long-term residents with "roots and resources" who have low appreciation of the areas' natural features and a high acceptance of landscape change. In the present study, the residents' responses also depended on their perceptions of the social climate, which may relate to the social aspect of place attachment. Previous studies demonstrate that positive experiences of participation in the process preceding a local environmental change (Pedersen & Johansson, 2012) and trust in regulatory authorities (Johansson, Karlsson, Pedersen, & Flykt, 2012) broaden the available coping alternatives, making the changes less threatening.

Although the conceptual models employed in this research should be interpreted with caution, as the datasets used for the analyses are not completely congruent and the data was carried out over a lengthy period of time. The conceptual models presented in this paper were based on an established, reliable HEI model. The models were also based on three significant sample sizes with reasonable response rates. The contribution of the present approach therefore has a strong ecological validity, concerning "real world" changes relevant to the individual participants rather than a predefined single change. The conceptual models presented should be regarded as an attempt to bring forward the discussion on how changes in the local environment are perceived by the individual at a more general level.

The variation in perception of change explained by the predictors was as expected low, with the main predictors of magnitude and proximity of the change evident. However, the statistical significance of the influence was high in several cases, which indicates the relevance of the factors that were studied.

A single study including different modes of change, as well as validated measurements of social, environmental, and individual influencing factors would be preferable, but has to our knowledge not yet been carried out. Future research should contribute to a better overall understanding of the perception of changes and further development of a useful theoretical framework by integrating place attachment and restoration theory. Validated established measurements from both these theoretical areas should be used in joint studies. It would be interesting to further clarify how rural populations consist of various groups with different expectations and needs.

## Implications

This research highlights the ongoing need to establish a link between those who live with real-world consequences of environmental design changes and those who are tasked with their design and implementation. In order to ensure that changes made to encounter global environmental problems do not interfere with rural residents' need for a healthy environment, designers and planners must understand the antecedents of human responses to environmental changes (Sell & Zube, 1986). Global and local threats must therefore be jointly considered in planning for such changes. Local residents should feel that they are paid attention to and involved, and those who are unlikely to speak up should not be ignored (Waldo, Ek, Johansson, & Persson, 2013). Planners must provide participation opportunities and treat local views seriously to ensure that the changes made will advance local sustainability. Qualities unique to a given area and valued by the residents as important to their needs and ties to the environment must be retained.

## References

Cox, T. (1988). Psychobiological factors in stress and health. In S. Fisher & J. Reason (Eds.), *Handbook of life stress, cognition and health* (pp. 603–627). New York, NY: Wiley.

Devine-Wright, P. (2009). Rethinking NIMBYism. *Journal of Community & Applied Social Psychology, 19*, 426–441.

Devine-Wright, P., & Howe, Y. (2010). Disruption to place attachment and the protection of restorative environments: A wind energy case. *Journal of Environmental Psychology, 30*, 271–280.

Folkow, B. (1987). Stress, hypothalamic function and neuroendocrine consequences. *Acta Medica Scandinavica, 723*, 61–69.

Hay, R. (1998). Sense of place in developmental context. *Journal of Environmental Psychology, 18*, 5–29.

Herzog, T. R., Maguire, C. P., & Nebel, M. B. (2003). Assessing the restorative components of environments. *Journal of Environmental Psychology, 23*, 159–170.

Hobfoll, S. E. (1989). Conservation of resources: A new attempt at conceptualizing stress. *American Psychologist, 44*(3), 513–524.

Johansson, M., Karlsson, J., Pedersen, E., & Flykt, A. (2012). Factors governing human fear of brown bear and wolf. *Human Dimensions of Wildlife, 17*(1), 58–74.

Kanner, A. D., Coyne, J. C., Schaefer, C., & Lazarus, R. S. (1981). Comparisons of two modes of stress measurement: Daily hassles and uplifts versus major life events. *Journal of Behavioral Medicine, 4*(1), 1–39.

Knez, I. (2005). Attachment and identity as related to a place and its perceived climate. *Journal of Environmental Psychology, 25*, 207–218.

Korpela, K., & Hartig, T. (1996). Restorative qualities of favorite places. *Journal of Environmental Psychology, 16*, 221–233.

Kudielka, B.M., & Kirschbaum, C. (2001). Stress and health research. In N. J. Smelser & P. B. Baltes (Eds.), *The international encyclopedia of the social and behavioral sciences* (Vol. 22, pp. 15170–15175). Oxford, UK: Elsevier.

Küller, R. (1991). Environmental assessment from a neuropsychological perspective. In T. Gärling & G.W. Evans (Eds.), *Environment, cognition, and action* (pp. 78–95). New York, NY: Oxford University Press.

Laumann, K., Gärling, T., & Stormark, K. M. (2001). Rating scale measures of restorative components of environments. *Journal of Environmental Psychology, 21*, 31–44.

Lazarus, R. S., & Folkman, S. (1984). *Stress, appraisal, and coping.* New York, NY: Springer.

Morgan, P. (2010). Towards a developmental theory of place attachment. *Journal of Environmental Psychology, 30*, 11–22.

Pedersen, E., & Johansson, M. (2012). Wind power or uranium mine: Appraisal of two energy-related environmental changes in a local context. *Energy Policy, 44*, 312–319.

Pedersen, E., & Persson Waye, K. (2004). Perception and annoyance due to wind turbine noise: A dose-response relationship. *Journal of the Acoustical Society of America, 116*(6), 3460–3470.

Pedersen, E., & Persson Waye, K. (2007). Wind turbine noise, annoyance and self-reported health and well-being in different living environments. *Occupational and Environmental Medicine, 64*, 480–486.

Pedersen, E., van den Berg, F., Bakker, R., & Bouma, J. (2009). Response to noise from modern wind farms in the Netherlands. *Journal of the Acoustical Society of America, 126*(2), 634–643.

Raymond, C. M., Brown, G., & Weber, D. (2010). The measure of place attachment: Personal, community, and environmental connections. *Journal of Environmental Psychology, 30*, 422–434.

Scannell, L., & Gifford, R. (2010). The relations between natural and civic place attachment and pro-environmental behavior. *Journal of Environmental Psychology, 30*, 289–297.

Sell, J. L., & Zube, E. H. (1986). Perception of and response to environmental change. *Journal of Architecture and Planning Research, 1986*(3), 33–54.

Soini, K., Vaarala, H., & Pouta, E. (2012). Residents' sense of place and landscape perceptions at the rural-urban interface. *Landscape and Urban Planning, 104*, 124–134.

Stedman, R. C. (2002). Toward a social psychology of place: Predicting behavior from place-based cognitions, attitude, and identity. *Environment and Behavior, 34*, 561–581.

Svensson, E. (2001). Construction of a single global scale for multi-item assessments of the same variable. *Statistics in Medicine, 20*, 3831–3846.

van den Berg, A. E., Koole, S. L., & van der Wulp, N. Y. (2003). Environmental preference and restoration: (How) are they related? *Journal of Environmental Psychology, 23*, 135–146.

Waldo, Å., Ek, K., Johansson, M., & Persson, L. (2013). *Vindkraft i öppet landskap, skog, fjäll och hav. Lokala förutsättningar för förankring* [Wind power in open landscape, forest, mountain and sea] (Report 6540, Final report to Vindval). Stockholm, Sweden: Naturvårdsverket.

# Newspaper Coverage of Water Restrictions in Melbourne, Australia, in Relation to Climate Change Adaptation From 2006 to 2010

Simon Chun Kwan Chui

Faculty of Architecture Building and Planning, University of Melbourne, Victoria, Australia

## Abstract

From 1997 to mid-2010, Melbourne, Australia, experienced a prolonged drought, threatening the city's water supply, with conditions similar to those predicted in climate change modelling. In response to the drought, water restrictions were enacted, limiting the use of water outdoors, including watering household gardens, resulting in a negative impact on the vegetation of suburban landscapes. This paper presents the findings from a content analysis of articles from Melbourne newspapers, identifying changes in the way the topics of climate change and drought adaptation were discussed within the public discourse at the time. The study found that, between 2007 and 2010, expressions of uncertainty and scepticism towards climate change had increased over time in some Melbourne newspapers; this is consistent with the politicisation of the topic and the transition from a scientific debate into a political debate. The study also found that the acceptance of the responsibility of households to adapt to the immediate drought was generally high, despite any differences of opinion there may be about the role of climate change in relation to the severity of the drought.

**Key words:** climate change, content analysis, drought adaptation, newspapers, water conservation

## Introduction

From 1997 to 2010, there was reduced rainfall and inflows into the water supply reservoirs of Melbourne, Australia (Melbourne Water Corporation, 2010). Long periods of above average temperatures resulted in dry soils, with subsequent precipitation soaking into the parched soil reducing runoff. Projected climate change with increases in average temperatures in the coming decades will likely lead to a long-term reduction in water availability with increasing frequency and intensity of droughts in Australia (Cai & Cowan, 2008), an issue identified in the Intergovernmental Panel on Climate Change (IPCC) *Fourth Assessment Report* (Solomon et al., 2007). During the 1997–2010 drought (hereafter referred to as "the recent drought"), increasingly severe water restriction rules were enforced to reduce water consumption. These restrictions limited the use of mains water for outdoor recreational and ornamental purposes.

The water restrictions in Melbourne reached a peak in severity in 2007 along with the severe El Niño drought event of that year, before easing somewhat in 2010 after the weather transitioned into wetter La Niña conditions in Australia (Melbourne Water Corporation, 2011). The El Niño Southern Oscillation causes reductions in rainfall in much of Australia, approximately every 2–7 years, lasting 1 or 2 years each time. However the period from 1997 to 2010 was unusual for its long term low rainfall, independent from El Niño events. At the time of writing this paper in late 2012, water storage facilities in Melbourne were still recovering, helped by the wetter conditions as well as improvements to the water supply infrastructure made during the drought.

Although the recent drought was one of the most severe recorded in Australian history, significant increases in scientific and political awareness of global climate change around the same time added to the local impact and significance of the drought. The year 2006 saw the release of the documentary film *An Inconvenient Truth*, directed by David Guggenheim and starring former Vice President of the United States, Al Gore (IMDb.com Inc., 2012). The documentary conveyed to the lay audience the key points of climate change science and delivered the message that action on climate change is not only necessary, but a moral obligation to protect our planet. Then, in 2007, the IPCC released its *Fourth Assessment Report*, further confirming and elaborating on the scientific evidence of anthropogenic climate change, including predictions of longer and more severe droughts in Australia. In that same year, the Nobel Peace Prize was jointly awarded to the IPCC and Al Gore "for their efforts to build up and disseminate greater knowledge about man-made climate change, and to lay the foundations for the measures that are needed to counteract such change" (Nobelprize.org, 2012).

The increase in Australian political awareness became evident during the federal elections of 2007, with the incumbent Prime Minister (John Howard) being successfully attacked by his opponent Kevin Rudd for his negative stance on the effects of climate (Friedman, 2007). This gave Rudd an election winning advantage in the midst of a record-breaking drought particularly with the media focus on the impact of climate change in Australia, in the wake of Al Gore's and the IPCC's work. This confluence of climatic, political, scientific, and cultural events combined to catapult climate change from a fringe issue into the forefront of Australian consciousness, with the drought being an integral part of this climate change discussion.

This paper looks at the discussion of the drought in Melbourne newspapers in relation to household outdoor water use. The combination of water restrictions and high summer temperatures caused damage to the vegetation in Melbourne, impacting negatively on the suburban landscape. The water restriction rules stipulated such water-saving measures as banning the watering of lawns, banning the use of sprinkler systems, and specific times and days when households may water their gardens with mains water. However, other responses to the drought were also available, for example the replacement of damaged plants with drought-tolerant alternatives or the redesigning of landscapes to improve moisture retention and reduce evaporation, or the use of rainwater or household grey water to substitute for mains water. These measures were encouraged by the state government and water suppliers at the time (savewater!, 2009). To the extent that these actions would reduce the negative impacts of future droughts, they may be considered a form of climate change adaptation where the need for mains water use in the private suburban landscape is reduced or eliminated, while maintaining or improving the function and attractiveness of the ornamental and recreational landscape.

The way in which climate change issues are framed in the media helps contribute towards the potential success of responses, by encouraging or discouraging consumers to take adaptive action to drought and climate change in and around their own homes. The research described in this paper looked at the extent to which newspapers in Melbourne supported drought and climate change adaptation by private households during the recent drought, identifying areas where future responses may be improved.

## Literature Review

Studies of newspaper reporting on climate change outside Australia have shown that temporary increases in the quantities of articles discussing climate change issues are generally associated with key events, most dramatically with extreme weather events (Boykoff, 2007; Boykoff & Mansfield, 2008; McComas & Shanahan, 1999; Ungar, 1992). Boykoff and Mansfield highlighted differences in reporting between different types of newspapers in the United Kingdom, with UK tabloids being more likely to present positions divergent from the scientific consensus on climate change in comparison to the average of all UK newspapers. McComas and Shanahan noted that coverage of climate change in the United States followed identifiable cycles, beginning with a focus on the dangers and consequences of climate change, moving to controversies among scientists, and declining when discussions moved on to the economics of dealing with global warming. Ungar (1992) highlighted the impact of the unusual droughts and heat waves of 1988 in the United States, in causing a dramatic increase in the quantity of climate change discussion in the news media at that time, and subsequent decline of this discussion following an unusually cold winter in 1989.

While no studies were found that looked specifically at newspaper discussions of household outdoor water use during droughts, discussions of climate change as a consequence of the 2007 El Niño drought event were evident. Results were expected to follow a similar cycle in this study, with increasing politicisation of the climate change issue over time. Qualitative analyses of the politicisation on the climate change issue in Australia exist (Bailey, MacGill, Passey, & Compston, 2012), but this study is the first known attempt at quantitative measurement of the public discourse specifically on this issue in Australia during 2007. The increased media attention on climate change issues as a consequence of the drought event may be used to encourage action on climate change, but the subsequent politicisation may become an obstacle. As noted above, 2007 also coincided with the Australian federal elections, as well as the release of the IPCC's *Fourth Assessment Report*, which provided additional impetus to the discussion of climate change in Australian newspapers.

## Methodology

This study analysed articles discussing water restrictions in mainstream Melbourne newspapers, to identify the ways in which the public discourse on water use in the suburban landscape has changed during the recent drought. Four newspapers were used in this study: *The Australian*, *The Age*, the *Herald Sun*, and the *Leader*. *The Australian* has a nation-wide circulation and tended to focus on national political and economic issues; *The Age* and the *Herald Sun* have most of their readership in the state of Victoria, where Melbourne is located, and thus have greater coverage of state-wide issues; while the *Leader* newspapers are a series of local newspapers covering metropolitan Melbourne focusing on community and local news. These newspapers were chosen for their large readerships (News Limited, 2010; Ryan, 2008) and for their reliable and readily accessible archives through the *LexisNexis Academic* database.

All articles from July 2006 to December 2010 containing the term "water restrictions," and variations thereof, were read by the researcher. Each article's position on climate change and drought adaptation was recorded, as well as the presence of discussions about specific water supply and water use topics. Articles that did not discuss water restrictions were discarded from this study. While letters to the editor were aggregated for each day's newspapers in the database, for this study each letter was counted as a separate article. In total, 472 articles were analysed for *The Australian*, 790 for *The Age*, 838 for the *Herald Sun*, and 1568 for the *Leader* newspapers.

The content analysis was completed by the researcher alone and although there were no other raters involved, the analysis was conducted in a rigorous manner; this analysis identified three groups of findings. First: the positions on climate change taken by the newspaper articles, in terms of whether the author presented (1) a position consistent with the scientific consensus on climate change, (2) a position sceptical of climate change, or (3) an expression of uncertainty. Secondly, positions on whether households have a responsibility to adapt to drought with regard to water restrictions are presented either as (1) the acceptance of consumer responsibility to reduce water consumption, (2) the denial of this responsibility, or (3) a conditional acceptance. Thirdly, specific adaptations discussed by the articles will be grouped based on the longevity of their effects. In this group, adaptations that are purely behavioural with no lasting water conservation effects, such as watering gardens at certain times to minimise evaporative losses, are considered short-term adaptations. Adaptations that require periodic renewal or maintenance, such as the use of soil-wetting agents, are considered medium-term adaptations. Adaptations that last indefinitely, for example choosing known drought-tolerant plant species for planting in the garden, are considered long-term adaptations.

# Findings

Table 1 and Figure 1 show the half-yearly totals and percentages for each category of position on climate change, showing how the proportions of articles expressing the scientific view of climate change, the sceptical view, or an uncertain view had changed over time. Articles that did not express any position on climate change (CC) were excluded. *CC science* included those articles that expressed a position that is consistent with the scientific consensus on climate change. *CC sceptic* included those articles that rejected the scientific consensus, and *CC uncertain* included those articles that expressed uncertainty about climate change or which presented both scientific consensus and sceptical positions. The three categories are mutually exclusive.

In *The Australian*, the proportions of articles expressing agreement with the scientific consensus declined somewhat over time, while the proportions of articles expressing an uncertain position increased. In the *Herald Sun*, the proportions of articles expressing agreement with the scientific consensus over time also declined, while the proportions expressing sceptical positions increased. In *The Age* and the *Leader* newspapers, on the other hand, the proportions of articles agreeing with the scientific consensus on climate change remained very high throughout the time period studied. Note that these are the proportions of articles for each position in each half-year period, and not the absolute numbers of articles.

This discrepancy between the newspapers on expressions of climate science and scepticism was similar to the findings by Boykoff and Mansfield for newspapers in the UK. This suggests an editorial decision by each newspaper to interpret events in a way that may differ from the others (Boykoff & Mansfield, 2008), and is a reflection of the politicisation of the climate change issue over time. The expressions of the scientific consensus on climate change were similarly high for all four newspapers in 2006 and early 2007, but proceeded to diverge from there. At that time in Australia, Prime Minister Kevin Rudd followed up on his election victory in 2007 by proposing an Emissions Trading Scheme that would put a price on carbon emissions in Australia and create a market for carbon emissions trading (Anonymous, 2009). Australia has a large coal-mining industry and has historically relied on coal for generating electricity, and Rudd faced significant political opposition to his ultimately unsuccessful Emissions Trading Scheme from the coal industry and others. This political conflict was reflected in the newspaper articles of the time as some authors in *The Australian* and the *Herald Sun* cast doubt and

**Table 1.** Water restrictions articles, position on climate change, half-yearly totals, excluding "no position"

**The Australian**

|  | CC science | | CC sceptic | | CC uncertain | | Totals |
|---|---|---|---|---|---|---|---|
|  | n | % | n | % | n | % | n |
| 2nd Half 2006 | 16 | 80.0% | 1 | 5.0% | 3 | 15.0% | 20 |
| 1st Half 2007 | 20 | 76.9% | 0 | 0.0% | 6 | 23.1% | 26 |
| 2nd Half 2007 | 15 | 93.8% | 1 | 6.3% | 0 | 0.0% | 16 |
| 1st Half 2008 | 14 | 77.8% | 0 | 0.0% | 4 | 22.2% | 18 |
| 2nd Half 2008 | 6 | 85.7% | 0 | 0.0% | 1 | 14.3% | 7 |
| 1st Half 2009 | 2 | 40.0% | 1 | 20.0% | 2 | 40.0% | 5 |
| 2nd Half 2009 | 0 | 0.0% | 0 | 0.0% | 1 | 100.0% | 1 |
| 1st Half 2010 | 3 | 60.0% | 1 | 20.0% | 1 | 20.0% | 5 |
| 2nd Half 2010 | 3 | 75.0% | 0 | 0.0% | 1 | 25.0% | 4 |
| Articles in total | 79 | 77.5% | 4 | 3.9% | 19 | 18.6% | 102 |

**The Age**

|  | CC science | | CC sceptic | | CC uncertain | | Totals |
|---|---|---|---|---|---|---|---|
|  | n | % | n | % | n | % | n |
| 2nd Half 2006 | 26 | 89.7% | 1 | 3.4% | 2 | 6.9% | 29 |
| 1st Half 2007 | 24 | 88.9% | 1 | 3.7% | 2 | 7.4% | 27 |
| 2nd Half 2007 | 11 | 73.3% | 1 | 6.7% | 3 | 20.0% | 15 |
| 1st Half 2008 | 10 | 90.9% | 0 | 0.0% | 1 | 9.1% | 11 |
| 2nd Half 2008 | 21 | 95.5% | 1 | 4.5% | 0 | 0.0% | 22 |
| 1st Half 2009 | 5 | 100.0% | 0 | 0.0% | 0 | 0.0% | 5 |
| 2nd Half 2009 | 10 | 100.0% | 0 | 0.0% | 0 | 0.0% | 10 |
| 1st Half 2010 | 6 | 100.0% | 0 | 0.0% | 0 | 0.0% | 6 |
| 2nd Half 2010 | 8 | 100.0% | 0 | 0.0% | 0 | 0.0% | 8 |
| Articles in total | 121 | 91.0% | 4 | 3.0% | 8 | 6.0% | 133 |

**Herald Sun**

|  | CC science | | CC sceptic | | CC uncertain | | Totals |
|---|---|---|---|---|---|---|---|
|  | n | % | n | % | n | % | n |
| 2nd Half 2006 | 11 | 68.8% | 0 | 0.0% | 5 | 31.3% | 16 |
| 1st Half 2007 | 9 | 69.2% | 0 | 0.0% | 4 | 30.8% | 13 |
| 2nd Half 2007 | 6 | 46.2% | 4 | 30.8% | 3 | 23.1% | 13 |
| 1st Half 2008 | 0 |  | 0 |  | 0 |  | 0 |
| 2nd Half 2008 | 6 | 60.0% | 4 | 40.0% | 0 | 0.0% | 10 |
| 1st Half 2009 | 1 | 100.0% | 0 | 0.0% | 0 | 0.0% | 1 |
| 2nd Half 2009 | 0 | 0.0% | 3 | 100.0% | 0 | 0.0% | 3 |
| 1st Half 2010 | 1 | 16.7% | 5 | 83.3% | 0 | 0.0% | 6 |
| 2nd Half 2010 | 2 | 66.7% | 1 | 33.3% | 0 | 0.0% | 3 |
| Articles in total | 36 | 55.4% | 17 | 26.2% | 12 | 18.5% | 65 |

**Leader**

|  | CC science | | CC sceptic | | CC uncertain | | Totals |
|---|---|---|---|---|---|---|---|
|  | n | % | n | % | n | % | n |
| 2nd Half 2006 | 3 | 100.0% | 0 | 0.0% | 0 | 0.0% | 3 |
| 1st Half 2007 | 3 | 50.0% | 0 | 0.0% | 3 | 50.0% | 6 |
| 2nd Half 2007 | 5 | 100.0% | 0 | 0.0% | 0 | 0.0% | 5 |
| 1st Half 2008 | 4 | 100.0% | 0 | 0.0% | 0 | 0.0% | 4 |
| 2nd Half 2008 | 0 |  | 0 |  | 0 |  | 0 |
| 1st Half 2009 | 2 | 100.0% | 0 | 0.0% | 0 | 0.0% | 2 |
| 2nd Half 2009 | 0 |  | 0 |  | 0 |  | 0 |
| 1st Half 2010 | 5 | 100.0% | 0 | 0.0% | 0 | 0.0% | 5 |
| 2nd Half 2010 | 0 |  | 0 |  | 0 |  | 0 |
| Articles in total | 22 | 88.0% | 0 | 0.0% | 3 | 12.0% | 25 |

*Notes.* "CC science" denotes the expression of a position consistent with the scientific consensus on climate change. "CC sceptic" denotes a position sceptical of climate change. "CC uncertain" denotes an uncertain position, or both sides presented.

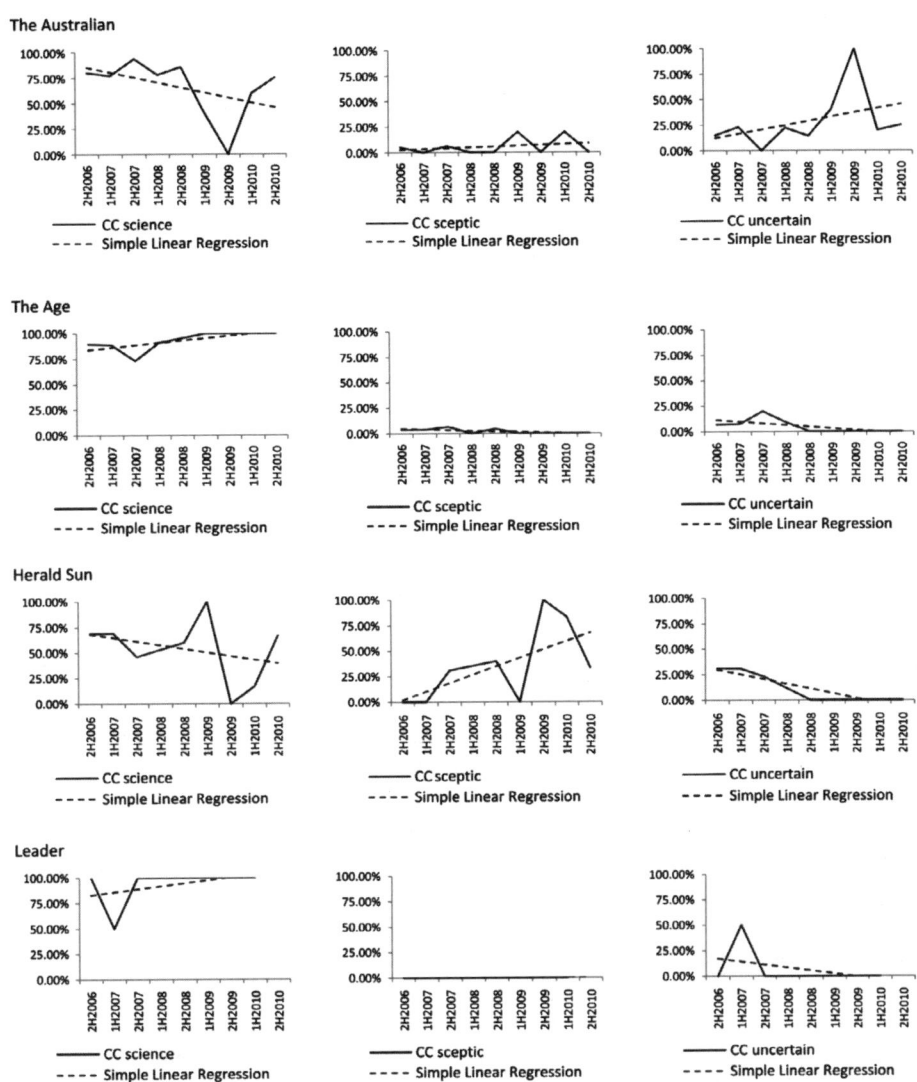

**Figure 1.** Water restrictions articles, position on climate change, half-yearly totals, excluding "no position."

*Notes.* "CC science" denotes the expression of a position consistent with the scientific consensus on climate change. "CC sceptic" denotes a position sceptical of climate change. "CC uncertain" denotes an uncertain position, or both sides presented.

**Table 2.** Water restrictions articles, consumer responsibility for adaptation, totals, excluding "no position"

| | The Australian | | The Age | | Herald Sun | | Leader | |
|---|---|---|---|---|---|---|---|---|
| | *n* | % | *n* | % | *n* | % | *n* | % |
| R accept | 63 | 33.16% | 202 | 55.96% | 301 | 61.30% | 560 | 81.04% |
| R deny | 49 | 25.79% | 32 | 8.86% | 66 | 13.44% | 20 | 2.89% |
| R compromise | 78 | 41.05% | 127 | 35.18% | 124 | 25.25% | 111 | 16.06% |
| Totals | 190 | 100.00% | 361 | 100.00% | 491 | 100.00% | 691 | 100.00% |

*Notes.* "R accept" denotes the opinion that consumers have responsibility to adapt to drought. "R deny" denotes consumers have no responsibility to adapt. "R compromise" denotes consumers having a conditional responsibility.

uncertainty onto climate science discussions in attempts to weaken the rationale for the Emissions Trading Scheme. On the other hand, authors in *The Age* tended to support action on climate change. The *Leader* newspapers tended to avoid the political debate altogether as the debate largely revolved around national economic policy, outside the scope of the community newspapers.

Table 2 shows the totals and percentages for each position on the consumers' responsibility for adaptation to drought for each newspaper, excluding all articles that did not express any position on consumer responsibility. *R accept* included those articles that expressed the position that consumers have a responsibility to adapt to drought, *R deny* included those articles that denied this responsibility, and *R compromise* included those articles that conditionally accepted responsibility for consumers to adapt to drought. This conditional acceptance was usually expressed as a desire for certain exemptions from the water restrictions or as the position that other groups of water users should make greater efforts to reduce their water usage before consumers should be required to take action. These categories are mutually exclusive. It is important to note that "adaptation" in this context refers to drought adaptation, not necessarily climate change adaptation, and that one can adapt to drought while simultaneously rejecting the position that climate change exists or that it will exacerbate droughts in Melbourne.

The *Leader* newspapers had the largest proportion of articles expressing acceptance of consumer responsibility, while *The Australian* had the smallest proportion. The articles from the *Leader*, being community newspapers, had the greatest focus on the household and community impacts of water restrictions, while *The Australian*, being a national newspaper, focused primarily on policy, economic, and political implications. In focusing on household issues, the *Leader* newspaper had the greatest proportion of articles expressing the position that households should abide by the water restrictions. In contrast, *The Australian* often framed the drought as a policy problem of managing water supply and demand and focused on the role of the federal and state governments with regard to the management of the water infrastructure, often expressing the position that consumers should not have to bear the responsibility of conserving water if the governments had managed water security more effectively. *The Age* and *Herald Sun* generally discussed water restrictions issues from both perspectives in their articles. However, despite generally widespread support for reducing water use during times of drought as responsible and considerate behaviour, it was easy for newspapers to avoid linking the drought to climate change. While *The Age* often discussed the drought in the context of climate change, the *Herald Sun* conspicuously did not, reflecting each newspaper's positions on their support for action on climate change.

Table 3 and Figure 2 show the half-yearly totals and percentages for each category of landscape adaptation longevity for each newspaper, counting only those articles that discussed water restrictions in relation to the household outdoor use of water. Specifically, timed irrigation, manual watering, and grey water use were considered as short-term adaptations, or *A Short*. Mulching and soil treatments were considered as medium-term adaptations, or *A Medium*. Rainwater tanks, drip irrigation, drought-tolerant plants, reductions in lawn sizes and the use of artificial plants were considered as long-term adaptations, or *A Long*. The three adaptation longevity categories were not mutually exclusive; an article may discuss any or none of the specific adaptations.

As noted earlier in this article, the height of the drought was in 2007, with conditions easing towards 2010. Consequently, far higher numbers of articles discussing drought adaptations were found in 2006 and 2007 than in 2009 and 2010. No clear trend favouring one category of adaptation over the others was found in any of the newspapers. In *The Australian*, which initially focused on the perceived mismanagement of water infrastructure as a contributing factor to the drought, the proportions of articles for both short- and long-term adaptations increased over time as the effects of policies promoting water conservation became more apparent. For *The Age*, the proportions for each category of adaptations remained fairly constant over time, while for the *Herald Sun* and for the *Leader* newspapers, all categories declined slightly over time as the severity of the drought eased. Given the support for action on climate change in *The Age*, it is consistent that they would continue to discuss water conservation even as the drought eased, as climate change projections indicated further reductions in water availability in Melbourne in the future. On the other hand, the coverage of water conservation topics in the *Herald Sun* and the *Leader* newspapers appeared to be proportional to the severity of the current drought only.

## Discussion

The findings show that there has been a divergence between the different newspapers in the way climate change was presented. While *The Age* and the *Leader* newspapers showed steadily high proportions of articles expressing opinions consistent with the scientific consensus, *The Australian* showed increasing uncertainty, and the *Herald Sun* showed increasing scepticism. Over the time period under study, the "climate debate" in Australia had become highly political over discussions of the scuttled Emissions Trading Scheme and the subsequent Carbon Tax negotiations (Bailey et al., 2012), both of which

**Table 3.** Articles discussing water restrictions, household outdoor water use, and landscape adaptations, by adaptation durability, half-yearly totals

**The Australian**

| | A Short | | A Medium | | A Long | | Articles |
|---|---|---|---|---|---|---|---|
| | n | % | n | % | n | % | n |
| 2nd Half 2006 | 13 | 25.5% | 0 | 0.0% | 9 | 17.6% | 51 |
| 1st Half 2007 | 15 | 34.1% | 2 | 4.5% | 7 | 15.9% | 44 |
| 2nd Half 2007 | 10 | 37.0% | 0 | 0.0% | 9 | 33.3% | 27 |
| 1st Half 2008 | 4 | 18.2% | 1 | 4.5% | 3 | 13.6% | 22 |
| 2nd Half 2008 | 8 | 47.1% | 2 | 11.8% | 6 | 35.3% | 17 |
| 1st Half 2009 | 2 | 28.6% | 0 | 0.0% | 2 | 28.6% | 7 |
| 2nd Half 2009 | 5 | 62.5% | 0 | 0.0% | 4 | 50.0% | 8 |
| 1st Half 2010 | 2 | 50.0% | 0 | 0.0% | 0 | 0.0% | 4 |
| 2nd Half 2010 | 1 | 50.0% | 0 | 0.0% | 1 | 50.0% | 2 |
| Articles in total | 60 | 33.0% | 5 | 2.7% | 41 | 22.5% | 182 |

**The Age**

| | A Short | | A Medium | | A Long | | Articles |
|---|---|---|---|---|---|---|---|
| | n | % | n | % | n | % | n |
| 2nd Half 2006 | 46 | 51.1% | 9 | 10.0% | 38 | 42.2% | 90 |
| 1st Half 2007 | 41 | 41.8% | 7 | 7.1% | 42 | 42.9% | 98 |
| 2nd Half 2007 | 9 | 33.3% | 2 | 7.4 | 9 | 33.3% | 27 |
| 1st Half 2008 | 3 | 13.6% | 1 | 4.5% | 8 | 36.4% | 22 |
| 2nd Half 2008 | 4 | 30.8% | 1 | 7.7% | 7 | 53.8% | 13 |
| 1st Half 2009 | 5 | 38.5% | 2 | 15.4% | 4 | 30.8% | 13 |
| 2nd Half 2009 | 5 | 29.4% | 3 | 17.6% | 10 | 58.8% | 17 |
| 1st Half 2010 | 5 | 29.4% | 2 | 11.8% | 7 | 41.2% | 17 |
| 2nd Half 2010 | 10 | 40.0% | 1 | 4.0% | 9 | 36.0% | 25 |
| Articles in total | 128 | 39.8% | 28 | 8.7% | 134 | 41.6% | 322 |

**Herald Sun**

| | A Short | | A Medium | | A Long | | Articles |
|---|---|---|---|---|---|---|---|
| | n | % | n | % | n | % | n |
| 2nd Half 2006 | 46 | 56.8% | 16 | 19.8% | 34 | 42.0% | 81 |
| 1st Half 2007 | 50 | 43.1% | 11 | 9.5% | 44 | 37.9% | 116 |
| 2nd Half 2007 | 17 | 45.9% | 9 | 24.3% | 12 | 32.4% | 37 |
| 1st Half 2008 | 7 | 29.2% | 3 | 12.5% | 11 | 45.8% | 24 |
| 2nd Half 2008 | 6 | 24.0% | 3 | 12.0% | 10 | 40.0% | 25 |
| 1st Half 2009 | 3 | 33.3% | 2 | 22.2% | 4 | 44.4% | 9 |
| 2nd Half 2009 | 6 | 31.6% | 3 | 15.8% | 7 | 36.8% | 19 |
| 1st Half 2010 | 7 | 43.8% | 2 | 12.5% | 3 | 18.8% | 16 |
| 2nd Half 2010 | 13 | 50.0% | 1 | 3.8% | 5 | 19.2% | 26 |
| Articles in total | 155 | 43.9% | 50 | 14.2% | 130 | 36.8% | 353 |

**Leader**

| | A Short | | A Medium | | A Long | | Articles |
|---|---|---|---|---|---|---|---|
| | n | % | n | % | n | % | n |
| 2nd Half 2006 | 31 | 34.1% | 9 | 9.9% | 34 | 37.4% | 91 |
| 1st Half 2007 | 99 | 50.3% | 11 | 5.6% | 61 | 31.0% | 197 |
| 2nd Half 2007 | 33 | 34.7% | 10 | 10.5% | 30 | 31.6% | 95 |
| 1st Half 2008 | 18 | 54.5% | 2 | 6.1% | 12 | 36.4% | 33 |
| 2nd Half 2008 | 12 | 37.5% | 9 | 28.1% | 17 | 53.1% | 32 |
| 1st Half 2009 | 5 | 33.3% | 1 | 6.7% | 4 | 26.7% | 15 |
| 2nd Half 2009 | 1 | 12.5% | 1 | 12.5% | 2 | 25.0% | 8 |
| 1st Half 2010 | 20 | 27.8% | 3 | 4.2% | 23 | 31.9% | 72 |
| 2nd Half 2010 | 5 | 11.4% | 0 | 0.0% | 10 | 22.7% | 44 |
| Articles in total | 224 | 38.2% | 46 | 7.8% | 193 | 32.9% | 587 |

*Notes.* "A Short" denotes discussion of short-term adaptations. "A Medium" medium term adaptations. "A Long" denotes long-term adaptations.

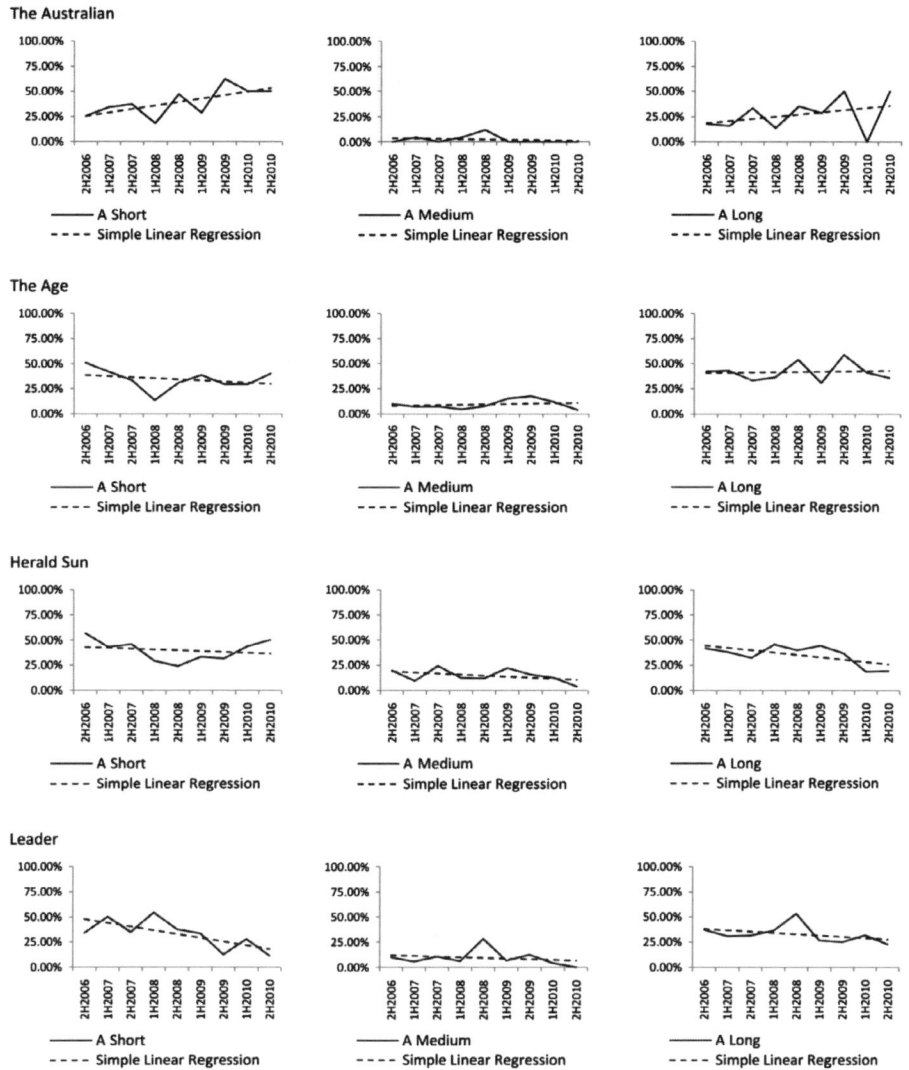

**Figure 2.** Articles discussing water restrictions, household outdoor water use, and landscape adaptations, by adaptation durability, half-yearly totals.
*Notes.* "A Short" denotes discussion of short-term adaptations. "A Medium" denotes medium-term adaptations. "A Long" denotes long-term adaptations.

were attempts to put a price on carbon emissions in order to encourage their reduction. Opponents of these climate change mitigation actions strongly challenged both the rationale behind climate change mitigation and the specifics of the schemes. Their tactics included highlighting misconceptions and known uncertainties in the climate change science, in attempts to strengthen opposition against these mitigation efforts. The divergent positions taken by the newspapers perhaps reflected the political leanings of each newspaper's editors and expected readership, and did not reflect the findings of scientific climate change studies. This obfuscation of climate science potentially impeded successful adaptation as it attempted to influence public opinion away from taking action on climate change.

While the newspapers showed a lack of consensus on climate change, the acceptance of consumer responsibility for conserving water during the drought was high in the state and local newspapers. Notable proportions of articles in *The Age* and the *Herald Sun* argued for a compromise position, but these focused on circumstances where the water restriction rules were believed to be a suboptimum method for conserving water, while ostensibly not questioning the underlying premise that it was necessary to conserve water during the drought. When faced with the immediate effects of drought, the newspapers quickly turned their focus towards conserving water and expanding the water supply, and while there was some debate over the most effective way to accomplish these, few articles denied that something needed to be done. The *Leader* newspapers, in particular, consistently urged its readers to comply with the water restrictions. Thus, we see in the newspapers both an effective short-term response to a drought crisis, and the politicisation and obfuscation of the climate debate on the part of some of the newspapers, hindering efforts to deal with the long-term threat of climate change.

The relationship between the acceptance of climate change science and opinions on drought-adaptation is not a simple one. One can simultaneously be sceptical of climate change and effectively adapt to future droughts if one denies the link between the two. However, the scientific evidence shows that higher temperatures will most likely increase the severity and frequency of droughts, given that recurring El Niño droughts are already part of the Australian cyclical climate. The data for the discussion of specific drought-adaptations in each newspaper must be understood in this light. For all newspapers, short-term adaptations were associated with water restrictions and drought. The short-term adaptive actions of timed irrigation, manual irrigation, and grey water use were specified in the water restriction rules. Medium- and long-term adaptations, on the other hand, have more to do with the expected duration of the current drought and the expected frequency of future droughts, issues that are associated with opinions on climate change. Actions such as installing rain-water tanks or replacing lawns require significant investments of time and money, and generally do not make sense if the assumption is that droughts will not be frequent or long-lasting in the future. However, there was no clear preference for long-term adaptations even for *The Age* and the *Leader* newspapers, which consistently presented positions consistent with the scientific consensus when discussing climate change.

While the recent drought in Melbourne presented an opportunity to focus people's attention on the need to adapt to the expected reductions in future water availability due to climate change, the stipulations of the water restrictions rules were such that much of the discussion of household outdoor water use in the newspapers revolved around short-term adaptations that had no lasting water conservation effects. The increasing politicisation of the climate change issue may have posed problems for framing drought adaptations as responses to climate change, but nevertheless the opportunity existed to strongly promote long-term drought adaptations as a suitable response to the recurring droughts of Australia. This would also have the effect of increasing the resilience of the Melbourne suburban landscape against future climate change.

## Conclusion

The period of reduced water availability from 1997 to 2010 undoubtedly had a significant impact on the people and landscape of Melbourne. The immediate effects of El Niño drought events, most severely in 2007, coupled with a longer-term reduction of inflows into Melbourne's reservoirs, resulted in the imposition of prolonged and onerous restrictions on outdoor mains water use, causing damage to lawns and vegetation across the city. Such conditions are likely to become more common in the future as a result of climate change, unless long-term drought adaptations are implemented, either by expanding the water supply infrastructure or by increasing the drought tolerance of the urban and suburban landscape, or both.

This article has used rigorous content analysis on a considerable number of articles in four different Melbourne newspapers; however it is acknowledged that the lack of inter-rater checks is a limitation that future research could address. The results showed increasing uncertainty and scepticism towards climate change in two of the four newspapers analysed. This appears to reflect the politicisation of the climate debate as discussions transitioned towards the economics of climate change mitigation. While the acceptance of the need for households to adapt to the immediate drought was very high in the local newspapers and somewhat high in the Victorian newspapers, it did not necessarily equate to an acceptance of the need to adapt to climate change. This could particularly occur where individuals may not accept that climate change is happening or that it will lead to more frequent and more severe droughts in the future. Despite the recent drought lasting over 10 years, and the expectations of future climate change, the newspaper discussion, on adaptations to drought in household outdoor areas, did not noticeably focus on adaptations that focused on long-term effects, even towards the end of the drought. Rather, the stipulations of the water restrictions rules meant that much of the discussion was on short-term behavioural adaptations that did conserve water at the time, but which did not increase the resilience of the Melbourne suburban landscape against future droughts and climate change.

While it may be hoped that the newspapers would serve to disseminate unbiased, factual, and helpful information on climate change and water conservation to encourage successful adaptation, in reality they merely served as arenas in which the political contest over climate change played out. Climate change is both a scientific and a political issue, and those engaging with the politics did not necessarily refrain from attempting to contest the science as well, thus obfuscating and confusing attempts to communicate climate science through newspapers. While it is difficult to prove any direct links between the portrayal of climate science in the mass media and people's water conservation behaviour, it is difficult to imagine that this obfuscation might help climate change adaptation in any way. For those engaging with newspapers or other forms of mass media, it seems necessary to be mindful that mass media is an arena for political contests as well as a way to communicate facts and information. Attempts to communicate climate science through the mass media may be inseparable from entering into conflicts over climate politics, and the avoidance of climate politics may prevent the communication of climate science altogether.

Subsequent to the easing of the drought from 2010 onwards, media attention on water conservation in household outdoor areas has also faded. The questions of how people and the media in Melbourne will react to the next El Niño event, and whether people will effectively adapt to the drying effects of climate change in the long term, must be left to future studies. However, despite the apparent short-term nature of the climate change news agenda, it is important to establish patterns of data and perhaps a range of environmental behaviours. It is therefore necessary to continue to research future droughts and the ways in which their effects can be mitigated at local, regional, and global levels. Newspapers provide a rich and valuable record of political, scientific, and economic information relating to climate change and as such provide a platform for analysis and longitudinal studies.

When the next El Niño drought occurs, will there be greater agreement with the scientific consensus on climate change? Will newspaper articles discuss long-term, climate-appropriate drought adaptations sooner and more frequently? Will the limitations of short-term drought adaptations be recognised? Such questions and the analysis of multi-decadal trends will reveal whether Melbourne is responding adequately to the challenge of climate change in the long term, and allow the differentiation of these long-term trends from the responses to the waxing and waning of a single drought.

# References

Anonymous. (2009, June 4). Coals from Newcastle: Plans for a carbon-emissions trading scheme may bring an early election. *The Economist*, p. 50.

Bailey, I., MacGill, I., Passey, R., & Compston, H. (2012). The fall (and rise) of carbon pricing in Australia: A political strategy analysis of the carbon pollution reduction scheme. *Environmental Politics, 21*(5), 691–711.

Boykoff, M. T. (2007). Flogging a dead norm? Newspaper coverage of anthropogenic climate change in the United States and United Kingdom from 2003 to 2006. *Area, 39*(4), 470–481.

Boykoff, M. T., & Mansfield, M. (2008). "Ye Olde Hot Aire": Reporting on human contributions to climate change in the UK tabloid press. *Environmental Research Letters, 3*(2), 024002.

Cai, W., & Cowan, T. (2008). The South-East Australia drought: Possible causes. *Water (Melbourne),* *35*(5), 95–97.

Friedman, T. L. (2007, May 4). The Aussie "big dry". *New York Times*, 23.

IMDb.com Inc. (2012). *An inconvenient truth (2006).* Retrieved from http://www.imdb.com/title/tt0497116/

McComas, K., & Shanahan, J. (1999). Telling stories about global climate change: Measuring the impact of narratives on issue cycles. *Communication Research, 26*(1), 30–57.

Melbourne Water Corporation. (2010). *Melbourne Water Annual Report 2009/10.* Melbourne, Australia: Author.

Melbourne Water Corporation. (2011). *History of Melbourne's Water Supply 1803–2008.* Retrieved from http://www.melbournewater.com.au/content/water_storages/water_supply/history_of_melbournes_water_supply.asp

News Limited. (2010). *Leader (Vic) | NewsSpace.* Retrieved from http://www.newsspace.com.au/communitynews/leader

Nobelprize.org. (2012). *The Nobel Peace Prize 2007.* Retrieved from http://www.nobelprize.org/nobel_prizes/peace/laureates/2007/

Ryan I. (Ed.). (2008). *State of the news print media in Australia: 2008 report.* Sydney, Australia: Australian Press Council.

savewater! (2009). *Saving water in the garden.* Retrieved from http://www.savewater.com.au/How-to-save-water/In-the-garden

Solomon, S., Qin, D., Manning, M., Chen, Z., Marquis, M., Averyt, K. B., . . ., Miller, H. L. (Eds.). (2007). *Climate change 2007: The physical science basis. Contribution of Working Group I to the Fourth Assessment Report of the Intergovernmental Panel on Climate Change.* Cambridge, MA: Cambridge University Press.

Ungar, S. (1992). The rise and (relative) decline of global warming as a social problem. *The Sociological Quarterly, 33*(4), 483–501.

# Vulnerability Assessment of Urban Populations in Africa

## The Case of Dar es Salaam, Tanzania

Regina John,[1] Nathalie Jean-Baptiste,[2] and Sigrun Kabisch[2]

[1]School of Urban and Regional Planning, Ardhi University, Dar es Salaam, Tanzania
[2]Department of Urban and Environmental Sociology, Helmholtz Centre for Environmental Research – UFZ, Leipzig, Germany

**Abstract**

Climate induced hazards jeopardise the social and economic livelihood of hundreds of millions of urban dwellers in Africa. Indeed, it is well recognised today, that African cities have to simultaneously deal with development challenges as well as the impact of extreme events. More frequent floods and recurring heat waves add stress on growing urban areas making them particularly vulnerable. This chapter focuses on the case of Dar es Salaam, Tanzania, and highlights two settlements that are frequently flooded with resulting disproportionate impact on exposed communities. We propose to understand the differential capacity of households to adapt and cope with floods, through a vulnerability framework which incorporates: asset, institutional, attitudinal, and physical dimensions. Preliminary data was collected through interviews, focus group discussions, reconnaissance visits, and participant observations. We also used a context-centred participatory approach that places attention on the circumstances of the poor and identifies local-based adaptation measures that can be included in strategic responses to prevent future threats.

**Key words:** community participation, Dar es Salaam, floods, vulnerability assessment

## Introduction

The variability and uncertainty of the environment and the increase in climate-related hazards in urban settlements are global challenges (Parry, Canziani, Palutikof, Van der Linden, & Hanson, 2007). These challenges particularly affect developing communities, which are simultaneously dealing with inadequate infrastructure, environmental degradation, and governance failure. Severe weather events (drought, flood, changes in rainfall patterns, sea level rise, and decrease in water availability) are expected to increase in the continent (Parry et al., 2007; United Nations Human Settlements Programme, 2010). High levels of urbanisation, characterised by expansive informal settlements and unregulated urban growth onto risky sites make them particularly vulnerable (Kebede & Nicholls, 2012).

Although Africa is considered a continent clearly threatened by the effects of climate change, its real impact, especially on a local scale, is still poorly understood. For this reason, a selected number of cities in West and East Africa were identified for further research within CLUVA (Climate Change and Urban Vulnerability in Africa), a research project funded through the Seventh Framework Programme.[1] Among the cities selected in CLUVA is Dar es Salaam, the largest coastal city in Tanzania, with almost 4.4 million inhabitants as per the 2012 National Population Census. In December 2011 this city experienced one of its worst flooding events in over five decades. As a result, several communities were severely affected. The flood caused major destruction of buildings, closure of businesses and schools, lack of water, loss of crops, massive evacuation, and temporary relocation as well as loss of lives. The rapid pace at which flooded communities are changing drives us to centre our attention on human experiences in the face of a disaster. This chapter thus informs those responsible for implementation and policy on specific vulnerability indicators and highlights local voices and their differentiated adaptive capacities.

## Vulnerability Assessment Approach

The term vulnerability carries different meanings depending on the perspective from which it is perceived and depending on different research traditions (Kabisch, Kunath, Schweizer-Ries, & Steinführer, 2012). Yet, in disaster studies and recently in climate change discourses, vulnerability is most often constituted by elements of exposure, susceptibility, coping, and adaptive capacity. Exposure describes the physical setting under threats. Susceptibility involves the preconditions to suffer harm due to some level of fragility or disadvantageous conditions, and finally, coping and adaptive capacities refer to

---

[1]   CLUVA is an international project which focuses on environment and climate change. It aims to develop context-centred methods to assess vulnerability and increase knowledge on managing climate-related risks. For more information see http://www.cluva.eu

R. John et al.
Vulnerability Assessment of Urban Populations in Africa
**235**

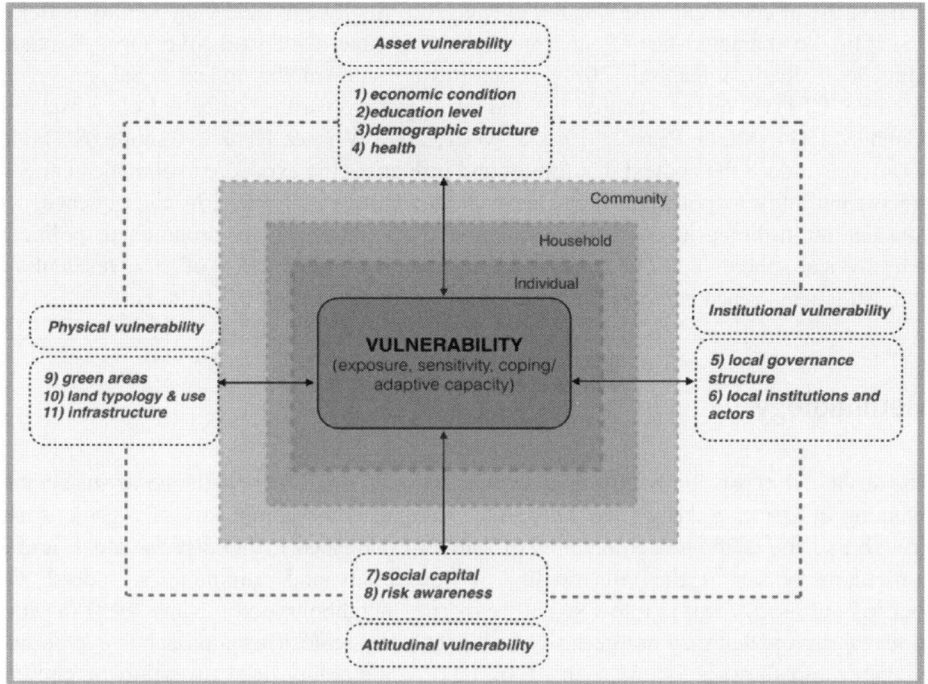

**Figure 1.** CLUVA vulnerability framework. (Source: Jean-Baptiste, Kuhlicke, Kunath, & Kabisch, 2011)

the ability to prepare for, cope with and recover from the impact of a hazard (Fuchs, Kuhlicke, & Meyer, 2011).

Assessing vulnerability in the African urban context implies understanding the processes of affectation and adaptation of individuals, communities and cities, while taking into account their exposure, susceptibility, and coping and adaptive strategies. In light of contextual particularities found in many African cities (e.g., population growth, the informal economy, attitude and perception of risks, complexity of land management, and lack of effectiveness of local authorities), it is necessary to highlight and interlink relevant indicators and/or perceptions enabling conditions of vulnerability and/or resilience.

Figure 1 proposes a model of vulnerability to the impacts of a disaster in the form of a collective umbrella integrating four specific dimensions of vulnerability: *asset, institutional, attitudinal,* and *physical.*

First, asset vulnerability encompasses the human livelihood and material resources of individuals and groups. Second, attitudinal vulnerability conveys the perception and risk management attitude of individuals and groups. Third, institutional vulnerability refers to the state of local authorities and civil action groups that operate to prevent, adapt, or mitigate the effect of extreme weather events. And finally, physical vulnerability is determined by the characteristics of either natural and/or man-made land cover (Jean-Baptiste, Kuhlicke, Kunath, & Kabisch, 2011). Assessment of vulnerability in Dar es Salaam – as in the other CLUVA cities – cannot be studied in isolation from contextual circumstances (Cannon, 1994; Adger, Paavola, Huq, & Mace, 2006; Wisner, Blaikie, Cannon, & Davis, 2004). It is indeed the context that frames and influences the exposure to climatic changes, the susceptibility to potential threats as well as adaptive responses. In consequence, we consider multi-dimensional factors stemming from the social, environmental, political, and physical spheres that either enhance or lessen the vulnerability of local residents in two settlements repeatedly affected by floods.

## Methodology

The sustained expansion of informal settlements presents a real challenge to sustainable planning in Dar es Salaam City. This study recognises the complexity of organic urban growth and the differentiated realities of settlers established in flood prone areas, and it particularly addresses the vulnerability of households and communities. Indeed, we focused our assessment at a low spatial scale (i.e., neighbourhood – Mtaa level) in order to reveal drivers that may not be easily visible at a city scale. This approach is explorative by nature and allows a context-centric framing of vulnerability, drawing mainly on circumstantial factors.

The study mixes data collection tools in order to obtain multiple clues drawing on all possibilities. We argue that combining numeric data (quantitative) generally requested by decision and policy makers, with nuanced explanations (qualitative) from focus group discussions, provides a complete picture as to the vulnerability and resilience of a group. Data was collected through interviews, focus group discussions (held with women, local leaders, and youth groups), reconnaissance visits, and participant observations. The interviews and discussions covered five main topics: (i) Socio-economic status of households in the flooding settlements-asset indicators (ii) Level of social networks, attitudes, norms, and hazard experience of the residents – attitudinal indicators (iii) Local governance structures including local institutions and their roles in adaptation to flood hazards – institutional indicators (iv) conditions of the built environment – physical vulnerability and (v) Households and communities coping and adapting strategies.

In Dar es Salaam settlements frequently flooded combine features such as: low lying topography, housing development densification as well as lack of infrastructure (i.e., poor drainage and waste management). The study was carried out in Magomeni Suna showed in Figure 2 and Bonde la Mpunga illustrated in Figure 3. These were selected as representative of communities experiencing recurrent flooding (exposure), comprising different development conditions (susceptibility) and featuring different responses to flooding (coping and adaptive strategies).

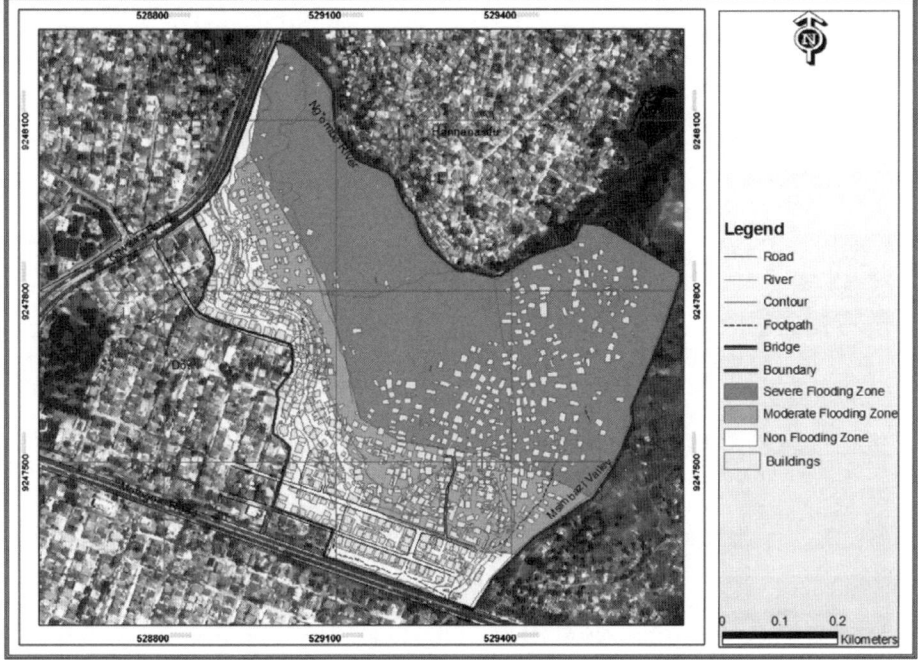

**Figure 2.** Map of the Magomeni Suna settlement.

## The Magomeni Suna Settlement

Magomeni Suna is a booming settlement situated in the Kinondoni Municipality about 5 km away from the city centre and covers an area of about 60 hectares. The settlement has two main land use categories: planned and unplanned. The North-East and Southern parts are unplanned low lying basins and are mostly exposed to the overflow of the Msimbazi and Ng'ombe rivers bordering the settlement. Our interview with Mtaa local leaders in 2012 revealed a population estimated at 9,450 inhabitants with approximately 2,500 households. 370 from 770 houses were counted in the most exposed flooding zone shown in Figure 2.

## The Msasani Bonde la Mpunga Settlement

Msasani Bonde la Mpunga is a saturated settlement from the Kinondoni Municipality located around 6 km away from the city centre. It covers an area of approximately

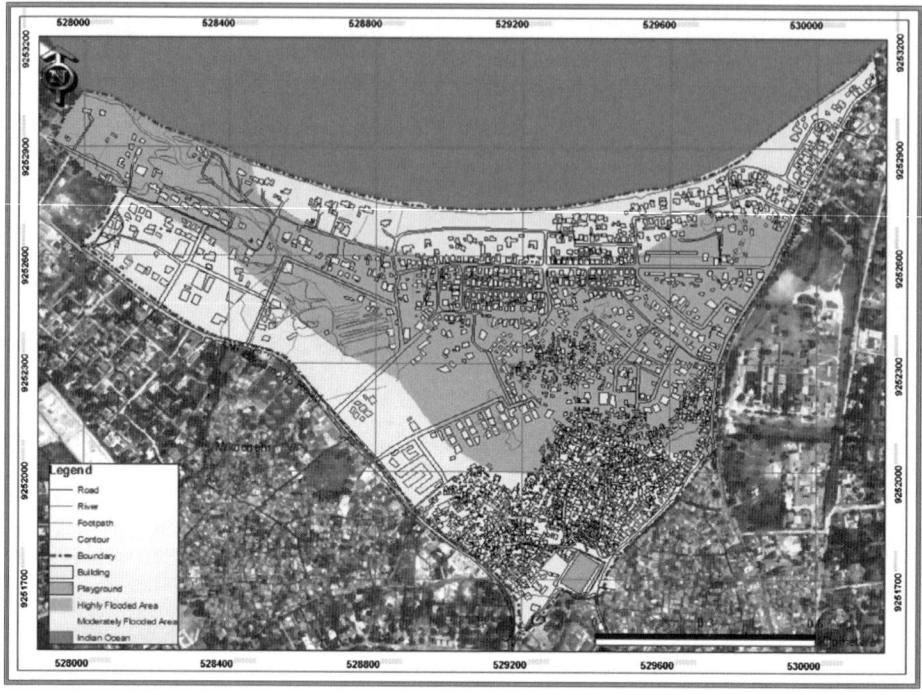

**Figure 3.** Map of Msasani Bonde la Mpunga settlement.

120 hectares and lies between 0 and 3 m above sea level. Bonde is valued today as prime land located in proximity with Dar es Salaam's central business district. Formally used as paddy fields, Bonde was declared hazardous land three decades ago due to being one of the cities main drainage basins (1979 Dar es Salaam Master Plan). Notwithstanding government policies, first settlers occupied the area during the mid 1980s and continued to grow, incorporating both commercial and residential land use. Our interview with local leaders indicated a total of 2,820 households in 2010. As shown in Figure 3, 68% of houses are located in the area highly susceptible to flooding (Kiunsi et al., 2009).

## Preliminary Findings

The preliminary findings discussed below are centred along five main points: asset, physical, attitudinal, and institutional vulnerabilities as well as adapting capacities.

R. John et al.
Vulnerability Assessment of Urban Populations in Africa

**239**

**Table 1.** Asset vulnerability in Magomeni Suna and Bonde la Mpunga

| Indicator | Magomeni Suna | Bonde la Mpunga |
|---|---|---|
| Employment nature | Largely informal | Formal and informal |
| Income levels | Generally low; TSh 5,000 (approx. US $3) | Mixed-low, medium, and high average for each category not yet established |
| Main economic activities | Small business and urban agriculture | Small business |
| Health situation | Prevalence of water borne diseases (bilharzia, cholera, dysentery, fungal infection) | Prevalence of water borne diseases (bilharzia, cholera, dysentery) |
| Education | Generally low (mostly standard seven leavers) | Mixed education levels (no education, primary, secondary, university) |

*Note.* Tsh = Tanzanian Shilling.

## Asset Vulnerability of Households

We considered the type of employment, income levels, main economic activities, and education levels as well as the current health situation in order to estimate the human and material resources of households in Magomeni Suna and Bonde la Mpunga. Table 1 shows a prevalence of low income activities through local-based small businesses (e.g., food vending, selling in retail shops) and urban agriculture (e.g., small-scale livestock and vegetable farming) in Magomeni Suna. Given this context, informal employment patterns accentuate households' vulnerability, particularly as those with unstable and poorly remunerated occupations have fewer economic and social resources to anticipate, survive, and recover from the effects of a massive flood.

## Local Governance Structure

In Dar es Salaam, the local government runs vertically starting from "Ten Cell" and "Mtaa" levels (lowest levels of government) to the "District" level. At each stage, decisions on how to best cope with floods are discussed and implemented. However, this vertical structure does not operate on its own as shown in Figure 4, there are other formal and informal institutions and actors operating within the settlements, playing different roles in adapting the impact of climate change induced floods.

The level of trust in the different institutions varies significantly. In Magomeni Suna among trusted institutions are the community environmental committee, religious groups,

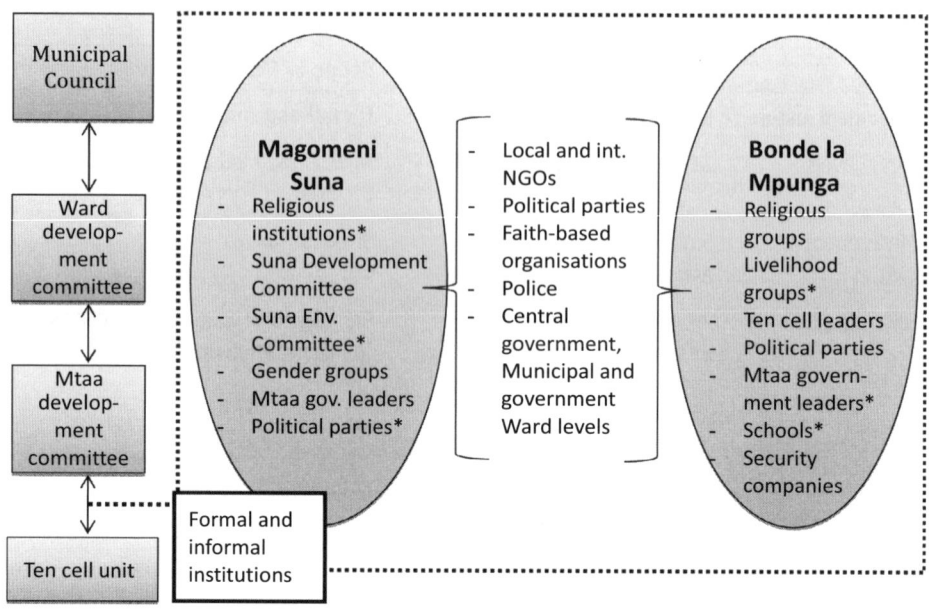

**Figure 4.** Governance structure of the local communities.
*Important stakeholders identified during a focus session conducted in July 2012. The session aimed at identifying and ranking stakeholders that were particularly relevant in terms of coping and adaptive capacities at Mtaa levels.

and political parties, in Bonde la Mpunga they are the livelihood groups, Mtaa government leaders and schools.

Two different scenarios appear in terms of relationships between the formal and informal institutions at the local level. These are competitive and complimentary scenarios. Competitive scenario exists when the level of trust between the community and the Mtaa government is low while the compatibility scenario is exhibited when there is a high level of trust. These two contrasting scenarios translate into different levels of vulnerability for households as well as communities. While under the competitive scenario the vulnerability is high due to lack of common goals to improve resilience, whereas the compatibility scenario enhances adaptive capacity of communities and thus causes less vulnerability.

## Social Networks and Risk Perception

Additionally, we explored the level of social networks and risk perception of households as indicators for measuring attitudinal vulnerability and adaptive capacity of the two

R. John et al.
Vulnerability Assessment of Urban Populations in Africa

**241**

settlements. Social networks related to ethnic, religious, livelihood, and gender groups were observed as important as they provide relief to their members in terms of moral, financial, or material support during and after flooding events.

We found social arrangements in the form of family/friend support groups to have significant importance in coping, as well as in restoring people's livelihoods. When the need to relocate arose, residents at risk mostly moved into their relatives and/or family members' residence in safer areas. Equally, when small businesses were compromised or destroyed, entrepreneurs relied on assistance and loans from relatives and friends for re-establishment capital. For instance, 10 local traders out of 15 interviewed in Magomeni Suna accessed credit from friends and relatives for re-establishing their retail shops after the flood of December 2011. Although these arrangements are largely informal, they play a vital role in terms of the recovery of households. The different social ties exhibited by households are due to strong traditions of assisting one another, particularly among the poor in urban areas (Kombe, 2010).

In terms of households and community risk perception, the results show that there is low level of risk perception associated with flooding in these communities. Flooding is not considered as a serious problem as residents have more important concerns such as meeting their basic daily needs. This is an outcome from and a response to urbanisation in poverty stricken situations, where households have limited choices and are struggling to maintain a healthy standard of financial and physical subsistence (Kombe, 2005). Moreover, it was concluded that collective memories of past flooding events trigger preparedness and thus helps reduce the vulnerability of the households and communities to flood hazards. However, Salick and Byg (2007) also noted that residents are more at risk due to their inability to precisely predict and prepare for future flooding events. This was observed in the two studied settlements where the intensity of more recent climatic events exceeds previously experienced ones.

# Characteristics of Built Environment

The physical exposure of individuals and communities are partly shaped by inadequate infrastructures that includes, deficient road access, inadequate water drainage as well as lack of solid waste management. Reconnaissance visits conducted in both settlements revealed arduous conditions for those housed in low lying basins and in proximity to the rivers bordering the settlements. Easy access and low cost of land were among the most common reasons given by residents for settling in these areas. Indeed, underprivileged households are restricted to low-priced parcels with no basic infrastructure and the use of substandard building materials. In both Magomeni Suna and Bonde la Mpunga, the vast majority of dwelling units had walls made of cement blocks and corrugated iron sheet roofs. Pit latrines are used as the primary sanitation system and solid waste management is buried or collected selectively. The built world in these communities determines the quality of the living environment which is implicitly related to physical fragility and/or resistance to damage.

**Table 2.** Households short and long term coping and adapting strategies

| Aspect of daily life | Before flooding | During flooding | After flooding |
|---|---|---|---|
| Housing | – Raising building foundation (L)<br>– Earth filling to elevate floor levels (L)<br>– Construction of protection walls in front of buildings (L) | – Improvised outlets to remove water from houses | – Repair damage to housing (S)<br>– Participate in community efforts to stabilise river banks by putting up bags of sands or car tires (S) |
| Mobility and overall safety | – Evacuate children, elders, and the sick to safer places (S) | – Temporary relocation (S)<br>– Stop sending children to schools (S)<br>– Improvise walk ways (S) | – Participate in community actions to unblock storm water drains (S) |
| Belongings/household material assets and businesses | – Prepare stands for hanging properties (S)<br>– Fix/hang items upon receiving signals/information for big rains (S) | – Place material items on raised levels (S)<br>– Relocate with some material assets (S)<br>– improvise outlets to remove water from houses<br>– Empty water with buckets (S) | – Wash the affected items (S)<br>– Repair damaged items (S)<br>– Borrow money from relatives and friends to replace the damaged stock of business items (SL) |

*Note.* L = long term. S = short term.

R. John et al.
Vulnerability Assessment of Urban Populations in Africa

**243**

## Households and Communities Coping and Adaptive Strategies

Vulnerable people individually and collectively develop their own means, resources, and strategies to cope with flooding both in short (S) and in long terms (L). Short term strategies are the temporary actions taken for survival when disaster strikes or shortly in the aftermath. Long terms strategies refer to those integrated to household's daily life to avoid damages on assets (properties and livelihoods). Both short and long term strategies aim to protect different aspects of affected households as indicated in Table 2. Different coping strategies identified, especially those related to protecting the house structures and properties, have significant cost implications, and thus accessible to only those wealthier households. The study's findings further implies that the continuous implementation of the various coping mechanisms, out with intervention on the flooding problem itself, may lead to further impoverishment of the communities because of the recurrent losses they experience.

## Conclusion

As suggested in the empirical findings, impacts of climate change directly affects the living conditions and livelihoods of the urban poor, especially in informal settlements, where the built environmental itself is one of the determinants of vulnerability. In the case of Dar es Salaam, the findings of the households' experiences with flood and general living conditions expose the fact that climate change only exacerbates existing vulnerabilities. Furthermore, it appears that adaptation to climate change is shaped by a number of factors, namely the socio-economic context of those exposed. In the two settlements studied, it is clear that the ability to recover and respond to flood is influenced by some socio-economic characteristics, specific institutional settings, and the built environment. Despite being subjected to successive floods over a number of years the regions under research have developed alternative and localised methods of adaptation as well as utilising the somewhat limited formal institutional support. Households in Magomeni Suna and Bonde la Mpunga have developed different structural (e.g., construction of protection wall, elevation of house foundation) and non-structural strategies (loans and support groups) for coping and adapting to floods.

Decision makers need to be well-informed about what works in cities such as Dar es Salaam as informal settlements continue to grow with increasing migration from rural areas. Ad hoc and hasty arrangements in response to floods, including efforts to relocate vulnerable communities, have been a challenging undertaking with little if any success. It is important to recognise that the impacts of climate change on African cities must be contextualised within the broader perspective of the human experience and threatened environments. Vulnerability reduction strategies in less privileged settlements should begin by recognising the capacities of the households and communities in responding to extreme events. Given the role that climatic events plays in shaping cities, it has never been more crucial for policy makers to acknowledge the differentiated realities of the urban poor. This call for a paradigm shift in policy making would enable the process of building climate resilient cities.

# References

Adger, W. N., Paavola, J., Huq, M., & Mace, J. (Eds.). (2006). *Fairness in adaptation to climate change*. Cambridge, MA: MIT Press.

Cannon, T. (1994). Vulnerability analysis and the explanation of "natural" disasters. In A. Varley (Ed.), *Disasters, development and the environment* (pp. 13–30). Chichester, UK: Wiley.

Fuchs, S., Kuhlicke, C., & Meyer, V. (2011). Editorial for the special issue: Vulnerability to natural hazards – the challenge of integration. *Natural Hazards, 58*(2), 609–619. doi: 10.1007/s11069-011-9825-5

Jean-Baptiste, N., Kuhlicke, C., Kunath, A., & Kabisch, S. (2011). *Review and evaluation of existing vulnerability indicators for assessing climate related vulnerability in Africa* (UFZ Report 07/2011). Leipzig: Germany: Helmholtz-Zentrum für Umweltforschung (UFZ).

Kabisch, S., Kunath, A., Schweizer-Ries, P., & Steinführer, A. (Eds.). (2012). *Vulnerability, risks, and complexity: Impacts of global change on human habitats*. Göttingen, Germany: Hogrefe.

Kebede, S. A., & Nicholls, J. R. (2012). Exposure and vulnerability to climate extremes: Population and asset exposure to coastal flooding in Dar es Salaam Tanzania. *Regional Environmental Change, 12*, 81-94.

Kiunsi, R., Kassenga, G., Lupala, J., Malele, B., Uhinga, G., & Rugai, D. (2009). *Mainstreaming disaster risk reduction in urban planning practice in Tanzania, AURAN Phase II* Project final report. Retrieved from http://www.preventionweb.net/files/13524_TANZANIAFINALREPORT 27OCT09Mainstrea.pdf

Kombe, W. (2005). Land use dynamics in peri-urban areas and their implications on the urban growth and form: the case of Dar es Salaam, Tanzania. *Habitat International, 29*(1), 113–135.

Kombe, W. (2010, November). *Dysfunctional cities, poor governance: The power of social regulation in African cities*. Paper presented at Our Common Future: Urbanisation in Poverty – from Exclusion to Inclusion, Essen, Germany.

Parry, M., Canziani, O., Palutikof, J., Van der Linden, P., & Hanson, C. (Eds.). (2007). *Climate Change 2007 (AR4): Impacts, adaptation and vulnerability. Contribution of Working Group II to the Fourth Assessment Report of the Intergovernmental Panel on Climate Change*. Cambridge, UK: Cambridge University Press.

Potts, D. (2009). The slowing of sub-Saharan Africa's urbanization: Evidence and implications for urban livelihoods. *Environment and Urbanization, 21*, 253–259.

Salick, J., & Byg, A. (2007). *Indigenous peoples and climate change*. Retrieved from http://www.ecdgroup.com/docs/lib_004630823.pdf

United Nations Human Settlements Programme (UN-HABITAT). (2010). *The state of African cities: Governance, inequality and urban land markets*. Nairobi, Kenya: Author.

Wisner, B., Blaikie, P., Cannon, T., & Davis, I. (2004). *At risk: Natural hazards, people's vulnerability and disasters*. London, UK: Routledge.

# Is Urban Sustainability Possible in the Face of Accelerated Property Development and Major Public Works?

## The Case of Recife, Brazil

Fátima Furtado,[1] Edinéa Alcântara,[2] and Onilda Bezerra[3]

[1]Architecture and Urbanism Department and Urban Development Programme (MDU), Universidade Federal de Pernambuco (UFPE), Recife, Brazil
[2]Urban Development Programme (MDU), Universidade Federal de Pernambuco (UFPE), Recife, Brazil
[3]Architecture and Urbanism Department, Universidade Federal de Pernambuco (UFPE), Recife, Brazil

---

**Abstract**

Some Brazilian cities are currently growing very fast because of the increased construction of skyscrapers, or public works for the 2014 World Cup. One example is Recife, a coastal city in northeastern Brazil. Regional development policy has encouraged growth and this is set to increase. Property values have risen steeply; urban accessibility and mobility have become major problems. The lack of drainage infrastructure and other elements needed to reduce the impact of heavy rains makes the region highly vulnerable to flooding and rising sea level, tendencies aggravated by climate change. How is the municipal management system equipped to deal with the city's growth and its present and future impacts? How could these be reduced through mitigation at the level of administration, turning a situation of vulnerability in Brazil's coastal cities into the potential for resilience? Recife is an example of the need to strengthen urban planning and city management in the face of climate change.

**Key words:** climate change, economic growing, governance, sustainable cities, urban sustainability

---

## Introduction

The central focus of this article, as reflected in its title, is the sustainability of cities in a context of accelerated property development and major public works. This is a desk based case study utilising Recife (Brazil) as a real-world, ethnographic, example of an area undergoing substantial urban and peri-urban development. The focus of the case study is not on the development of new innovative, methodological research philosophies but takes a qualitative approach to the research relating to socio economic, cultural, political, and environmental sustainability dilemmas Brazilian society faces in a time a rapid change.

This is a crucial issue for all countries, particularly those experiencing economic growth and new dynamism, such as the BRICs. In the case of Brazil, the last decade has brought significant changes in the political, social, and economic context, and its large cities are accordingly facing enormous transformations. This article discusses two central questions:

(1) What is the direction of such transformations in terms of urban sustainability?
(2) Is the urban population in control of the transformation process?

When one considers that the majority of the world's population now lives in cities, making them the main centers' of production and consumption, it is clear that urban environments are the key to the survival of the human species.

Latin America is the most highly urbanised of the continents, and Brazil the most urbanised country within it. The unsustainability of Latin American conurbations, and the causes of this, has been widely discussed in the literature (ONU-Habitat, 2012; Ribeiro, 2012). The challenge for countries such as Brazil with a high level of growth is to plan and manage large cities to take advantage of economic growth by promoting interventions to overcome the existing situation of socio-spatial inequality and environmental imbalance, thus ensuring their sustainability. But is this proving to be possible?

This article will discuss the difficulties faced in the attempt to achieve sustainable urban environments with reference to two important and interrelated aspects of economic growth:

- Large-scale public works,
- The heating up of the property market in Brazilian cities.

The city of Recife and its metropolitan region (RMR) makes for a good example, because it is the capital of Pernambuco, the state with the highest level of growth in the Northeast, which is in turn the fastest-growing region in Brazil.[1]

---

[1]   Brazil's GNP increased by 8.3% in 2010 (Boletim Conjuntura Econômica, Etene). Pernambuco's GNP grew by 15.78 in the same year, attaining R$87 billion. During the last four years, public investments in the state grew by a factor of 2.5. (http://www.grandesconstrucoes.com.br/br/index.php?option=com_conteudo&task=viewMateria&id=425)

F. Furtado et al.
Is Urban Sustainability Possible? The Case of Recife, Brazil

**247**

The initial picture suggests there will be gains and losses in different aspects of sustainability, generally with greater gains in economic terms and to a certain extent socially, but with resulting environmental costs; in other words, short-term gains at the cost of medium and long-term harms.

## Brazilian Cities in a Context of Economic Growth

There has been much discussion in Brazil regarding the nature of its economic development and the consequences for Brazilian society and the environment, especially the urban environment. Whenever the topic is global sustainability or sustainable development, from whatever ideological point of view, cities are seen as having a major impact on environmental resources, if not the greatest. This includes those who are generally sceptical or critical of discourse relating to the, perceived or otherwise, effects of sustainability as a concept.

Brazil's recent levels of growth have made it the sixth largest economy in the world, but the country is not finding it easy to reduce social inequality or mitigate the impact on the environmental structures of Brazilian cities. This damage to urban sustainability will tend to increase, since the development model adopted by state and federal governments, including Pernambuco, focusses on strengthening industry with a view to creating jobs and increasing tax revenue. The car industry and the construction industry are having a particularly large impact on cities. The government stimulus includes changes to fiscal policy to make it easier for people to buy a car and their own home. As a result, the urban and peri-urban areas of the RMR are seeing the construction of trunk roads, city road projects, and thousands of housing projects aimed at the working and lower middle classes.

Brazil's current development model has affected the sustainability of its large cities for the worse in two ways: the preference for individual rather than public transport, generally involving burning fossil fuels; and significant changes in urban land use and occupation, heavily influenced by the interests of civil construction and the private building industry.

The discovery of major oil fields along the Brazilian coastline (known as "Pré-sal") has also bolstered the preference for individual transport, and as a result no significant measures have been taken to reduce greenhouse gas emissions from this source. Between 2001 and 2011 the number of cars in Brazil's 12 major cities grew from 11.5 million to 20.5 million (Rodrigues, 2012). Around half of Brazilian households currently possess a car or motorbike, however the government's strategies to encourage car and home ownership can only serve as an inducement for the population, especially in poorer regions where vehicle ownership is low, to increase the number of vehicles on Brazilian roads. This increasing trend has not only worsened the existing urban mobility crises in large cities but seems likely to continue to grow, resulting in increased logistical and environmental issues (PNAD, 2009).

The other key national development strategy (also a response to the global economic crisis) has been to stimulate the civil construction industry with a view to strengthening the

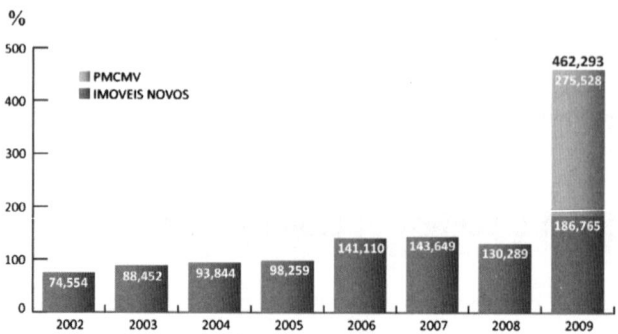

**Figure 1.** Programa Minha Casa Minha Vida (PMCVC). (Source: Ministry of Finance, 2010, p. 59)

internal market. The two main planks of the strategy were the Growth Acceleration Programme (PAC, Programa de Aceleração do Crescimento), created in 2007, and the My House My life Programme (PMCMV, Programa Minha Casa, Minha Vida), the Brazilian government housing programme to finance building, inaugurated in 2009. Figure 1 shows the impact of the PMCMV on the volume of new house building.

These two stimuli to economic growth have made a significant contribution to Brazil's continued growth during the global economic crisis, but they have ALSO had a considerable impact on urban sustainability.

The progress of contemporary society is not being matched by appropriate changes to build the material basis needed for sustainability. The process of urbanisation in Brazilian cities is fragmented and gives priority "to making room for cars and the growth of real estate capital, while neglecting the essence of the modern condition, which is to provide for man's basic needs" (Somekh, 2010, p. 13).

The Observatório das Metrópoles (Metropolitan Observatory, part of Brazil's National Institute of Science and Technology, INCT) has developed an index of urban well-being (the IBEU), based on three indicators:

(1) Quality of public services,
(2) Housing conditions,
(3) Urban mobility.

In 2009, the Recife Metropolitan Region (RMR) had the second worst IBEU in the country (INCT, 2010).

Urban mobility is a major contributor to low indices of urban well-being. A study by IPEA (2013a, 2013b), carried out by Pereira and Schwanen (2013), analysed data from the National Household Sampling Survey (PNAD) between 1992 and 2009. The study showed that the average journey time from home to work is greater in major Brazilian cities than in comparable conurbations in other countries with over 2 million inhabitants. In São Paulo and Rio de Janeiro, the journey to work takes 31% longer. The data shows that urban transport has worsened in the major Brazilian conurbations since 1992, resulting in increased journey times. This seems to be linked to a combination of factors, including population growth, increased urban areas, higher vehicle numbers, and levels of congestion. This was one of the main reasons around 2 million people took to the streets in June 2013 to demand improved mobility.

The next section discusses the ways the RMR has been affected by this development model, taking its history into account as well as its specific geographical and environmental characteristics.

## The Case of Recife, Brazil

Recife is a coastal city in the northeast of Brazil with 1,537,704 inhabitants (IBGE, 2011, p. 36). It was founded in 1,537 and its principal role was as a commercial port to transfer sugarcane production to the European market of the time. This was colonisation based on the exploitation and export of natural resources, and the city developed within that model.

Deforestation, land reclamation, mineral extraction, and cutting into hillsides for construction, together with the intensive and persistent process of land use and appropriation for the city, radically transformed and defined its current aspect. Recife's high level of inequality can be seen in the many favelas that form part of its urban fabric. Such settlements doubled between 1975 and 1990, when they made up 15% of the urban land area and 26% of the built-up area, containing around 56% of the city's dwellings (Souza, 1990 *apud* Souza, 2007).

Recife's flat topography and location at sea level, the occupation of hills through cutting away their slopes, land reclamation in mangrove areas and floodplains, inadequate drainage networks, and the precariousness of maintenance and operational services have combine to make the city one of the most vulnerable, especially to flooding and to the increasing sea level. The low income population is most vulnerable because they live on low-lying land, so they would be the first to be affected. In periods of high rainfall the city's roads and drainage systems enter a state of collapse, providing an indication of what may happen in the future.

In the RMR, the low priority given to public transport affects the movement of around 2.3 million people. Journeys to work take longer than in New York, Tokyo, and Paris. (Diário de Pernambuco, 2013; IPEA, 2013a, 2013b) The Sistema Estrutural Integrado (SEI, Integrated Structural System), transport model in Pernambuco, which aims to integrate the travelling public's daily movements, is rendered ineffective by the lack of coordinated traffic flow. The high number of cars on the roadsresults in scheduled buses being unable to fulfil their journeys, with a loss of almost 30% of timetabled buses per day. The lack of bus lanes is an important factor, with less than 10% of dedicated coverage. In real terms this means that of 560 km of roads used by buses, there are only 35 km with bus lanes. The Empresa Metroplitana (EM) which runs 10% of the RMR's public transport, records a loss of 150 journeys per day due to traffic jams. As a result of the ongoing public transport issues there is an annual R$30 billion shortfall due to reduced demand. This has a detrimental effect on the SEI who has responsibility for transporting 900 thousand passengers or 40% of all journeys within the RMR. The Greater Recife Transport Consortium estimates that IN 2011, 184 thousand journeys were lost, in 2012 this figure increased to 216 thousand; in 2013 till June, 114 thousand journeys were lost (Jornal do Comércio, Cadernos Cidades, Recife, 15.09.2013).

This scenario is representative of the mobility situation in Recife and its poor state. The political strategy seems to be focussed on car users and this areas' expected growth through mobility projects such as the Via Mangue. Although this may help private traffic congestion by providing alternative routes it does little to specifically address the public transport issue, the economic and environmental impacts on the bus companies and commuters, and the overall experience of moving across the city.

## Large Projects in the RMR

Against the background of environmental vulnerability, the RMR has hosted a number of large-scale projects. The biggest of these, the Suape port complex (CPIS), began more than 30 years ago to the south of the RMR, but the pace of activity has picked up sharply since 2000. The current level of investment is around US$17 billion, with more than 100 ventures already running and another 35 being set up. A petrol refinery, three petrochemical plants, and the largest dockyard in the southern hemisphere are currently all being built there. To the north of the RMR, projects currently being implemented include a Fiat car plant, the Hemobrás blood derivatives factory, and new hospitals, some large-scale, to make up a pharma-chemical agglomeration.

In order to stimulate the growth of the RMR to the west, the "Cidade da Copa" is being built through a public-private partnership with Norberto Odebrecht Construction to host part of the World Cup in 2014. To improve links between these three areas of development a major road-building scheme is being carried out, the "Arco Viário Metropolitano"; that includes several complementary schemes to increase capacity in the road system (CONDEPE/FIDEM, 2010).

## The SUAPE Industrial Port Complex

The Port of Suape was located in an area of high ecological significance and beautiful landscape, and the scale and pace of development there have provoked considerable controversy. In 1975, a group of scientists published a manifesto outlining the dangers of modifying the landscape and environment by building a port and industrial complex on such a scale. This manifesto emphasised the long-term social costs and the fact that the project's own studies had chronically underestimated "the importance of the environment, natural landscape, ecological balance, and the immeasurable richness that Suape represents for Pernambuco" (Cavalcanti, 2008, p. 16). This advocacy for urban sustainability was roundly criticised by the media as well as the government.[2] In a country that needs economic growth it is easy to justify any large project on the basis of economic development and as a way of combating poverty.

Today it is clear that the predicted jobs for local residents were never created, because investment in training for local workers was inadequate. Workers from other states currently migrate to work in the port and its associated industries. Nor were the recommendations and conclusions of the environmental studies carried out during the planning application put into practice. The damage caused by construction (removal of mangroves, dredging, and land reclamation) were not compensated for at other locations as agreed. Measures intended to maximise positive impacts were not carried out, nor were measures to mitigate negative impacts. As a result, few positive steps were taken overall to preserve environmental quality in the Suape Port area (de Almeida, 2003). Indeed, the Suape Industrial Port Complex received an R$2.5 million fine in 2013 when it was proved that its activities were destroying fisheries (Globo G1, 2013). The presence of the port stimulated other large-scale projects in housing and tourism, such as the Mobility Residential Project Paiva Beach Complex, resorts, and other tourism projects.

## Urban Mobility Projects

With a view to improving mobility in the RMR, works have been planned to create bus lanes and build viaducts.[3] Most of these will be funded by PAC Mobility (Growth Acceleration Programme), which has allocated approximately R$2.9 billion for Recife. The majority of the projects being implemented favour individual transport, such as the 5.1-km Via Mangue. This a major municipal project in Recife that aims to improve primarily private traffic flow by building large trunk roads above the Pina mangroves. Five low-income communities along the route are being re housed in verticalised housing projects. The cost is about R$433 million, which means the cost per kilometre is very high at R$85 million.[4]

---

[2]    Moura Cavalcanti, then state governor, declared: "I will not allow the subtleties of landscape... to take precedence over empty stomachs (Jornal da Cidade, 1975 *apud* Cavalcanti, 2008, p. 12).

[3]    Bus Rapid Transport (BRT North-South), BRT East-West, the Via Mangue, the East-West Caxangá Corridor, expansion of the international airport and the maritime terminal.

[4]    The Habitat-UN document "ESTADO DE LAS CIUDADES DE AMÉRICA LATINA Y EL CARIBE 2012: Rumbo a una nueva transición urbana" (Cities in Latin America and the Caribbean in 2012: towards a new urban transition) includes a photo of Recife on the cover showing the contrast between the buildings in the background and the Pina mangroves, where the Via Mangue will be built.

The most controversial of these projects involves building four viaducts to cross the city's main ring road, the. Agamenon Magalhães. The stated aim of the project is to improve traffic flow along this key avenue; however there are no known studies of the impact on the roads the viaducts will feed, which are already filled to capacity. What is more, if the number of cars continues to increase at the current rate, these viaducts will exceed capacity within five years. The benefits in terms of mobility appear SMALL when set against the impacts on local communities, maintaining cultural identity, public safety, and the urban landscape.

As a result of pressure from civil society, as well as the chaos that would potentially arise during the 2014 World Cup if the works had not been completed on time, Pernambuco's state government has called a halt to the project, albeit temporarily.

## Cidade da Copa (World Cup City)

Alongside the big building projects associated with the Port of Suape, several more have resulted from the selection of Recife as one of the hosts of the 2014 FIFA World Cup. Major cultural or sporting events are expected to bring urban renewal, where new urban projects are built to replace precarious or inadequate existing infrastructure. It is also expected that the influx of people and goods will bring new business to the city. However, the historical pattern seen throughout the world generally necessitates legislative change. The physical investment and urban improvements notwithstanding, such events are often associated with legal concessions allowing the occupation of environmentally protected areas and changes to land use and occupation. This results in large changes in the urban environment (Greene, 2003; Lungo, 2004; Smolka & Mullahy, 2007).

To the west of the RMR, a large multi-use area is being built to host this mega event, including the stadium itself (Arena Pernambuco), the Smart City (a planned residential district), and a major hospital, together with various projects to improve mobility. The private sector is also planning, negotiating, and implementing large-scale investment throughout the city, in some cases in partnership with the State of Pernambuco, including more residential districts, parks, hotels, marinas, and large-scale sporting facilities. The Cidade da Copa Smart City is described as the first ever example in Latin America of a suburb "... planned and conceived throughout in conjunction with high technology. The project promotes security and environmental sustainability. It balances urban development with the presence of natural resources".[5] This is a typical example of projects that could only be made possible by changing the city's planning and environmental legislation, which will in turn tend to threaten the sustainability of the peri-urban area of the RMR. The project will alter the socio-spatial reality of this place and neighbouring areas. An area formerly defined as being of social interest, earmarked for social housing projects, was rezoned to allow densities best suited for upper middle class and high income residents (INCT, 2012).

---

[5]   http://www.odebrechtnacopa.com.br/cidadedacopa/, the official Odebrecht site for Cidade da Copa.

Numerous incidents have been reported in several Brazilian cities where individual rights have also been violated and local residents expelled, to carry out works related to the 2014 World Cup (Amorim, 2013; Comitês Populares da Copa, 2013; INCT, 2012; ONU, 2011; Amorim, 2013).

## Other Property Development Projects

Apart from these projects directly linked to the Port of Suape or the 2014 World Cup, the RMR's trend to property growth is reinforced by unrelated projects. Experts and other social groups have objected to the changes in the city's landscape and the excessive verticalisation the new legislation permits. One of the consequences is that the buildings are now so high that at the beginning of the afternoon the city's main beach, Boa Viagem, is no longer reached by the sun. Two examples are the pair of tower blocks built in a spot with one of the best views in the city, known as the "Twin Towers," and the Projeto Novo Recife (New Recife Project), a complex of 13 tower blocks for residential use, hotels, business, culture and leisure. The latter will constitute a massive COLLECTION of buildings, EACH forty storey's high. The likely impact of such a project has led the public and some public institutions to resist it on the grounds that it will reduce ventilation in other areas, privatise one of the city's most attractive views, adversely affect urban infrastructure and mobility, and ruin the landscape of the place. The "Occupy Estelita" campaign involved three day-long gatherings of citizens at the site to protest, in an attempt to influence decisions concerning the production of space in their city.

Some researchers, for instance Lapa (2011), warn that planned districts (like the Cidade da Copa) will do nothing to mitigate Recife's excessive density, arguing that its growth should be primarily based on revitalising neglected central areas, and secondarily by creating new centres. Furthermore, Lapa considers that the system of public-private partnerships that made projects such as the Cidade da Copa possible may leave the public authorities hostage to the strength and power of real estate capital.

With regard to the public authorities, it can be seen that changes made to planning legislation that allows such projects have weakened protections for biodiversity, landscape, and natural and cultural heritage, making them incapable of effectively conserving "places of memory and collective identity" (Lapa, 2011, p. 46). Moreover, the majority of the population is unaware that such legislative changes have been made; or they may be accepted on the basis of the argument that jobs will be created and tax revenues will increase. The planning permission and enforcement processes lack structure and institutional strength, quite apart from actual distortion by political and economic interference. The city is receptive to economic growth in the form of property development which means in practice there is "a tacit agreement between property developers and public administrators based on the argument that a significant contribution will be made to job creation and increasing local government revenues" (Lapa, 2011, p. 46). Furthermore, this type of growth may be seen as a double-edged sword where economic development is created through a profusion of commercial and service activity that brings material wealth and dynamism to the city, but the quality of the new infrastructure is compromised, particularly in environmental terms. Additionally the city's cultural and natural heritages lose their character, as do the spaces in which the population goes about its daily life. As a result, vulnerability is increased both in socio-cultural terms and in relation to the physical and natural environment.

To sum up, there is a real possibility that Recife is withdrawing from the paradigm of sustainability. The population is largely unaware of the city's Master Plan, so no pressure is exerted by civil society to demand its implementation. On the other hand, urban projects are not properly discussed with society, on the grounds of getting things done quickly. As a result, the knock-on effects of these projects are not brought to light. In many cases, the information given to experts, the university sector, and the population itself is more akin to marketing material than proper technical documents. This makes it hard for society to evaluate such projects.

## Conclusion

The process of urbanisation in Brazilian society has not produced sustainable cities, and the country's major cities are characterised by serious economic and social inequality. They also suffer from problems associated with the disappearance of living urban and peri-urban structures that are of strategic importance for their continued existence, as well as from further environmental imbalances caused by an excess of by-products, atmospheric emissions, and waste.

The model of development in place in Brazil during the previous decade (2001–2010) led to a series of gains in economic and social terms, but since it was not that different from the existing model, it seems like "more of the same," aggravating environmental and social problems in cities. This is an obstacle to their sustainability, particularly as regards the major civil engineering projects that underpin the current growth of the RMR, creating pressure on urban land and a mobility crisis, above all in cities getting ready for sporting mega-events such as the 2014 World Cup and the 2016 Olympic Games.

The case of RMR demonstrates that although such projects help to reduce poverty, the major works associated with Pernambuco's recent upsurge in growth have a substantial negative impact on the environment, on local communities and on the quality of life in the city. In the case of the Suape port complex, many families have been relocated without new dwellings being ready for them on time, and this still continues to occur. (Movimento Ecossocialista de PE, 2012a, 2012b, 2012c). Rural and riverside communities were moved to apartments in urban areas, a typology completely foreign to their *modus vivendi*, showing flagrant lack of respect for their identity and culture. For example in Abençoada por Deus, Recife (Alcântara, 2011; Alcântara & Monteiro, 2010, 2011), when residents were removed with minimal compensation to allow mobility and drainage works in the

F. Furtado et al.
Is Urban Sustainability Possible? The Case of Recife, Brazil

255

community of the Coque, Recife (Coque Vive, 2013), and also to allow works for the 2014 World Cup in São Lourenço da Mata and other cities (Amorim, 2013; Comitês Populares da Copa, 2013; INCT, 2012; ONU, 2011; Portal2014, 2012).

The Suape complex has brought a series of negative consequences, such as soil displacement, the eradication of vegetation, removal of mangroves, relocation of communities, undermining the local culture, and a potential for pollution that places local ecosystems at risk and compromises environmental services and the landscape of the place.

Large road-building and housing projects, including those associated with mega-events, are causing the destruction of permeable urban areas, particularly green areas, as well as altering microclimates and reducing natural drainage. Indices for green areas calculated by the Pelópidas Silveira Institute show a percentage of 12.5%, half the 25% stipulated by planning law (Instituto Pelópidas Silveira, 2013). As a result, there is an increase both in runoff from water that is no longer absorbed by the ground, and in local temperatures, which would be reduced by vegetation if it were present. This leads to hot spots which make outdoor activities difficult at times when the sun is most intense, with increases between 7 °C and 9 °C caused by the absence of vegetation and higher building density (Barros & Lombardo, 2012; Moreira & Galvíncio, 2007; Moreira & Nóbrega, 2011; Oliveira et al., 2011). In Recife, the reduction of natural drainage causes major problems through flooding, landslides, and by aggravating mobility problems (a vicious circle).[6] From a spatial point of view, such projects increase pressure on urban land prices, leading in turn to excessive verticalisation and building density. Recife is 21st in the world ranking for cities with tall buildings, and it is the third most highly verticalised city in Brazil, second only to São Paulo and Rio de Janeiro (Diário de Pernambuco, 2011). All this undermines the balance of the city's morphology and structure, as well as aggravating its existing socio-spatial inequality.

This scenario, for all the reasons above, suggests that it is very difficult for the RMR to achieve sustainability. The one positive factor is that to some extent poverty and social inequality can be shown to have actually reduced during the current cycle of growth, and can be argued that it has the potential to make the city more sustainable at least in that respect. However, the spatial implications of inequality itself harm the environmental balance of the RMR, reducing its political and social sustainability. The true threat to the city's sustainability is thus not only economic in nature; it is above all a problem of *governance*, as shown in the choice of an environmentally erroneous model of urban development in association with a form of planning and urban administration divorced from collective interests. Recife has seen a number of protests and demonstrations in defense of the common good and public spaces, including legal action against the previous mayor with a view to building a city focussed on the needs of its people (Alcântara et al., 2013). Nonetheless, there are 28 high-impact projects awaiting approval by Recife's Urban

---

[6]    Traffic in Recife has increased almost threefold over 22 years, with 64% of this attributable to cars. (DETRAN, 2012) It is estimated that if the annual growth rate of 7 % is maintained, the number of cars will double by 2020.

Development Council (Conselho de Desenvolvimento Urbano, CDU) which has recently been moved from the Urban Planning Secretariat to Urban Control and Mobility. This is a telling sign of the weak link between the city's development and any planning process. Rather than a longer-term vision, the city is conceived in a fragmented way with a focus on making individual projects happen.

The sustainability of the RMR depends on major changes in the city's planning process whereby economic growth can go hand in hand with quality of life while preserving its environmental and cultural heritage. The most worrying aspect is the process by which decisions affecting the city's future are made, with little concern for the environment and little transparency or accountability, contrary to the legal requirements of the Cities Statute and the Brazilian constitution itself. (Amorim, 2013; Comitês Populares da Copa, 2013; ONU, 2011).

Such changes should include urgent, extremely short-term measures for environment conservation, and longer-term measures to improve the quality of municipal governance. The first group of measures must include:

- Greater concern for the environment when it comes to mobility and emissions, giving priority to non-motorised journeys and making them viable, or also public transport with clean technology;
- Guaranteeing the protection and conservation of the city's living structures, maintaining ground permeability to reduce runoff and increasing non-built-up areas;
- Social policies to promote citizenship through the preservation of the city's memory and culture and an environmentally appropriate approach.

The changes needed to improve the city's governance should guarantee that:

- The planning process considers the short, medium, and long term without making concessions to the very short-term interests underlying the corporate decisions of the civil construction sector in Pernambuco;
- Planning is protected against political and economic management failures and is guided by collective interests;
- New mechanisms must be created to allow society to participate in choosing the city's future course, going far beyond the current system of councils, committees, and participatory budgets, which are at the mercy of political failures of management and even party political manipulation;
- Planning must become more transparent, which will mean changing existing government planning mechanisms to ensure they are widely disseminated and can be easily read and understand by ordinary citizens;
- The process should include monitoring mechanisms to convert the administration's objectives into goals whose fulfilment can be easily checked by society;
- Society should be informed of the outcome of the decisions taken and their consequences.

F. Furtado et al.
Is Urban Sustainability Possible? The Case of Recife, Brazil

257

All this will require considerable effort, which depends on more than political will and government action: the population must mobilise and organise, in awareness of the part played in the broader context of a worldwide project by Recife's transformation to become more sustainable and resilient. It is still too soon to assess the recent demonstrations that brought the people onto the streets; but they have already led to rapid changes and show clear evidence of popular empowerment or at any rate, signs that something significant is happening in Brazil.

# References

Alcântara, E. (2011). *Solidariedade em Comunidades de Baixa Renda: Análise das práticas cotidianas e da relação com o lugar a partir do sistema da dádiva* [Solidarity in low income communities: Analysis of daily practices and the relationship with the place from the donation system] (Unpublished doctoral dissertation). Universidade Federal de Pernambuco, Recife, Brazil.

Alcântara, E., Beech, T., Furtado, F., Lancellotti, A., & Cazuza, L. (2013). Cyberactivism in the struggle for more sustainable cities – a resource for urban social resilience? *Annals. AESOP-ACSP Joint Congress*. 15–19 July 2013, Dublin.

Alcântara, E., & Monteiro, C. (2010). *Em que a vida na favela é melhor do que em um conjunto de apartamentos? O Caso de Abençoada por Deus, Recife* [CD-ROM]. In Encontro Nacional da Associação Nacional de Pós-Graduação d Pesquisa em Ambiente e Sociedade, 5. Anais. Florianópolis: UFSC. 1–13.

Alcântara, E., & Monteiro, C. (2011). *Valores Culturais e Possibilidades na Produção do Lugar: O caso de Abençoada por Deus, Recife* [CD-ROM]. In Encontro da Associação Nacional de Pós-Graduação e Pesquisa em Planejamento Urbano e Regional Integração Sul-Americana, Fronteiras e Desenvolvimento Urbano e Regional, 15, Anais. Rio de Janeiro, 1–20.

Amorim, E. (2013). *Mais de 2.000 famílias são removidas por obras da Copa em PE*. Retrieved from http://esportes.terra.com.br/futebol/copa-2014/mais-de-2000-familias-sao-removidas-por-obras-da-copa-em-pe,4cfb2688e59b0410VgnVCM4000009bcceb0aRCRD.html

Barros, H. R., & Lombardo, M. A. (2012). A relação entre ilhas de calor urbana, ocupação do solo e morfologia urbana na cidade do Recife. *Revista Geonorte, Edição Especial 2*, 2(5), 65–76.

Cavalcanti. (2008). *Desenvolvimento a todo custo e a dimensão ambiental: O conflito do complexo industrial-portuário de Suape, Pernambuco*. Retrieved from http://www.unicap.br/humanitas/wp-content/uploads/2010/06/Cl%C3%B3vis-Final3.pdf

Comitês Populares da Copa. (2013). *Megaeventos e Violações de Direitos Humanos no Brasil. Dossie da Articulação Nacional dos Comitês Populares da Copa*. Retrieved from http://www.google.com.br/url?sa=t&rct=j&q=&esrc=s&source=web&cd=7&ved=0CGEQFjAG&url=http%3A%2F%2Fwww.apublica.org%2Fwp-content%2Fuploads%2F2012%2F01%2FDossieViolacoesCopa.pdf&ei=kjE3UrPTPITk8gTgioDQCQ&usg=AFQjCNH7LxxwCxivFtd40-rvSaqE6UgPsg&sig2=umGgHB14LCPk-L9SNCG7Tw&bvm=bv.52164340,d.eWU

CONDEPE/FIDEM. Governo de Pernambuco. Secretaria de Planejamento e Gestão. (2010). *Oeste Metropolitano Diagnóstico para o Desenvolvimento Sustentável. Recife*. Retrieved from http://www.ajaconsultoria.com.br/pdf/produto4.pdf

Coque Vive. (2013). *Despejo #3*. Retrieved from http://vimeo.com/73375864

de Almeida, L. P. (2003). *Análise da Efetividade dos Estudos Ambientais: O Caso do Complexo Industrial Portuário de Suape* [Analysis of the effectiveness of environmental studies: The case of the SUAPE industrial port complex] (master dissertation). Universidade Federal de Pernambuco, Recife, Brazil. Retrieved from http://www.liber.ufpe.br/teses/arquivo/20041109154947.pdf.

DETRAN. (2012). Retrieved from http://www.detran.pe.gov.br/index.php?option=com_content &view=article&id=36&Itemid=72

Diário de Pernambuco. (2011). *Uma cidade verticalizada. Recife esté em 21 lugar no ranking mundial de edifícios de grande porte. No país, fica atrás apenas de SP e RJ* [A vertical city. Recife is 21st in the world ranking of large buildings. In the country, behind only the SP and RJ]. Retrieved from http://www.skyscrapercity.com/showthread.php?t=1318895 and http://www.vermelho.org.br/pe/ noticia.php?id_noticia=147146&id_secao=91

Diário de Pernambuco. (2013). *Recife entre as capitais com maior tempo de deslocamento de casa para o trabalho.* Retrieved from http://blogs.diariodepernambuco.com.br/mobilidadeurbana/2013/ 03/recife-entre-as-capitais-com-maior-tempo-de-deslocamento-de-casa-para-o-trabalho/

Globo G1. (2013). *CPRH multa Complexo de Suape em R$ 2,5 milhões por crime ambiental.* Retrieved from http://g1.globo.com/pernambuco/noticia/2013/09/cprh-multa-complexo-de-suape-em-r-25-milhoes-por-crime-ambiental.html

Greene, S. J. (2003). Staged cities: Mega-events, slum clearance, and global capital. *Yale Human Rights and Development Law Journal, 6,* 161–187.

IBGE. (2011). *Censo Demográfico 2010. Sinopse do Censo e Resultados Preliminares do Universo* [Population census 2010. Synopsis of the census and preliminary results]. Retrieved from http:// www.ibge.gov.br/home/presidencia/noticias/imprensa/ppts/0000000402.pdf

INCT Observatório das Metrópoles Núcleo Recife. (2010). *IBEU – Índice de Bem-Estar Urbano. Ribeiro, L. C. Q. (coord.). Instituto NacionaL de Ciência e Tecnologia (INCT), FINEP, UFPE, MDU.* Retrieved from http://www.google.com.br/url?sa=t&rct=j&q=&esrc=s&source=web&cd= 2&ved=0CDEQFjAB&url=http%3A%2F%2Fwww.observatoriodasmetropoles.net%2Fdownload%2 Findice_bem_estar_urbano.pdf&ei=t_Q2Upe6NY7Y8gTXiYHoDw&usg=AFQjCNHtw9nadrxOK VsP9rH3 DL0aC09Lhw&bvm=bv.52164340,d.eWU

INCT Observatório das Metrópoles Núcleo Recife. (2012). *Projeto Metropolização e Megaeventos: Os impactos da Copa do Mundo 2014 e das Olimpíadas 2016. Relatório Parcial Recife – Abril de 2012. Souza, M. A; Ramalho, A. M. (org). Instituto NacionaL de Ciência e Tecnologia (INCT), FINEP, UFPE, MDU.* Retrieved from http://www.observatoriodasmetropoles.net/download/ Relat_Recife2012.pdf

Instituto Pelópidas Silveira. (2013). *Estudo aponta ilhas de calor no Recife, zonas em que a população pode ter saúde prejudicada.* Jc3.uol. Retrieved from http://jc3.uol.com.br/blogs/blogjamildo/canais/ noticias/2013/05/27/estudo_aponta_ilhas_de_calor_no_recife_zonas_em_que_a_populacao_pode_ ter_saude_prejudicada_152171.php

IPEA. (2013a). *Ricos e pobres perdem cada vez mais tempo no trânsito.* Retrieved from http:// www.ipea.gov.br/portal/index.php?option=com_content&view=article&id=17212

IPEA. (2013b). *IPEA: deslocamento em SP e RJ é 31% mais demorado que outros países.* Retrieved from http://noticias.terra.com.br/brasil/ipea-deslocamento-em-sp-e-rj-e-31-mais-demorado-que-outros-paises,e9d1bc95d467d310VgnCLD2000000ec6eb0aRCRD.html

Lapa, T. A. D. (2011). *Grandes Cidades Constroem-se com Edifícios Grandes?* Editora Universitária UFPE.

Lungo, M. (2004). *Grandes proyectos urbanos: una visión general.* San Salvador: UCA Editores.

Ministry of Finance. (2010). *Economia Brasileira em Perspectiva* [Brazilian economy in perspective]. Retrieved from http://www.fazenda.gov.br/divulgacao/publicacoes/economia-brasileira-em-perspectiva/economia_brasileira_em_perspectiva_pt_ed3_jan2010.pdf

F. Furtado et al.
Is Urban Sustainability Possible? The Case of Recife, Brazil

**259**

Moreira, E. B. M., & Galvíncio, J. D. (2007). Espacialização das Temperaturas à Superfície na Cidade do Recife, utilizando Imagens TM - Landsat 7. *Revista de Geografia, 24*(3), 101–115. Retrieved from http://www.revista.ufpe.br/revistageografia/index.php/revista/article/viewFile/150/98

Moreira, E. B. M., & Nóbrega, R. S. (2011). Identificação do fenômeno ilhas de calor na área urbana do Recife-PE, através do canal infravermelho termal do satélite landsat 5. In *Annals. XV Simpósio Brasileiro de Sensoriamento Remoto - SBSR, Curitiba, PR, Brasil* (pp. 1–8). Retrieved from http://www.dsr.inpe.br/sbsr2011/files/p1164.pdf

Movimento Ecossocialista de PE. (2012a). *Fórum Suape Espaço Socioambiental. Remoção dos posseiros do Engenho Tiriri em SUAPE (Cabo de Santo Agostinho – PE) – Parte 08.* Retrieved from http://forumsuape.ning.com/video/remo-o-dos-posseiros-do-engenho-tiriri-em-suape-cabo-de-santo-7

Movimento Ecossocialista de PE. (2012b). *Fórum Suape Espaço Socioambiental. Remoção dos posseiros do Engenho Tiriri em SUAPE (Cabo de Santo Agostinho – PE).* Retrieved from http://www.youtube.com/watch?v=I0OjfVyaYzY

Movimento Ecossocialista de PE. (2012c). *Remoção dos posseiros do Engenho Tiriri em SUAPE (Cabo de Santo Agostinho – PE) – Parte 06.* Retrieved from http://www.mespe.com.br/video/remo-o-dos-posseiros-do-engenho-tiriri-em-suape-cabo-de-santo-5

Oliveira, J. C. F., Oliveira, T. H., & Galvíncio, J. D. (2011). Análise Espaço-Temporal da Cobertura Vegetal através do IVDN no Bairro de Boa Viagem, Recife-PE e Entorno. *Revista Brasileira de Geografia Física, 3*, 575–588. Retrieved from http://www.revista.ufpe.br/rbgfe/index.php/revista/article/viewFile/223/192

ONU. (2011). *Copa 2014, Olimpíadas 2016 e Megaprojetos – Remoções em Curso No Brasil.* Retrieved from http://www.google.com.br/url?sa=t&rct=j&q=&esrc=s&source=web&cd=3&ved=0CDwQFjAC&url=http%3A%2F%2Fwww.rets.org.br%2Fsites%2Fdefault%2Ffiles%2Fdossie-relatoria-remoc3a7c3b5es-megaeventos-brasil-2011.pdf&ei=kjE3UrPTPITk8gTgioDQCQ&usg=AFQjCNGJrOhjM5DpBSqmnrdREjgcl6zWZw&sig2=j32pus13hVBfQehadyGvrw&bvm=bv.52164340,d.eWU

ONU-Habitat. (2012). *Estado de las ciudades de América Latina y el Caribe 2012: Rumbo a una nueva transición urbana.* Nairobi. Retrieved from http://www.onuhabitat.org/index.php?option=com_docman&task=cat_view&gid=362&Itemid=18

Pereira, R. H. M., & Schwanen, T. (2013). *Tempo de Deslocamento Casa-Trabalho no Brasil (1992-2009): Diferenças entre regiões metropolitanas, níveis de renda e sexo.* Rio de Janeiro, Brazil: IPEA. Retrieved from http://www.mobilize.org.br/midias/pesquisas/tempo-de-deslocamento-casa-trabalho-no-brasil.pdf

PNAD. (2009). *Pesquisa Nacional por Amostra Domiciliar realizada pelo IBGE.* Retrieved from http://www.ibge.gov.br/home/estatistica/populacao/trabalhoerendimento/pnad2009/pnad_sintese_2009.pdf

Portal2014. (2012). *Governo inicia desapropriação para obra viária da Arena Pernambuco. Processo irá remover 120 imóveis no bairro da Várzea, na zona oeste do Recife.* Retrieved from http://www.portal2014.org.br/noticias/10088/GOVERNO+INICIA+DESAPROPRIACAO+PARA+OBRA+VIARIA+DA+ARENA+PERNAMBUCO.html

Ribeiro, L. C. Q. (2012). *Brasil urbano: Continuidade ou transição do modelo de desenvolvimento?* Retrieved from http://observatoriodasmetropoles.net/index.php?option=com_k2&view=item&id=382%3Abrasil-urbano-continuidade-ou-transi%C3%A7%C3%A3o-do-modelo-de-desenvolvimento%3F&Itemid=164&lang=pt

Rodrigues, J. M. (2012). *Metrópoles em Números. Crescimento da frota de automóveis e motocicletas nas metrópoles brasileiras INTC. Observatório das Metrópoles. 2001/2011.* Retrieved from http://www.google.com.br/url?sa=t&rct=j&q=&esrc=s&source=web&cd=2&ved=0CDEQFjAB&url=http%3A%2F%2Fobservatoriodasmetropoles.net%2Fdownload%2Frelatorio_automotos.pdf&ei=G_w2UrqQG4bI9gTg7YCoBA&usg=AFQjCNFPMnDPbxRY0NlCwr7KfcDDqQHn0A&bvm=bv.52164340,d.eWU

Smolka, M., & Mullahy, L. (2007). Una década de cambios: retrospectiva del Programa para América Latina y el Caribe. In M. Smolka, & L. Mullahy (org.), *Perspectivas urbanas: temas críticos em políticas del suelo em América Latina*. Cambridge, MA: Lincoln Institute of Land Policy.

Somekh, N. (2010). Apresentação [Presentation]. In F. Ascher (Ed.), *Os novos princípios do urbanismo*. São Paulo, Brazil: Romano Guerra.

Souza, M. A. A. (2007). *Política habitacional para os excluídos: O caso da Região Metropolitana do Recife. Habitare. Coleção 7. Capítulo 4*. Retrieved from http://www.habitare.org.br/pdf/publicacoes/arquivos/colecao7/capitulo_4.pdf

# Authors

**Dr. Edinéa Alcântara**
Urban Development Programme (MDU)
LEPUR
Universidade Federal de Pernambuco
Brazil
edinealcantara@gmail.com

**Dr. Onilda Bezerra**
Lecturer at the Architecture and
Urbanism Department
Universidade Federal de Pernambuco
Brazil
onibezerra@yahoo.com.br

**Prof. Vera Helena Moro Bins Ely**
Professor at the Architecture and Urban
Design Department
Federal University of Santa Catarina
Florianopolis
Brazil
Tel. +55 483721-4059
vera.binsely@gmail.com

**Sofia Arrias Bittencourt**
Undergraduate architecture and urban
design student
Federal University of Santa Catarina
Florianopolis
Brazil
Tel. +55 483209-2446
sofia.ab@gmail.com

**Dr. Lineu Castello**
Federal University Rio Grande do Sul
(UFRGS)
UniRitter-Mackenzie Universities
CNPq (Brazilian National Research
Council)
Rua Marquês de Pombal 1385/201
Porto Alegre

CEP: 90540-001
Brazil
Tel. +55 51 9996-7615
Fax +55 51 3342-1572
lincastello@terra.com.br

**Simon Chun Kwan Chui**
University of Melbourne
Level 2, 33 Lincoln Square South
Building 223
Carlton South 3053
Victoria
Australia
Tel. +61 3 8344-4000 ext. 57558
Fax +61 3 8344-5532
schui@student.unimelb.edu.au

**Daniel de Carvalho Moreira**
School of Civil Engineering
Architecture and Urban Design
University of Campinas (UNICAMP)
Campinas SP
Brazil
Tel. +55 019 3521-2920
damore@fec.unicamp.br

**Dr. Renato Tibiriçá de Saboya**
Professor at the Architecture and Urban
Design Department
Federal University of Santa Catarina
Florianopolis
Brazil
Tel. +55 483721-3721-4860
rtsaboya@gmail.com

**Marcella S. Deliberador**
School of Civil Engineering
Architecture and Urban Design
University of Campinas (UNICAMP)
Campinas SP
Brazil

Tel. +55 019 99140-0230
marcelladeliberador@yahoo.com.br

**Dr. Edward Edgerton**
School of Social Sciences
Psychology Division
University of West Scotland
High Street, Paisley
PA1 2BE
Scotland, UK
Tel. +44 141 848-3799
edward.edgerton@uws.ac.uk

**Prof. Fátima Furtado**
Associated Professor
Planning Studies (DPU/UCL)
MDU/UFPE
Laboratory of Peri-urban Studies
LEPUR
Brazil
fgfurtado@hotmail.com

**Fernando Giuliani**
Assistant Professor
School of Psychology
Central University of Venezuela
Caracas
Venezuela
Tel. +58 414 251-7846
fernandogiuliani58@gmail.com

**Norhuzailin Hussain**
Department of Landscape Architecture
Faculty of Design and Architecture
Universiti Putra Malaysia
43400 Serdang
Selangor
Malaysia
Tel. +60 38946-4054
zailin@upm.edu.my

**Nathalie Jean-Baptiste**
Department of Urban and Environmental

Sociology
Helmholtz Centre for Environmental
Research – UFZ
Permoserstr. 15
04318 Leipzig Germany
nathalie.jean-baptiste@ufz.de

**Maria Johansson**
Environmental Psychology
Department of Architecture and Built
Environment
Lund University
P.O. Box 118
SE-221 00 Lund
Sweden
Tel. +46 (0) 46 222-7169
maria.johansson@mpe.lth.se

**Regina John**
School of Urban and Regional Planning,
Ardhi University
Dar es Salaam
Tanzania
Tel. +255 754 398 694
lyakurwa_gina@yahoo.co.uk

**Dr. Anna Jorgensen**
Department of Landscape
The University of Sheffield
The Arts Tower
Western Bank
Sheffield, South Yorkshire
S10 2TN
UK
Tel. +44 (0)11422-20621
a.jorgensen@sheffield.ac.uk

**Sigrun Kabisch**
Department of Urban and Environmental
Sociology
Helmholtz Centre for Environmental
Research – UFZ
Permoserstr. 15
04318 Leipzig

Germany
sigrun.kabisch@ufz.de

**Doris C. C. K. Kowaltowski**
School of Civil Engineering
Architecture and Urban Design
University of Campinas (UNICAMP)
Campinas SP
Brazil
Tel. +55 019 3521-2390
doris@fec.unicamp.br

**Dr. Ray Lucas**
Senior Lecturer
Manchester Architecture
Research Centre (MARC)
School of Environment, Education
and Development
The University of Manchester
Oxford Road
Manchester
M13 9PL
UK
raymond.lucas@manchester.ac.uk

**Dr. Gesine Marquardt**
Head of the Junior Researchers' Group
Architecture Under Demographic Change
Technische Universitaet Dresden
Faculty of Architecture
01062 Dresden
Germany
Tel. +49 (0) 351 463-34724
Fax. +49 (0) 351 463-35578
gesine.marquardt@tu-dresden.de

**Natalia Naoumova**
Architecture and Urban Planning
Department
Federal University of Pelotas
Rua Benjamin Constant 1359
Pelotas
96010-020
Brazil

Tel. +55 53 3284-5500
naoumova@gmail.com

**Marialena Nikolopoulou**
Kent School of Architecture
Centre for Architecture and Sustainable
Environment
University of Kent
CT2 7NR Canterbury, Kent
UK
Tel. + 44 (0) 1227 82-7779
m.nikolopoulou@kent.ac.uk

**Dr. Maria Nordström**
AEM
Swedish University of Agricultural
Sciences/SLU
Box 88
SE-230 53 Alnarp
Sweden
Tel. +46 70 296-8900
maria.i.nordstrom@slu.de

**Eja Pedersen**
Environmental Psychology
Department of Architecture and Built
Environment
Lund University
P.O. Box 118
SE-221 00 Lund
Tel. +46 (0)46 222-3241
eja.pedersen@arkitektur.lth.se

**Paula R. P. Pereira**
School of Civil Engineering,
Architecture and Urban Design
University of Campinas (UNICAMP)
Campinas SP
Brazil
Tel. +55 019 3885-2070
paulapzr@hotmail.com

**Prof. Adriana Portella**
Professor in Architecture and Urbanism
Federal University of Pelotas

Brazil
Tel. +55 53 3303-8423
adrianaportella@yahoo.com.br

**Dr. Louise Ritchie**
Institute of Older Persons' Health
& Wellbeing
University of the West of Scotland
Hamilton
ML3 0JB
Scotland
UK
Tel. +44 169828-3100
louise.ritchie@uws.ac.uk

**Dr. Ombretta Romice**
Senior Lecturer
IAPS Past President
Urban Design Studies Unit
Department of Architecture
University of Strathclyde
Level 3, James Weir Building
75 Montrose Street
Glasgow, G1 1XJ
Scotland, UK
Tel. +44 (0)141 548 3006
ombretta.r.romice@strath.ac.uk

**Euclides Sánchez**
Senior Professor
Institute of Psychology
Central University of Venezuela
Caracas
Venezuela
Tel. +58 414 302-7590
eusanche@gmail.com

**Mariana Colin Stelzner**
Undergraduate architecture and urban
design student
Federal University of Santa Catarina
Florianopolis
Brazil
Tel. +55 483721-4059
marianacolins@gmail.com

**Kevin Thwaites**
Department of Landscape
University of Sheffield
Arts Tower
Western Bank
Sheffield S10 2TN
UK
k.thwaites@sheffield.ac.uk

**Carolina Vasilikou**
Kent School of Architecture
Centre for Architecture and
Sustainable Environment
University of Kent
CT2 7NR
Canterbury, Kent
UK
Tel. +44 0758033-3929
Fax +44 01227 82-4689
kv46@kent.ac.uk

**George Weeks**
111 Knatchbull Road, Flat B
London
SE5 9QU
UK
Tel. +44 07870 45 4655
george.weeks@cantab.net

**Esther Wiesenfeld**
Senior Professor
Institute of Psychology
Central University of Venezuela
Caracas
Venezuela
Tel. +58 414 3322-1183
esther.wiesen@gmail.com

**Sinval Xavier**
Professor in Civil Engineer
Federal University of Rio Grande
Brazil
sinval.xavier@pelotas.com.br
Tel. +55 533303-8423

# Index

# Advances in People-Environment Studies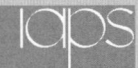

Roderick J. Lawrence, Hulya Turgut, & Peter Kellett (Editors)

# Requalifying the Built Environment
## Challenges and Responses
### Volume 4

2012, x + 234 pp., ISBN 978-0-88937-430-0
US $77.00 / £ 44.00 / € 54.95

**How global change is impacting on the social, physical, and economic structure of cities and their inhabitants**

In recent decades significant financial and professional resources have been invested in urban regeneration, housing renovation, and the revitalization of old neighborhoods, with considerable impacts on the social, physical, and economic structure of cities and their inhabitants.

The first objective of this volume is to present the key issues related to these changes, which were discussed at an international symposium of experts organized by the International Association for People-Environment Studies and Housing and CSBE (Culture and Space in the Built Environment) Network in Istanbul. The second objective is to show how concepts and methods in the field of people-environment studies can be successfully applied to study complex questions related to the revitalization of the built environment.

The contributions in this volume are centered around the following main themes:

- Key issues concerning heritage and cultural identity
- The institutional, economic, and political contexts of revitalization
- Implementation and how to address the key challenges

This volume will be useful to researchers, graduate students, teachers, and professional practitioners in housing design and construction, the maintenance and upgrading of existing buildings and urban areas, conservation management, and the broad field of housing studies.

## Table of Contents:

Hogrefe Publishing
30 Amberwood Parkway · Ashland, OH 44805 · USA
Tel: (800) 228-3749 · Fax: (419) 281-6883
E-Mail: customerservice@hogrefe.com

Hogrefe Publishing
Merkelstr. 3 · 37085 Göttingen · Germany
Tel: +49 551 999 50-0 · Fax: -111
E-Mail: customerservice@hogrefe.de

Hogrefe Publishing c/o Marston Book Services Ltd
160 Eastern Ave., Milton Park · Abingdon, OX14 4SB · UK
Tel: +44 1235 465576 · Fax +44 1235 465555
E-mail: direct.orders@marston.co.uk

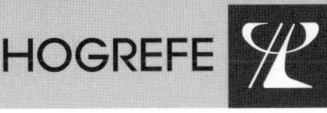 **HOGREFE**

Order online at **www.hogrefe.com**
or call toll-free **(800) 228-3749** (US only)

# Advances in People-Environment Studies IAPS

Sigrun Kabisch, Anna K. Kunath, Petra Schweizer-Ries, & Annett S. Steinführer (Editors)

# Vulnerability, Risks, and Complexity
## Impacts of Global Change on Human Habitats

Volume 3
2012, x + 322 pp., ISBN 978-0-88937-435-5
US $94.00 / £ 54.00 / € 66.95

**State-of-the art research on the interrelations between the social, built, and natural environment**

This volume offers state-of-the-art research on the interrelations between the social, built, and natural environments.

It will be useful to scholars in cross-cutting areas of urban, hazard, planning, governance, and sustainability research in relation to socio-psychological perspectives. Readers will benefit from new theoretical as well as empirically based research findings in the emerging field of social-science vulnerability studies. The contributions in this volume cover six broad research fields:
- Reflections on vulnerability and risks in complex environments
- Coping with climate change and natural hazards
- Social dimensions of vulnerability and risks
- Participation and strategies of risk reduction
- Strengthening pro-environmental behavior
- Place making and urban design

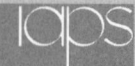

## Table of Contents:

Hogrefe Publishing
30 Amberwood Parkway · Ashland, OH 44805 · USA
Tel: (800) 228-3749 · Fax: (419) 281-6883
E-Mail: customerservice@hogrefe.com

Hogrefe Publishing
Merkelstr. 3 · 37085 Göttingen · Germany
Tel: +49 551 999 50-0 · Fax: -111
E-Mail: customerservice@hogrefe.de

Hogrefe Publishing c/o Marston Book Services Ltd
160 Eastern Ave., Milton Park · Abingdon, OX14 4SB · UK
Tel: +44 1235 465576 · Fax +44 1235 465555
E-mail: direct.orders@marston.co.uk

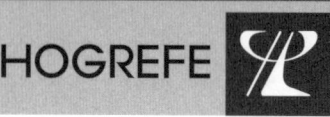

**HOGREFE**

Order online at **www.hogrefe.com**
or call toll-free **(800) 228-3749** (US only)

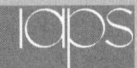
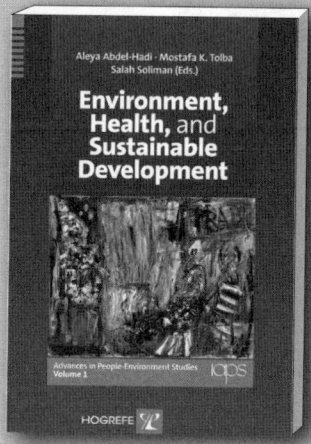
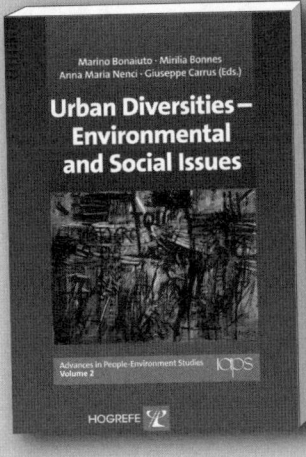
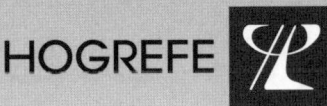

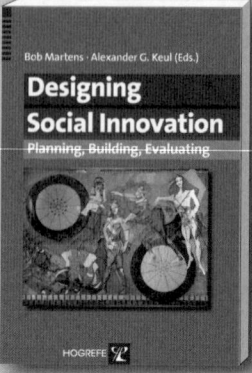
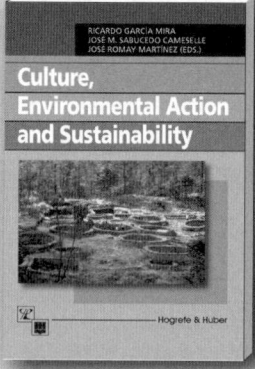
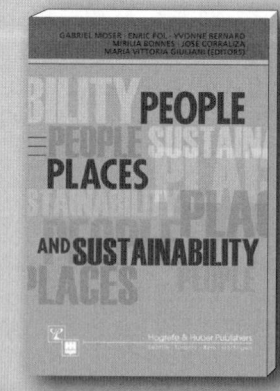
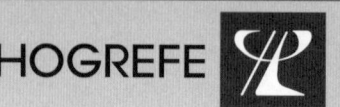

# Towns and Cities in the Future

There are many factors that will influence the appearance of a town or city in the future, such as new economic trends and political attitudes, the introduction of new technologies and changing patterns of population growth. Such ingredients determine whether a town or city will expand or decline and the manner in which it will do so. By understanding the ways in which these factors have operated in the past and are affecting our lives now, town planners are able to anticipate future problems and to design the kind of facilities that will be needed to cater for the living patterns of the future.

In this book a number of towns and cities around the world are examined in order to understand why and how towns and cities might change in the future.

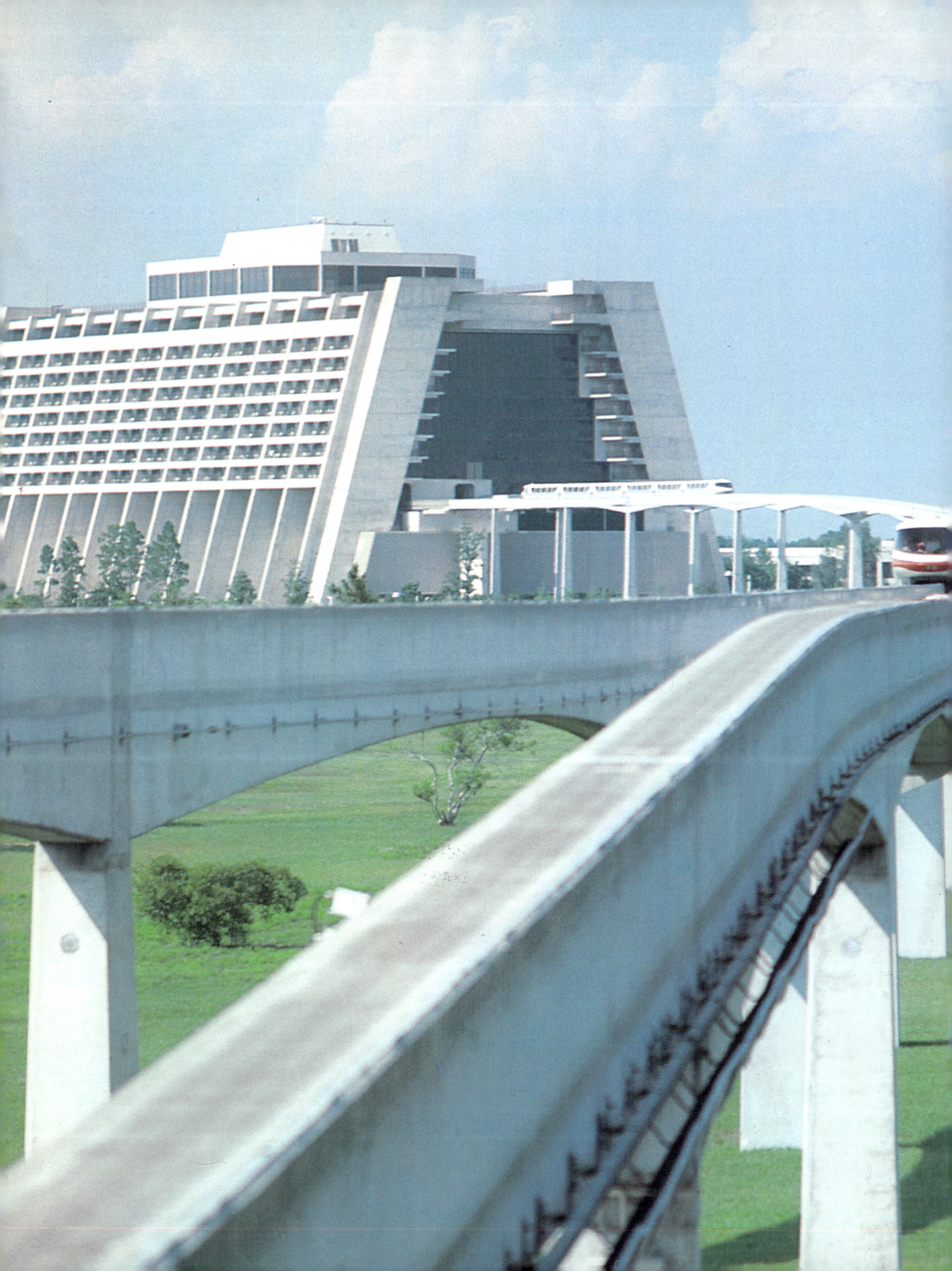

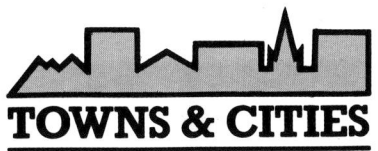

## TOWNS & CITIES

# TOWNS AND CITIES
# IN THE FUTURE

Laurie Bolwell & Cliff Lines

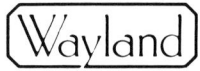

# Towns & Cities

**How Towns Work**
**How Towns Grow and Change**
**Living in Towns**
**Town and City Problems**
**The Parts of a City**
**Towns and Cities of the Past**
**Towns and Cities in the Future**
**Towns and Cities of the World**

**Cover Picture:** Futureworld, Epcot Centre; Orlando, USA.
**Frontispiece picture:** Disneyworld; Florida, USA.

First published in 1986 by
Wayland (Publishers) Ltd
61 Western Road, Hove
East Sussex BN3 1JD, England

© Copyright 1986 Wayland (Publishers) Ltd

**British Library Cataloguing in Publication Data**
Bolwell, L.H.
   Towns and cities in the future.—(Towns &
   cities)
   1. Cities and towns—Juvenile literature
   I. Title    II. Lines, C.J.    III. Series
   307.7′64    HT151

ISBN 0-85078-921-4

Phototypeset by The Bath Press, Avon
Printed in Italy by G. Canale & C.S.p.A., Turin
Bound in the UK at The Bath Press, Avon

# Contents

# Chapter One
# Expanding Cities

## Introduction

Towns and cities are living things. They change over time. Some grow and become very rich and powerful. Others lose their wealth and decline. We know of some cities that were once very powerful but have now disappeared almost without trace. The photograph shows Leptis Magna in North Africa. It was one of the greatest cities in the Roman Empire, but for many centuries it has just been a series of ruins. What do you think towns and cities will be like in the centuries to come? In the final section of this book you will be asked to design your own cities of the future!

Most of today's towns and cities will continue to exist in the next century, but they will not remain unchanged. One hundred years ago London had no electricity, there were no cars in the city, and radio and television had not been invented. The London of 2086 will be very different from the city we know

*The magnificent buildings of Leptis Magna, now in ruins, were built in the first and second centuries* AD.

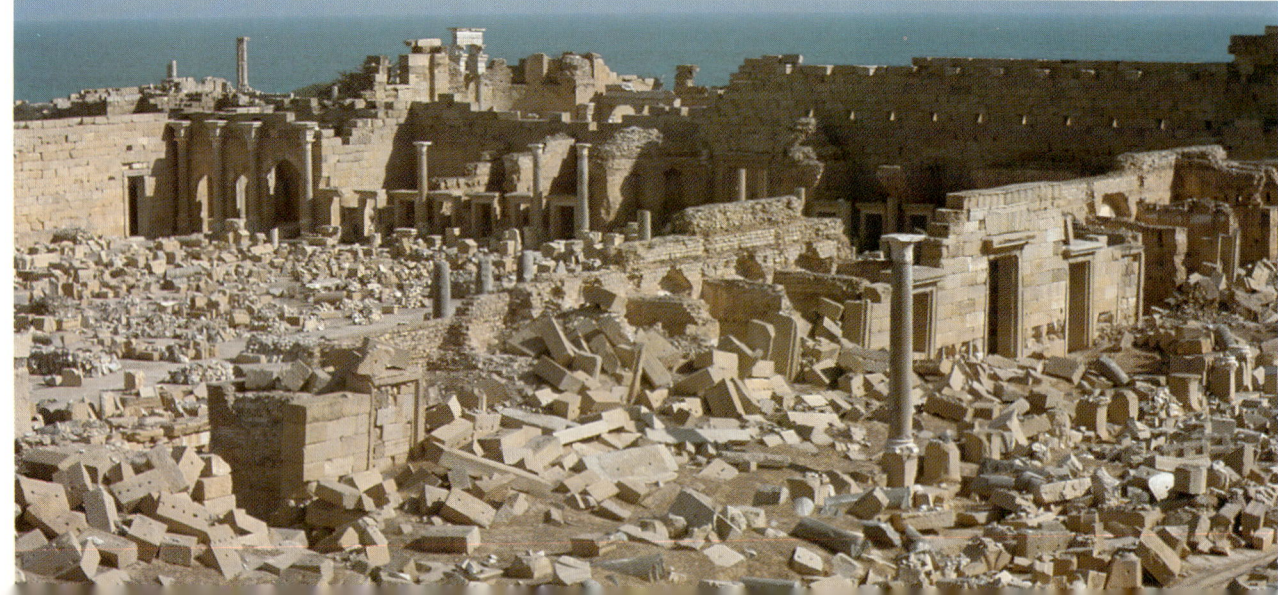

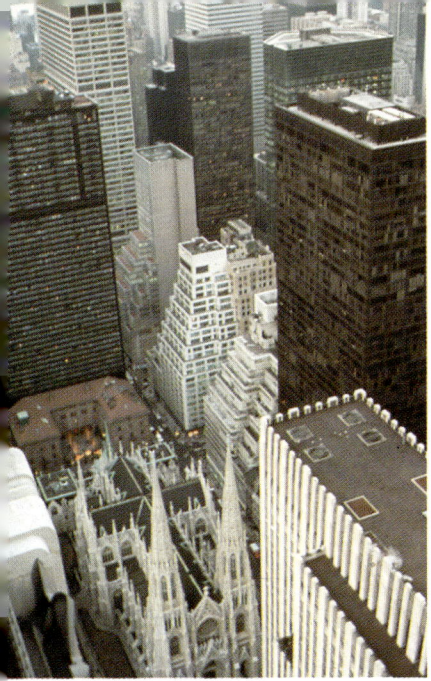

*The passage of time has seen skyscrapers and high-rise apartments spring up around St Patrick's Cathedral, in New York.*

*Some of the futuristic buildings on show at the Expo exhibition in Montreal, Canada.*

today, even if Big Ben will still be standing and the royal family still living in Buckingham Palace.

There are many things that affect the growth and appearance of a city. If changes are very rapid they are difficult to deal with. Town planners throughout the world are trying to shape the ways in which towns and cities develop. The population of the world is growing very rapidly and planning will become even more important, for many towns and cities are already threatened with overcrowding.

Within every town and city in the world, different groups of people have different styles of living. Ways of life change very rapidly too. Some people become much better off as certain industries prosper, others lose their jobs and become poor because their industries are no longer needed. As new inventions (such as computers, videos and space satellites) have come into general use, they have also changed the ways in which people live.

We are all very interested in what might happen in the future. There is concern about the quality of urban life in one hundred years time. So new ideas are planned and tried out. Some of these ideas are designed to tackle problems which may arise in years to come. Other plans envisage futuristic cities which would be quite different from those we know today.

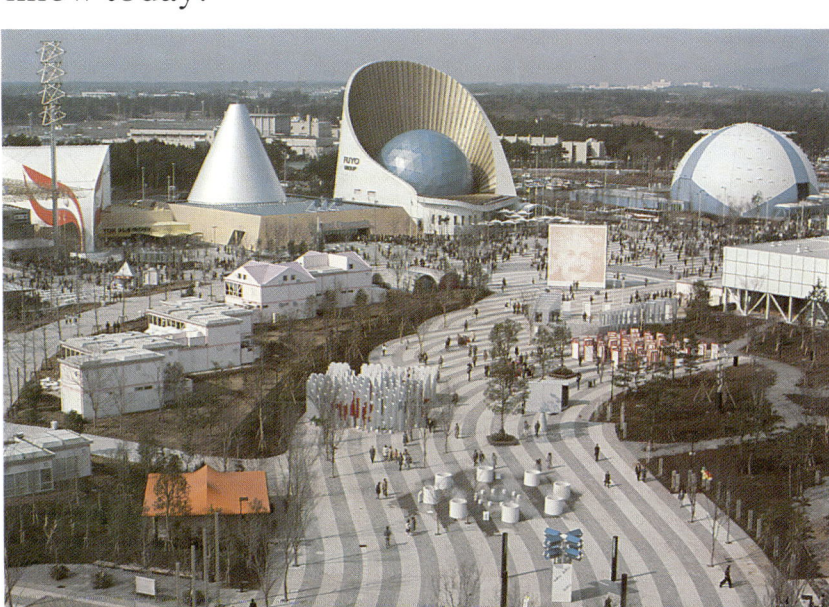

# Cities spreading outwards

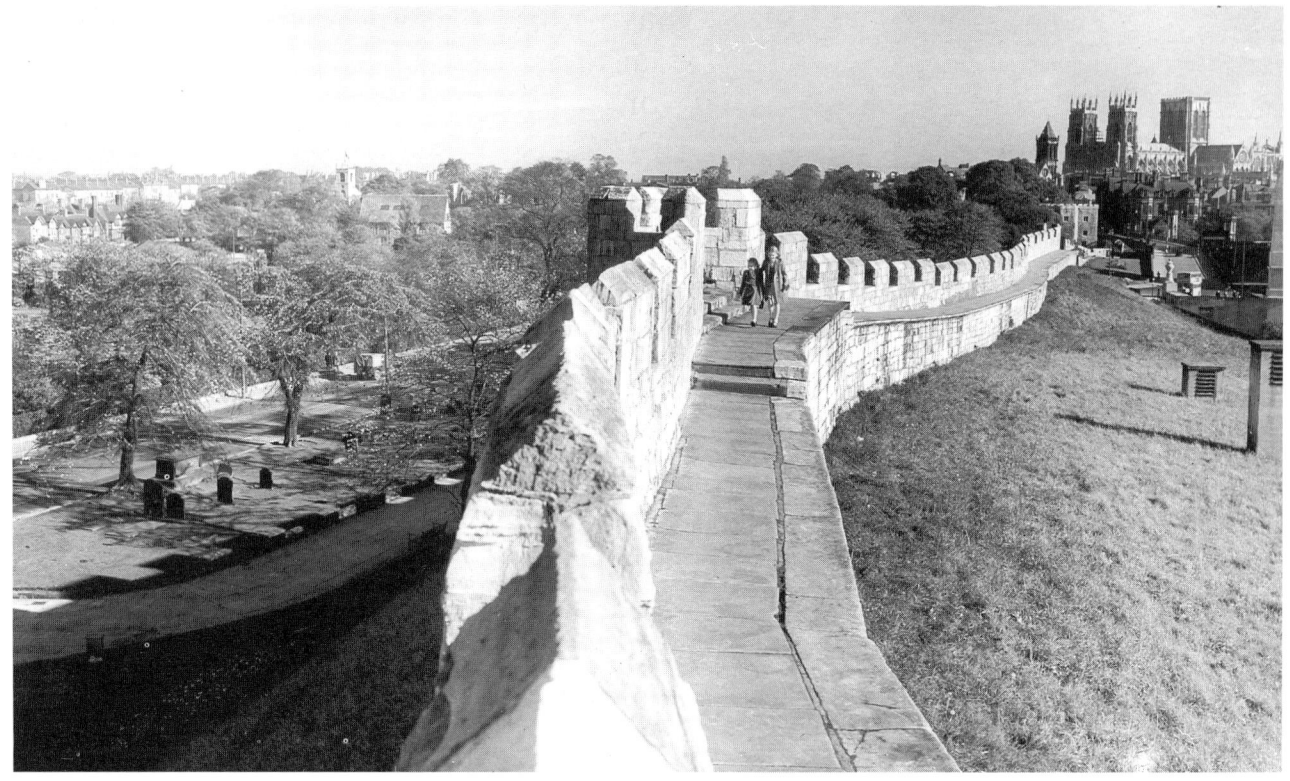

Towns and cities act like magnets, attracting large numbers of people from the countryside to live in them. Some large cities, such as London and New York, also attract people from other parts of the world. People choose to live in towns and cities because they provide more opportunities for work and entertainment, as well as the chance of a higher standard of living than in country districts.

In medieval times, about 600 years ago, towns in Britain were very small and surrounded by a wall for protection. These walls and their gates can still be seen near the centre of such cities as Norwich, Canterbury and York. They remind us of a time when most people lived in the countryside and not in towns. Today, many of these towns have become industrial and commercial centres and, as their

*The view from the medieval wall at York across the city's outlying residential districts.*

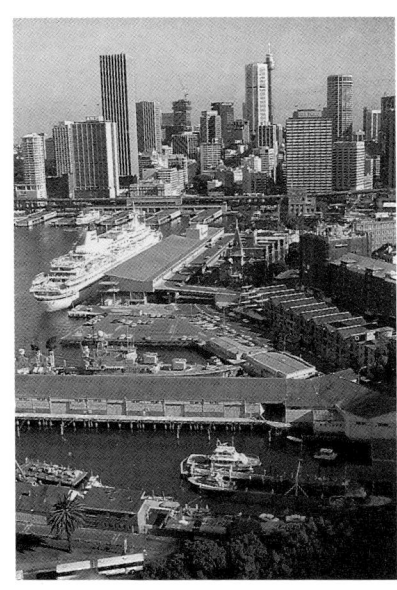

*The port of Sydney, with its business district in the background.*

populations have increased, they have spread outwards over the surrounding countryside. The building of railways and improvements in road transport have made it possible for people to live in suburbs and travel long distances into the city centre to work, shop and be entertained. The outer suburbs of York are five kilometres (three miles) from the medieval wall.

New cities have also grown up in those countries which took in large numbers of foreign settlers. These cities continued to grow outwards as more and more immigrants arrived from overseas. In 1788, eleven ships from England landed soldiers, officials and convicts in Australia to form a settlement at a place they named Sydney Cove. From these small beginnings, Sydney has spread across the surrounding countryside so that today it covers about 1,800 square kilometres (695 square miles). One Australian in every five lives in Sydney, which has a population of over three million people. The city continues to grow in size as new settlers and Australians from country districts move in.

*The rate of Sydney's growth has increased steadily during its 200-year history.*

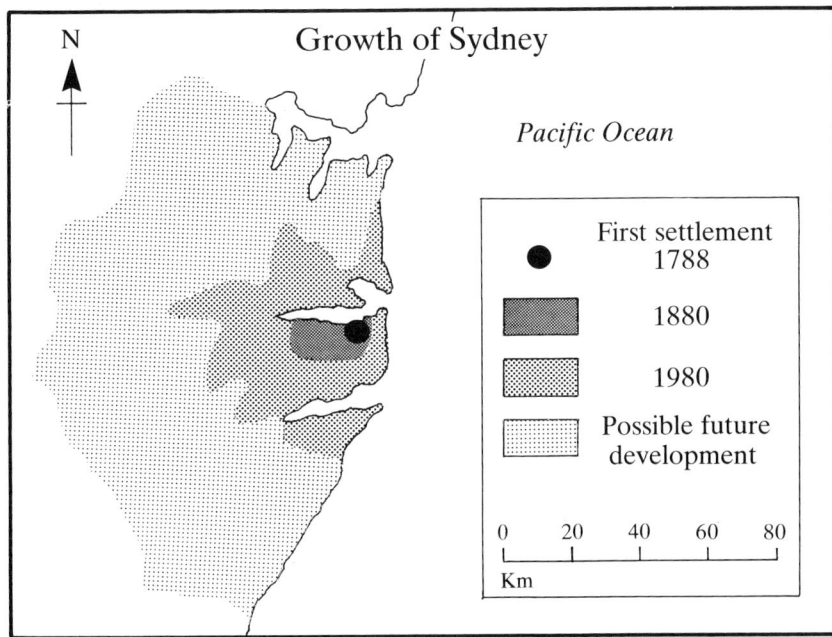

# Rapidly growing cities

## Aberdeen

In recent years Aberdeen has become the oil capital of Europe. When oil was discovered under the North Sea, the port of Aberdeen was ideally placed to handle supplies for the drilling rigs. It also became the base for oil companies and other industries connected with oil exploration. The city has grown rapidly since 1970, as workers and their families have been attracted to the area by its employment prospects and its promise of high wages.

Although many new houses have been built in Aberdeen, its average house prices have increased much more quickly than those in other parts of Britain. New industrial estates have sprung up and seven large hotels have been erected. A new bridge spans the River Dee and the airport has new buildings and a busy heliport to serve the oil rigs.

When Shell and Esso first opened joint offices in the city, they were situated above a bookshop. Now they occupy five large buildings and several smaller branches in different parts of the city. Recent discoveries of new oil and gas fields should help Aberdeen to expand still further in the future.

*An aerial view of Shell's offices at Tullos, Aberdeen.*

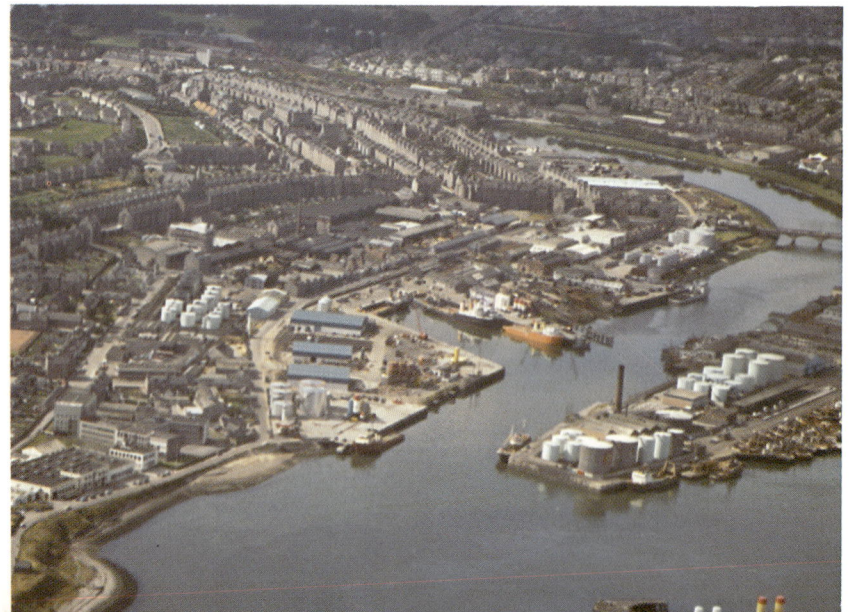

*An oil terminal at Aberdeen, in Scotland.*

## Dallas

Dallas in Texas, like Aberdeen, is a boom city whose wealth has largely come from the state's many oil-fields. In the last twenty years its population has more than doubled, making it the seventh largest city in the United States. People move to Dallas because it has a warm climate all through the year. It also has the reputation of being a city where people who work hard, especially in business or selling property, can become rich very quickly.

The city has grown upwards at its centre, as well as spreading outwards. Some of its skyscrapers can be seen in the opening shots of the TV programme *Dallas*. Wealthy citizens live on the north side of Dallas, where the houses are large and have swimming pools. The rich can spend their money in huge shopping malls which have skating rinks and indoor gardens.

*The First International Building in Dallas, one of the city's most famous sky-scrapers.*

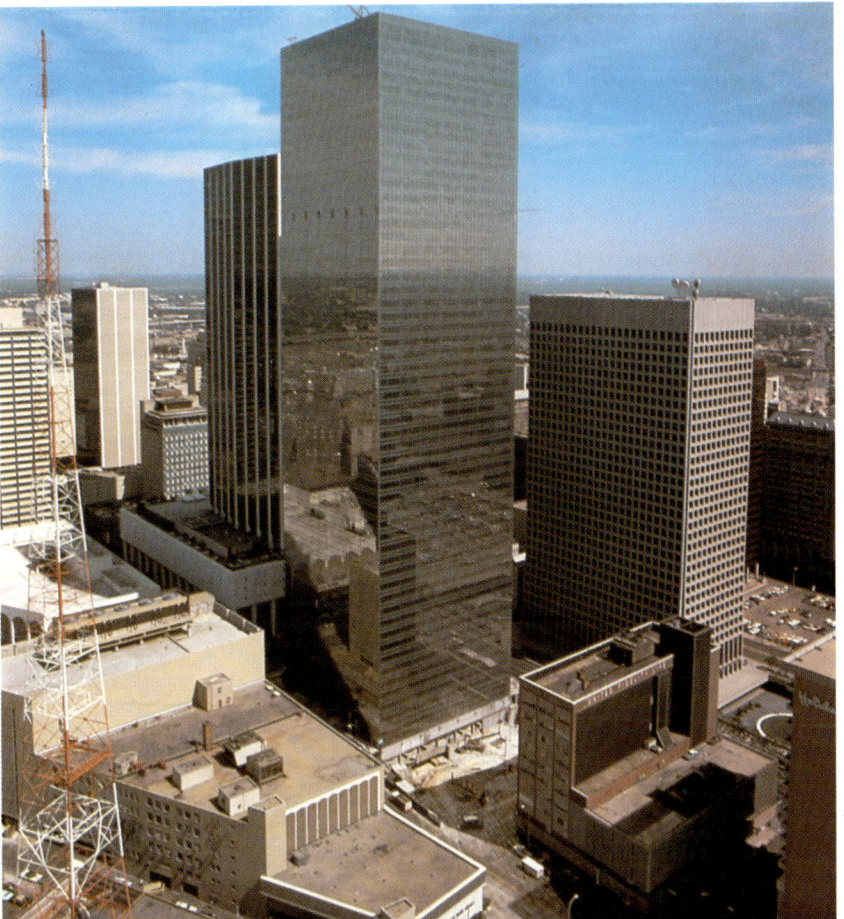

# Megalopolis

In a few parts of the world, a number of cities have grown up very close to one another and with only limited stretches of countryside between them. A region of this kind, where many towns and cities are linked together by roads and railways, is called a megalopolis (a Greek word meaning 'a very large city').

The best known megalopolis is in the north-east of the United States, stretching between the states of New Hampshire and Virginia. In this region there is an almost continuous chain of large cities that includes Boston, New York, Philadelphia, Baltimore and Washington. In addition, the area contains over a dozen smaller cities that help to give it a population of over fifty million. The concentration of people, wealth, industry and business in

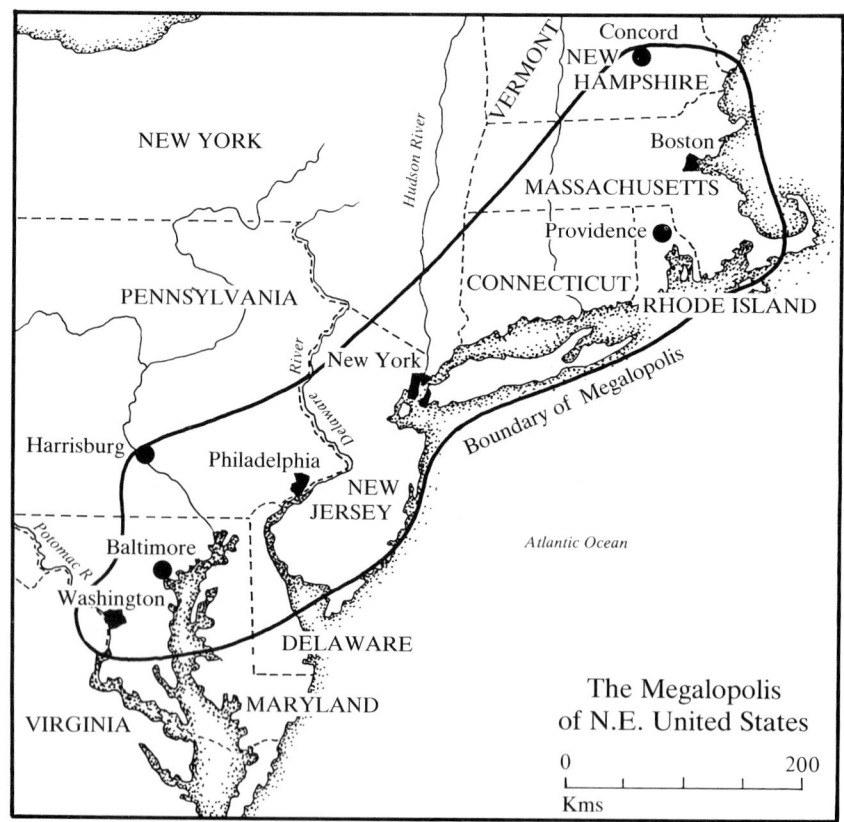

*The huge region covered by the megalopolis in the north-east of the USA.*

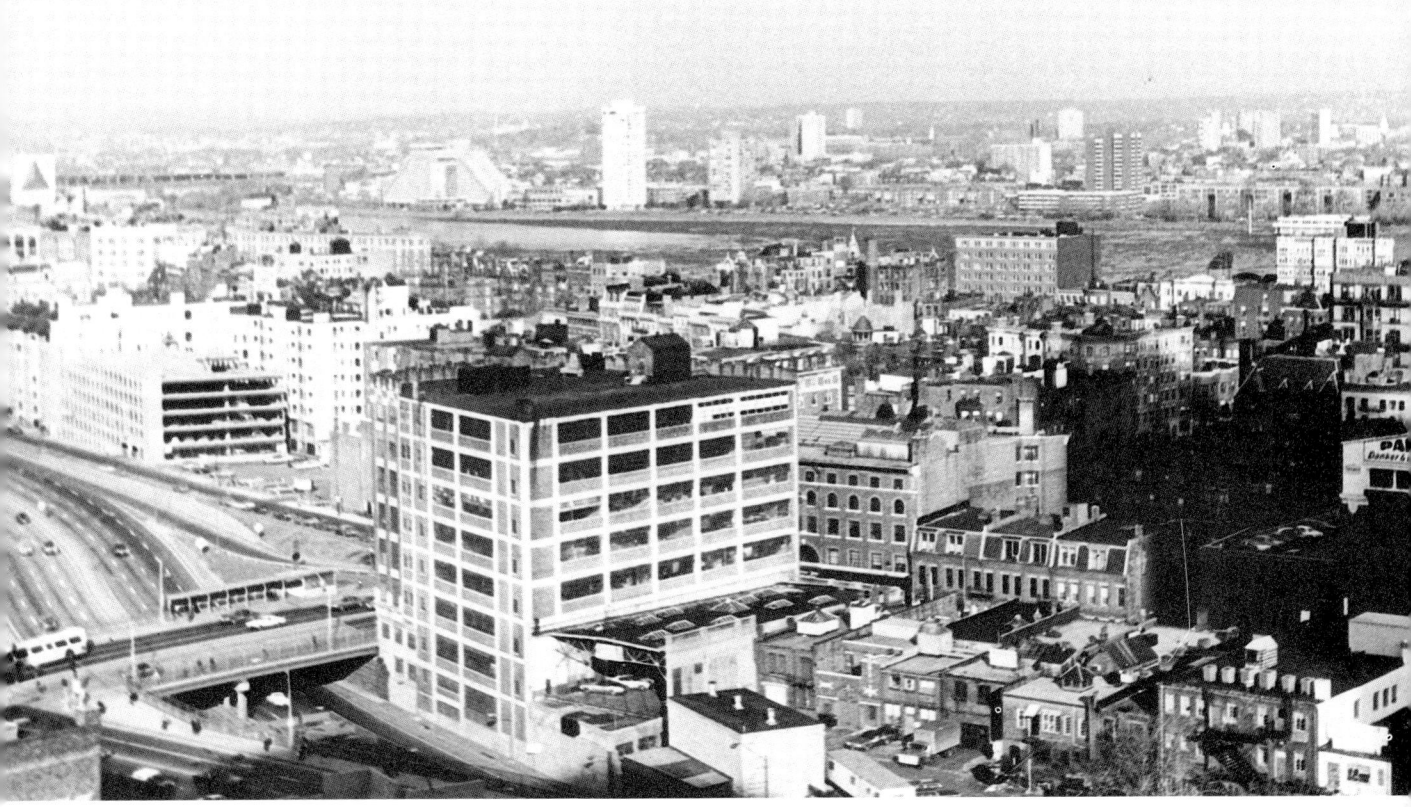

*A panoramic view of the industrial areas of Boston, Massachusetts, in the USA.*

this part of the United States has no equal anywhere else in the world.

A smaller megalopolis is growing up rapidly in California, between San Diego on the Mexican border and San Francisco. Los Angeles, which spreads along the coastal lowlands for over 100 kilometres (62 miles), lies within this region.

In Britain, a megalopolis has begun to develop from London north-westwards to the West Midlands, Stoke-on-Trent, Manchester and Liverpool. When the Channel Tunnel has been built, this megalopolis could be linked to the towns and cities of northern France. Another megalopolis has grown up in Japan, along the southern coastline of the main island, Honshu. At present it stretches from Tokyo to Osaka, Kyoto and Kobe and is the focus of industrial and commercial life in Japan.

As air, road and rail links are improved, clusters of other towns and cities in different parts of the world will connect up to form new megalopolises.

# Chapter Two
# Cities in decline

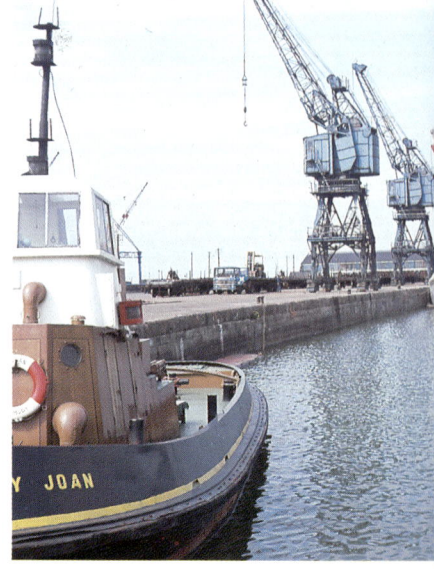

*The docks at Grimsby, which have suffered from the decline in the fishing industry.*

## Industry goes away

The town of Merthyr Tydfil in Mid Glamorgan, Wales, was at one time the iron-making capital of the world. Today, it is a small town of about 60,000 people in which iron is no longer made. The town has been in decline for more than one hundred years and unemployment in the area is high with little prospect of immediate improvement.

Even within the last twenty years, some important towns in England have declined as old industries have disappeared. Grimsby, in Lincolnshire, was once a very famous fishing port. A large fleet of trawlers landed supplies of fish that were sold in the market on the docks and sent to all parts of England by rail. More recently, some of the catch has been transported in refrigerated lorries and the rest processed in frozen-food factories. Since 1973, when Britain joined the European Community (the 'common market') each member nation has only been allowed to catch a quota, or set amount, of fish each year. At the same time, Iceland has banned foreign ships from the rich fishing grounds around its coasts. As a result, the fishing trade has declined and the main industry that supported the people of Grimsby has been very hard hit.

Some people who live near Consett, in County Durham, call it a 'ghost town'. This is because its main industry has closed down. A few years ago Consett, like Merthyr Tydfil, was an iron-making town. Recently, British Steel closed the town's iron

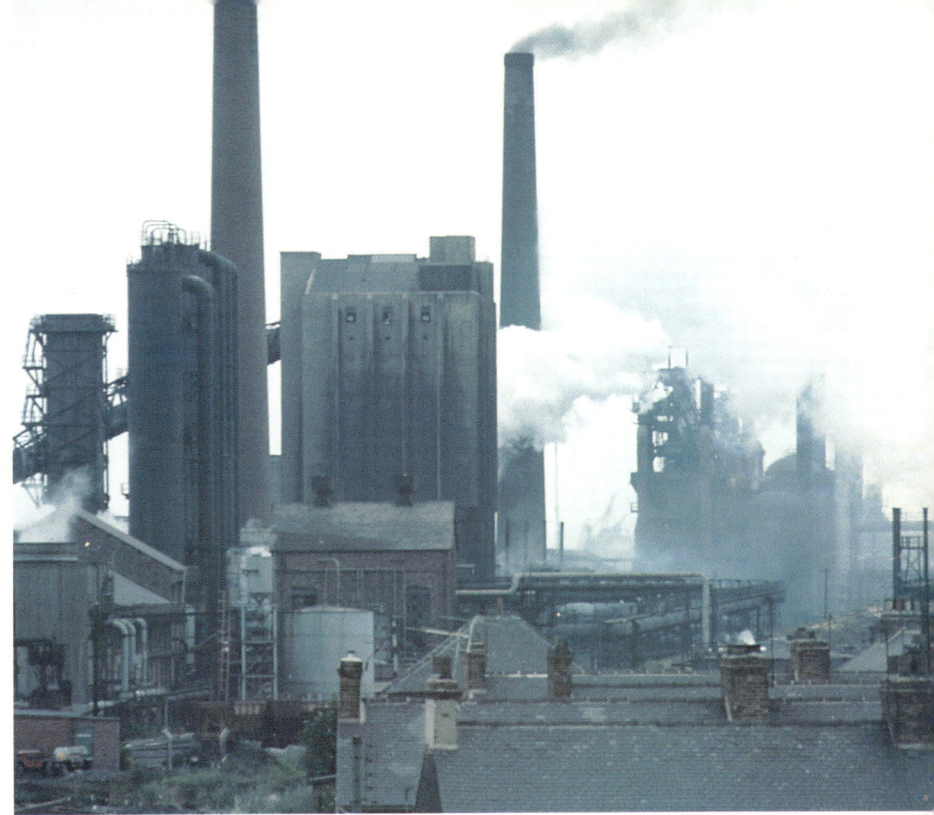

*Consett steel works in north-east England, shortly before they were finally closed down.*

*Bodie, a gold-mining ghost-town, lies deserted in California, USA.*

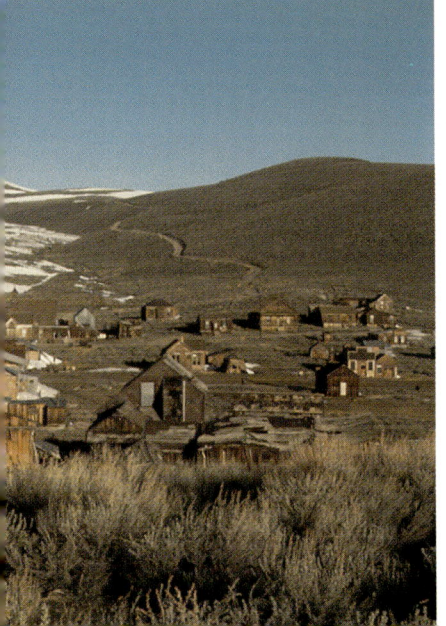

foundry and the people who worked there lost their jobs. Some of them moved away to look for work. Many shops closed in the town, because people could no longer afford to buy many things. Now, the young people in Consett feel that they have no future unless they leave the town and look for work elsewhere. So Consett is following the pattern of decline seen in Merthyr Tydfil many years ago.

In Australia, Canada, New Zealand and the United States, tourists make trips to 'ghost towns' that were once the centres of gold and silver mining. Some American towns (such as Tombstone, which was so famous in the days of the cowboys) are now either ruins or carefully preserved shells for the tourists to see.

As industries continue to change over the next hundred years and robots take over the jobs once performed by men and women, more industrial towns will fall into decline. Some people think that English seaside towns will also die out. Can you think of some reasons why this might happen?

# Inner city decay

The oldest parts of towns and cities are those nearest the centre. In Britain, there are many city centres that are ancient and picturesque, like the centre of Lincoln. However, around the shopping and business centres of most cities there is usually an area which is old and decaying called the inner city.

In the inner city many of the houses are old and out of date. A large number of them do not have the facilities that we have come to expect in modern homes. But these old buildings are still needed by those people who cannot afford their own homes or are unable to rent houses of better quality. So the inner city is usually characterized by its overcrowding and by its concentration of the poorest groups of people in society. In the USA this is usually the part of the city in which the most recently arrived immigrants and native black communities are found.

In the old days, there were also many industries situated in the inner city. Some of these were very specialist trades that were not found in any other parts of the city. In London and New York, the fashion trade – the 'rag trade' – was especially important in these areas, as were paper and printing works. Some of the industries were carried on in tiny workshops and factories that were as old as the houses around them. In many countries, the planners have redeveloped the inner city areas and many of the old works and houses have been knocked down. They have been replaced by modern office blocks, to which workers travel from the suburbs where they live. As a result, there is less work for the people who live in the inner city and unemployment in the area has risen.

Some large towns and cities grew because they

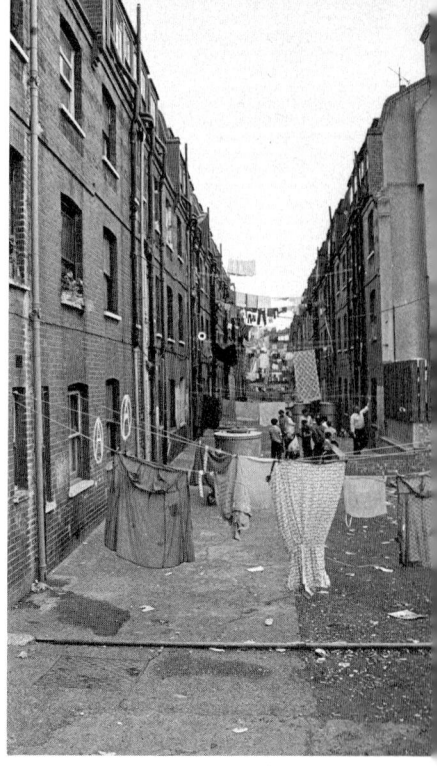

*Typical inner-city housing in London. New investment and building programmes are needed to replace such homes.*

*The old, built-up inner-city regions of Glasgow, in Scotland.*

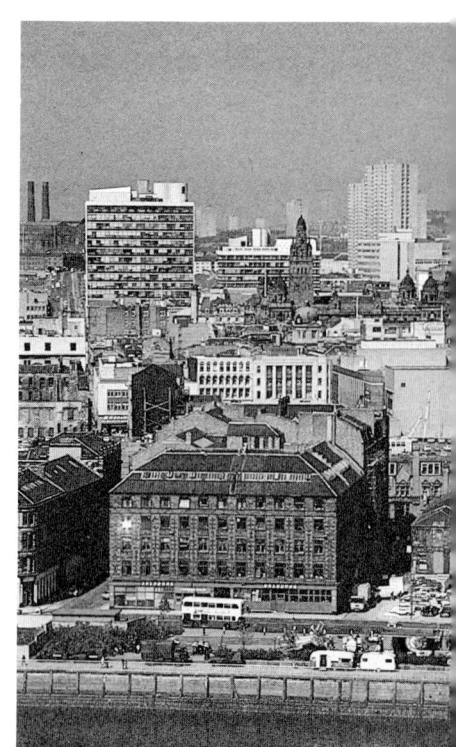

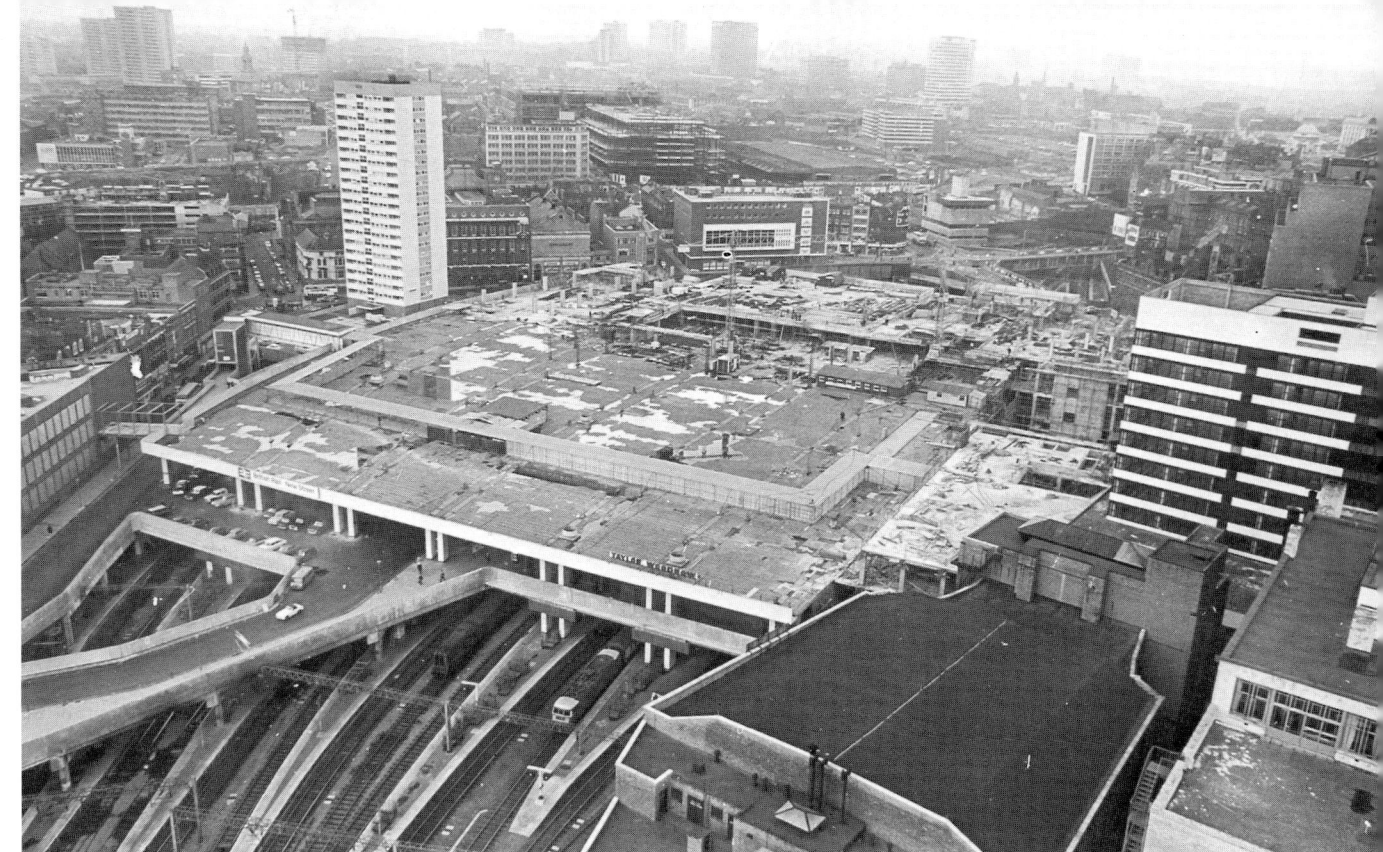

*Central Birmingham, in England, with its mixture of old housing, office blocks and redevelopment schemes.*

were ports. They gained their wealth from overseas trade. Usually, the docks were right in the heart of the city. The pattern of shipping has now changed and container terminals have been built outside the old dockland areas. Consequently, the docks have been closed and the offices and warehouses built alongside them are empty and derelict.

In addition to the shabby appearance of the inner city, its old roads are often narrow and twisting and therefore not suitable for large lorries. This means that traffic congestion is a further problem.

What will happen to these old city areas? In London, the docklands have already been taken over and redeveloped so that they might be useful in the future. Waterside hotels have been built for tourists, together with expensive private housing and office blocks. But the local residents complain that this type of rebuilding does not provide them either with homes that they can afford or with well-paid jobs. What do you think?

# When rich foreigners leave

At certain times in their history, some towns and cities become famous for the number of wealthy people who live in them. At present, a city like Monte Carlo attracts the rich and the famous.

In the past many Europeans used force to make large fortunes abroad and to claim territory for their countries. When Britain possessed a huge and powerful Empire, wealth and treasure from throughout the world were brought back to London. We can still see some of these treasures, which have been collected in museums. Some Britons made their fortunes in the colonies and built large houses and memorials in the cities in which they lived.

Calcutta was one of the great centres of the textile industry in the Empire. When India and Pakistan became independent, many British people left, taking their money with them. Some factories closed down, large mansions were left empty, and monuments built by the British were neglected and left to rot. The old buildings and decaying monuments

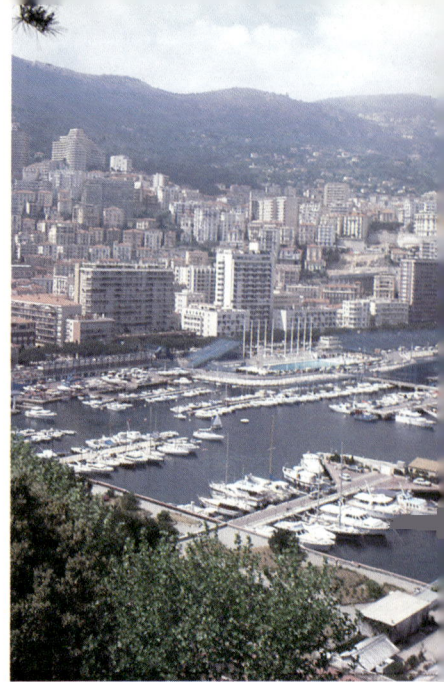

*The luxury homes and expensive yachts belonging to the residents of Monte Carlo.*

*The Marble Palace in Calcutta, a Victorian mansion built by the British.*

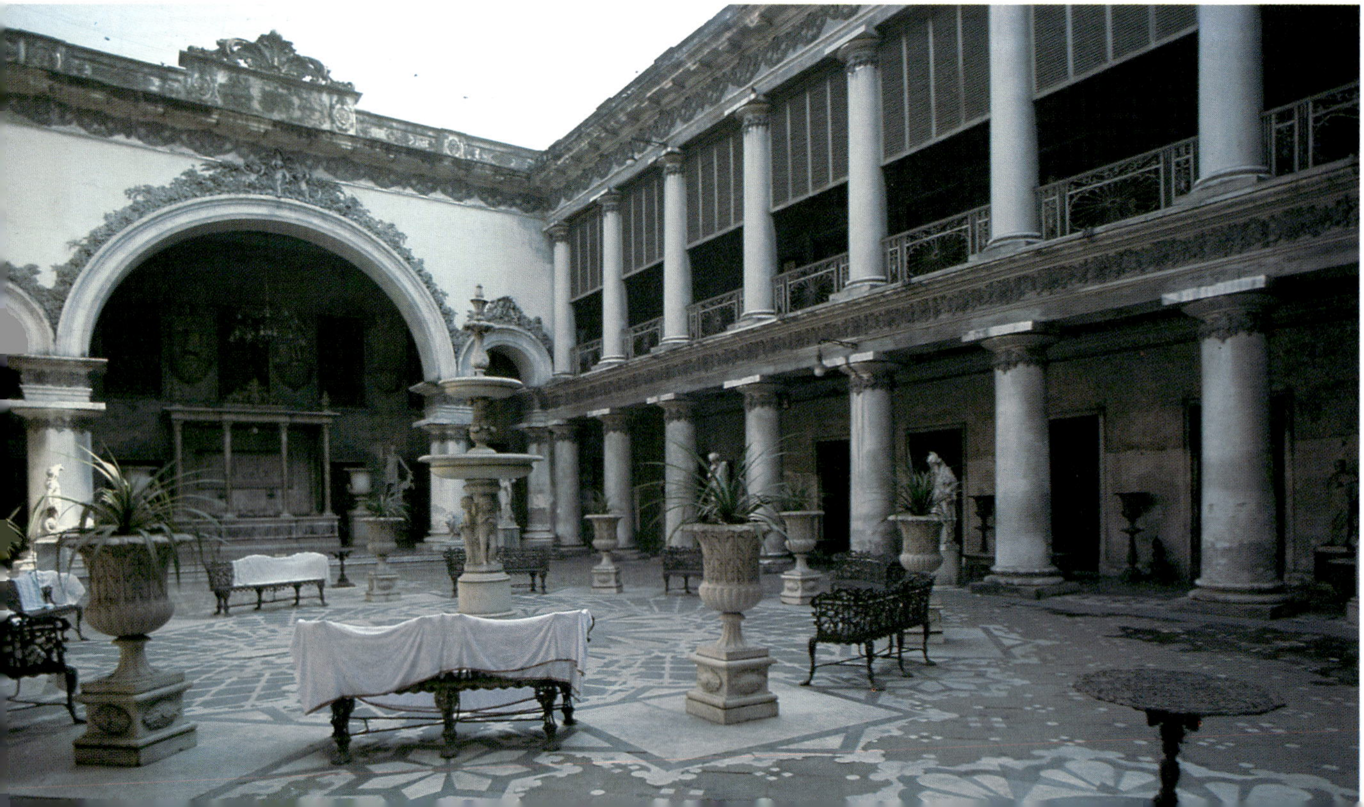

are still symbols of the fact that the land was once ruled by the British.

For thirty years, South Vietnam fought unsuccessfully to defeat the communists of the North. Vietnam had been a French colony and, for some years after independence, the French army stayed to help in the war. Later, the Americans took over the task. The well-paid American army brought a great deal of money into Vietnam and this created a 'false economy', one that was not natural to the country but based on the presence of the Americans. Cities like Saigon (now Ho Chi Minh City) became wealthy and important. When the defeated Americans left South Vietnam quite suddenly, the new lifestyle of the cities was destroyed. Many of the businesses created especially for the Americans, such as luxury shops, nightclubs and restaurants, were forced to close. Factories which produced items for the Americans no longer had customers to sell to. When the communists took over, they decided that the Western style of city life was unsuited to their country and they moved many people to the countryside to work. The cities tried to change back to their original character and to restore native industries.

When some countries became independent, the new and inexperienced governments were unable to keep up the level of trade and industry that had once existed. They were not given enough support by rich countries and a number of new nations became poorer. One result of this has been that they have not been able to spend a great deal on their towns and cities. For example Accra, the capital of Ghana, was the chief city of the British colony called the Gold Coast. But Ghana has very little money today and there are signs of decay in Accra. If the rich nations do not help the poorer ones, many cities of the Developing World may suffer from neglect in the future.

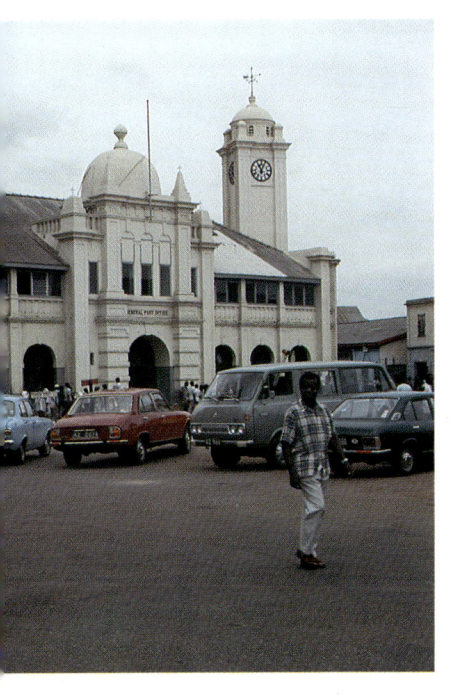

*A General Post Office in Ghana, with its typical colonial style of architecture.*

# Chapter Three
# Planning for change

## New towns and cities

After the Second World War, the people of Britain were determined to rebuild their country. The soldiers who had been fighting in the war needed new housing, while thousands of families had been left homeless by the heavy bombing the country had suffered. Furthermore, there had already been a shortage of houses before the war began. So many people in Britain needed somewhere to live.

The obvious solution to this problem was to build some new towns. It was decided that they should be about the size of country towns, which were felt by many people to be nice places to live in. So a ring of new towns was built around London and a number of others were constructed in areas of the country where new housing was very badly needed, such as the Midlands.

**Below** *Central Milton Keynes, an English new town, under development in 1975. It was designed to provide over one million square feet of covered shopping space for some 150 different shops.*

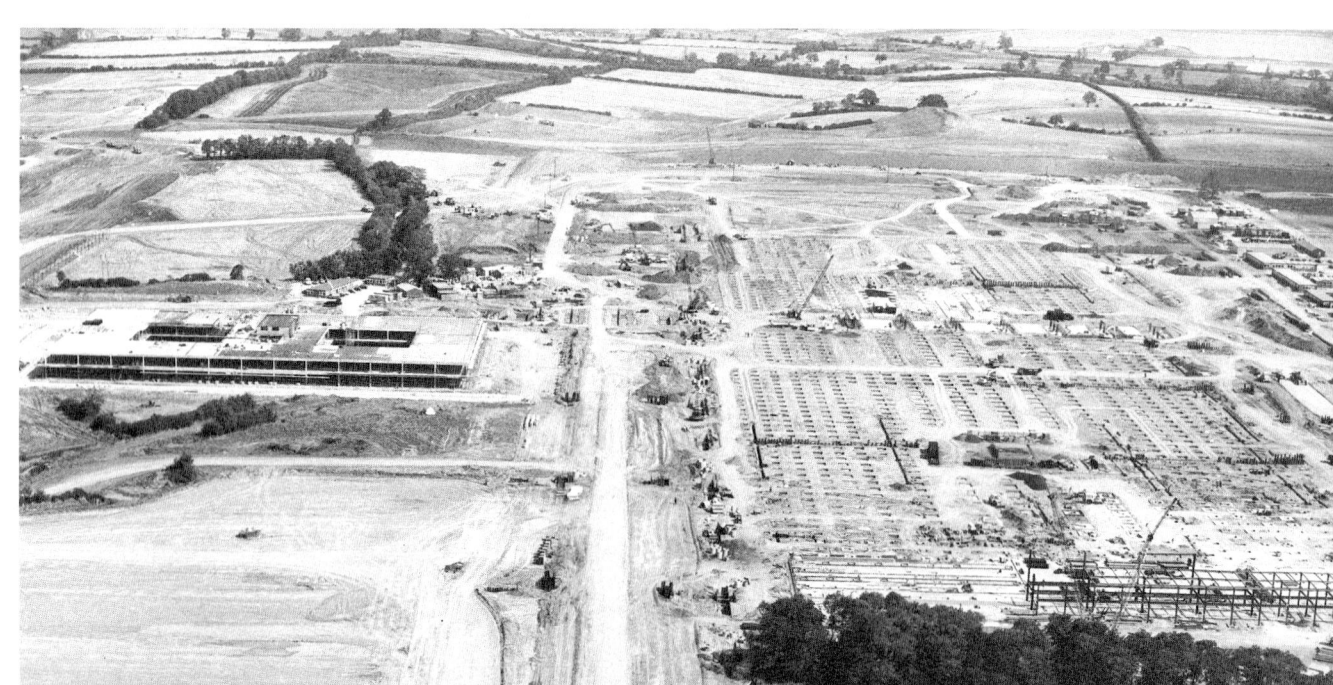

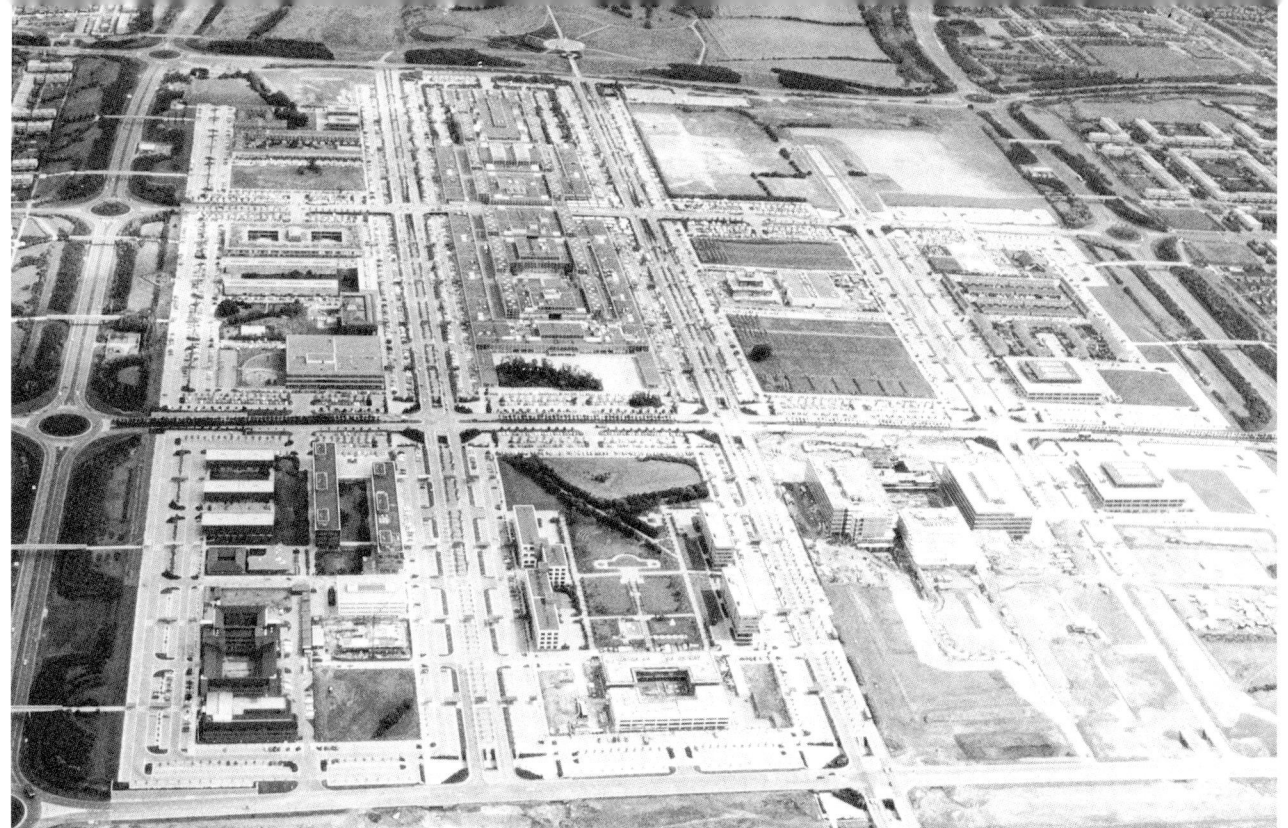

**Above:** *Milton Keynes in 1985, with the main shopping building in the central background.*

The new towns were intended to be 'self-contained'. This meant that they had their own shopping centres and industrial estates. As a result, people could work in their home town and did not need to commute to London or other large cities. The new towns were also designed to be 'socially balanced', so that there would be housing for many different groups of people. In this way, it was hoped the new towns would become more than very large council estates.

The first new towns that were built, like Basildon, were meant to be quite small. Their construction was begun before the majority of people owned cars, so no pedestrian precincts were created to keep traffic away from shoppers. As living patterns altered, the original plans had to be changed. The design of Washington new town, for example, was revised to make it a motorway city, with the motorway forming a spine right through the town. Milton Keynes was designed as a large modern city to hold 300,000 people.

# A regional city

The people of Holland had a problem. They already had more people living on every square mile of land than did most countries of the world. Now their big cities were growing so fast that they were likely to join up to make one huge urban sprawl. This would eventually mean that good farmland would disappear. The future did not look promising.

The Dutch planners came up with the idea of a 'ring city', which they called Randstadt. The new city was designed to include a number of regions: the Hague, where the government is located; Rotterdam, the chief port of the country; and Amsterdam, which is the chief business and tourist centre. Randstadt was to be a new conurbation, in which the cities would grow together to form a large urban ring. The ring of cities would surround some of the best farmland in Holland, which would then be carefully preserved. In this way, the worst effects of rapid city growth would be avoided.

However, the Dutch planners have been surprised by subsequent events. The populations of the cities have not grown as quickly as expected, so that the largest cities have still not grown together. So the 'ring city' plan will be an idea which can be used in the next century, instead of this one.

The Dutch planners were also worried that if a large number of people were sent to the outlying towns in order to keep the farmland areas intact, the old cities might decline. If factories were moved to the outer edges of the ring, cities like Amsterdam and Rotterdam would be weakened. The loss of people would also mean fewer customers for the sports and entertainment facilities in the old cities. Now that the planners have realized that the need to move people out is not so urgent, new factories and facilities have been built within the ring itself.

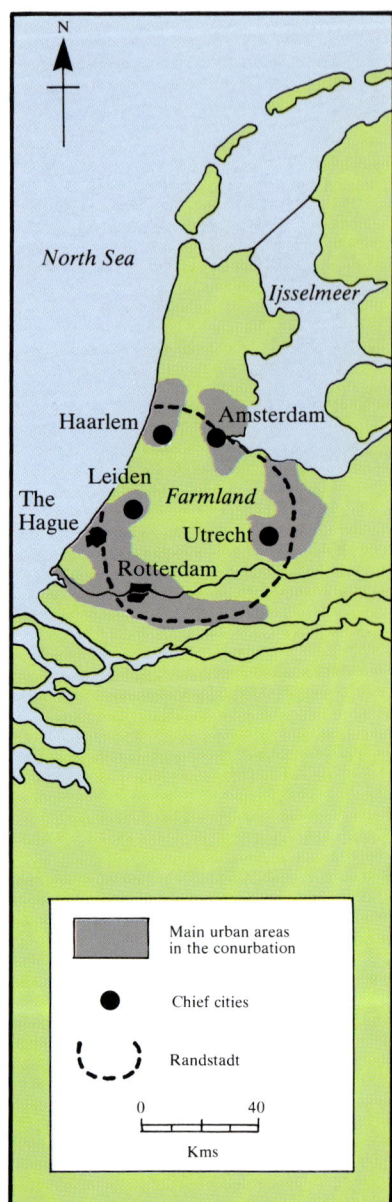

*The urban ring that makes up the regional city of Randstadt, in Holland.*

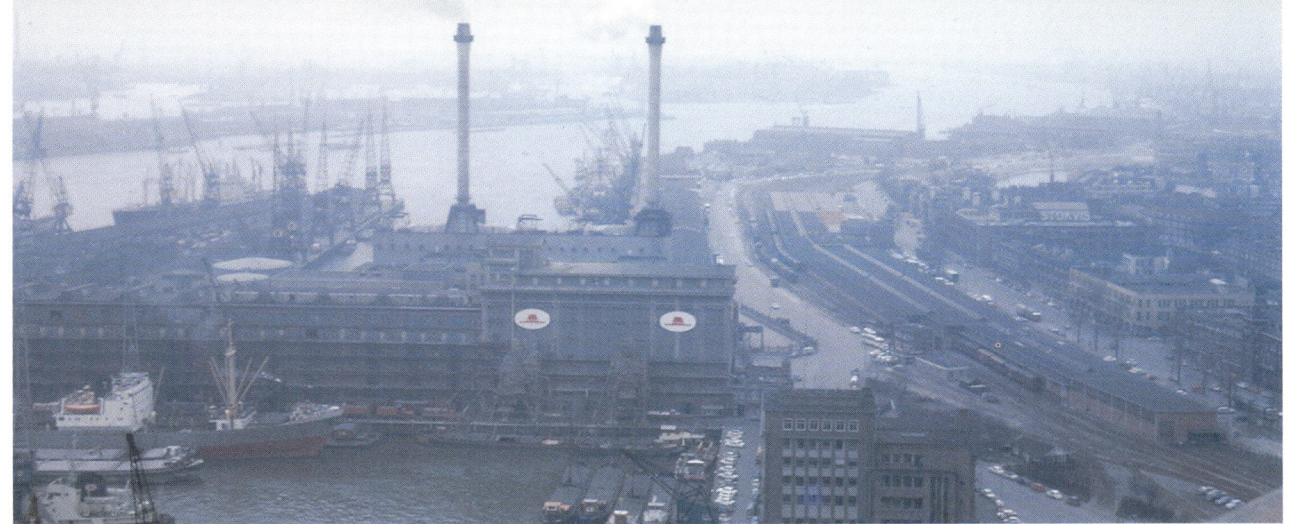

*A view of the Dutch port of Rotterdam, as seen from the city's Euromast.*

Within Randstadt, new residential areas are replacing old-fashioned houses. The better-quality houses from the past are being repaired and modernized. Traffic-free zones have been set up to make the old city centres more attractive. Some of the old streets of the Hague, for example, have been turned into picturesque shopping precincts.

In these ways, the Dutch hope to have a large efficient city in the future. However, within the regional city of Randstadt, the separate old cities will keep their own individual characters. So Amsterdam will be just as attractive to foreign visitors in the future, without it becoming a mere museum.

*One of the pedestrian precincts in the old area of The Hague.*

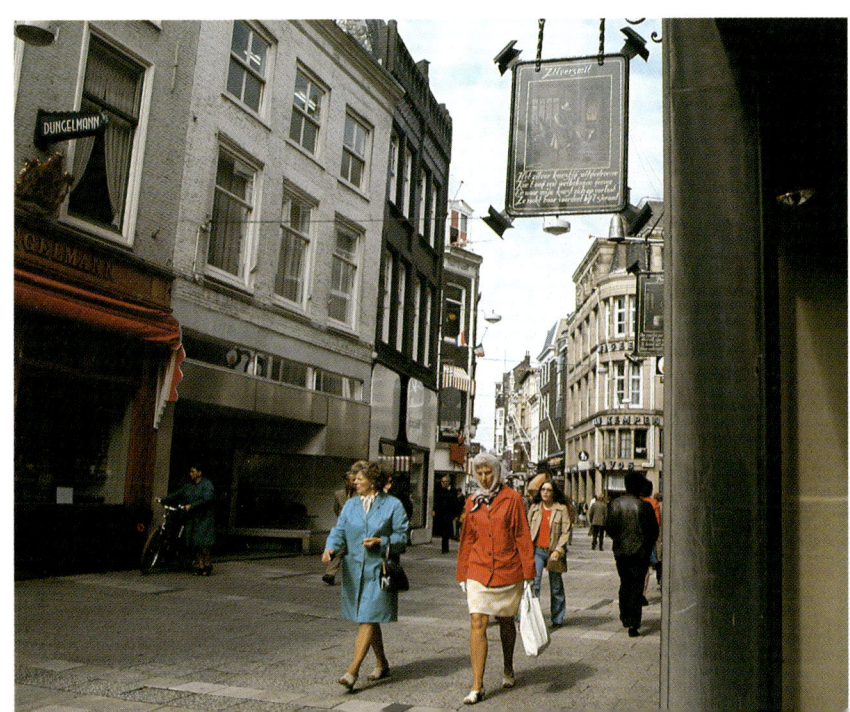

# Planning capital cities

This is an aerial photograph of part of Paris, the capital city of France. Paris is by far the largest city in France and is very crowded. There is a great deal of traffic congestion in the city and people are packed into densely-populated residential areas. In addition, many people who live outside Paris travel in to the city to work and so add to the crowds and the traffic jams. In the photograph all the main roads lead to a central point – the Arc de Triomphe. Where do you think the worst traffic jams are found?

The city now has a population of over eight million people. Throughout the year, thousands of tourists visit Paris and add to the crowds. As the city grows and gets busier, the town planners have a very difficult job to do.

The expansion of Paris is not a new event. From the time of the Middle Ages to about 120 years ago,

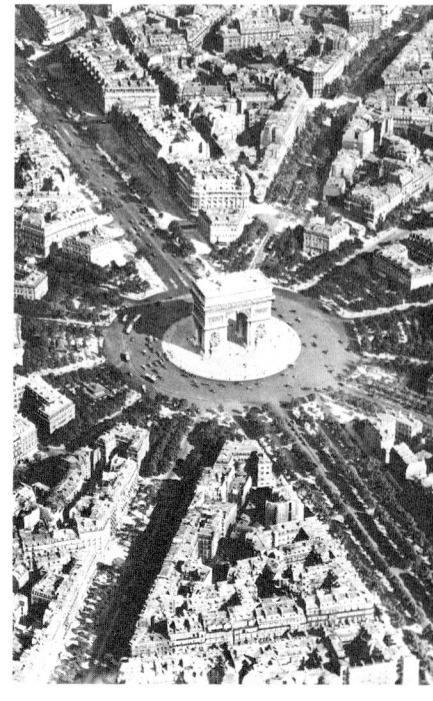

*The Arc de Triomphe in Paris, the meeting-point of twelve roads.*

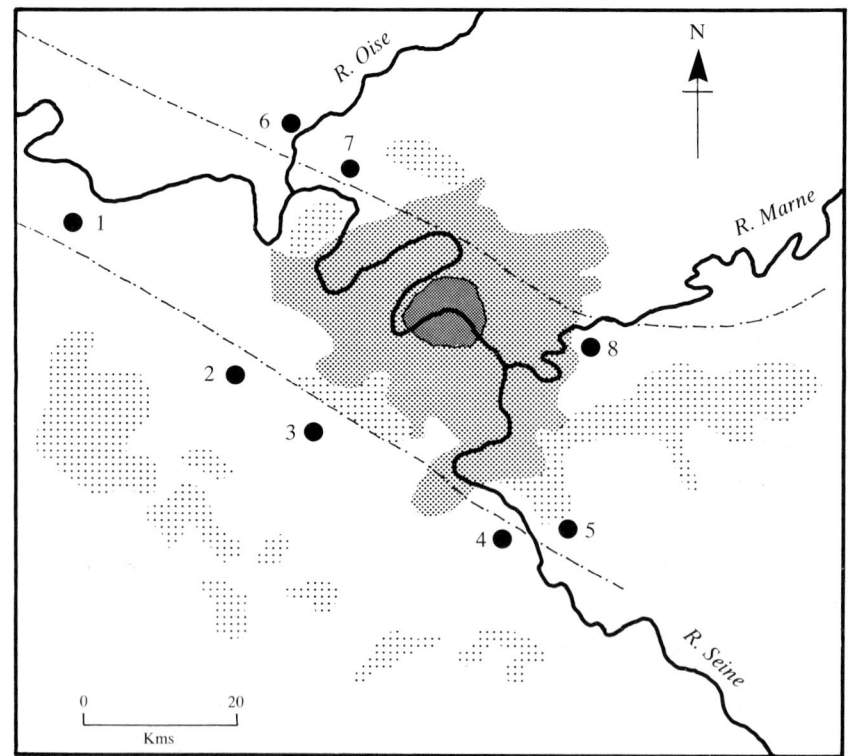

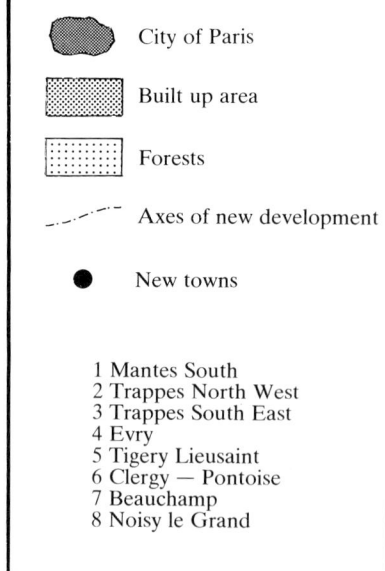

| | |
|---|---|
| City of Paris |
| Built up area |
| Forests |
| Axes of new development |
| ● | New towns |

1 Mantes South
2 Trappes North West
3 Trappes South East
4 Evry
5 Tigery Lieusaint
6 Clergy — Pontoise
7 Beauchamp
8 Noisy le Grand

*This map shows how the new towns are being developed around Paris.*

the growth of the city was controlled by building new city walls at greater and greater distances from the centre. The people of Paris were squeezed inside these walls and became used to living in overcrowded conditions. In the nineteenth century the old walls were pulled down, as were many old houses nearby. The space was used to make wide new roads, called *boulevards*, which opened up the city. New walls were also built, but people soon moved outside them to the new suburbs.

A new plan has been worked out to cope with the present growth of Paris. Instead of adding more buildings to the edges of the city, new towns have been planned. These towns are being built along two axes (lines) which run along two sides of the city. In each of the eight new towns there will be modern facilities and shopping centres. This will mean that people will no longer have to travel into Paris for everything they want. New underground and surface railways now take commuters to work and a new motorway (*the périphérique*), takes travellers around Paris instead of through it. So Paris is approaching the next century better equipped to cope with its evergrowing volume of people, businesses and traffic. At the moment, the city planners are confident that they have made the right decisions and the future of Paris seems bright.

*An aerial view of Clergy-Pontoise, one of the new towns near Paris.*

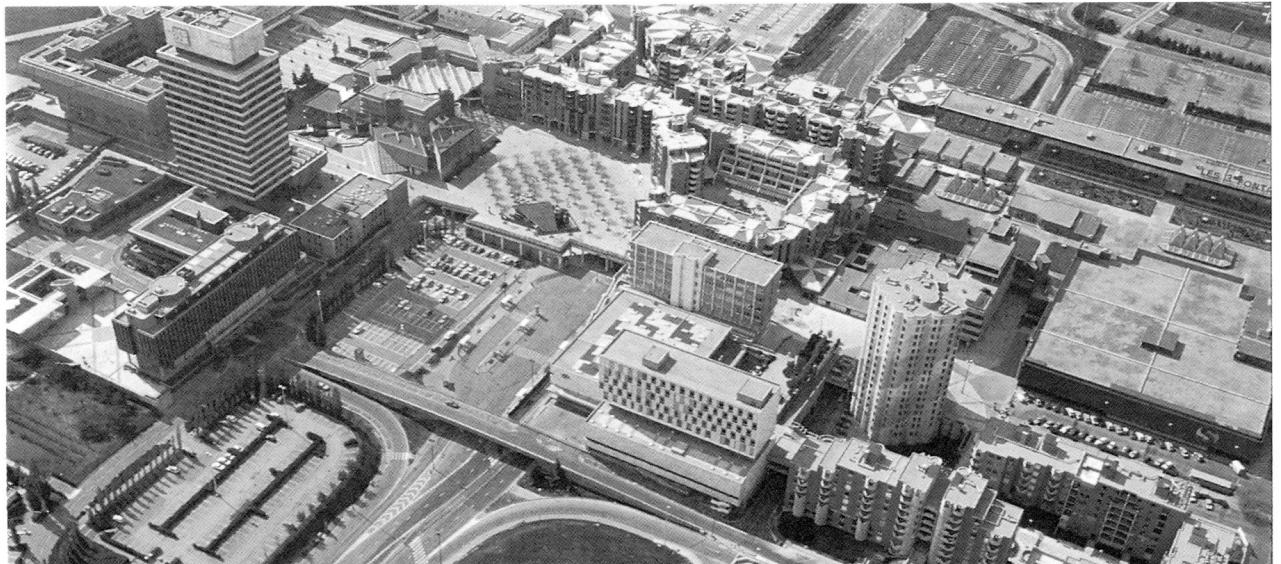

# Chapter Four
# Changing lifestyles

## Places to live

In the 1960s, there was an urgent need for more new homes to be built in Britain's cities to replace the old ones that were no longer fit to live in. Architects and planners tried to solve the problem quickly by building high-rise blocks of flats. These tower-blocks provided hundreds of homes on very small areas of land. Today, many of these high-rise blocks, in cities such as Glasgow, Liverpool and London, are empty, in a bad state of repair or are waiting to be pulled down. It has been realized that people prefer to live in smaller blocks of flats or in houses. The high-rise developments are being replaced by small, planned estates. These have their own shops, schools and other facilities for the residents.

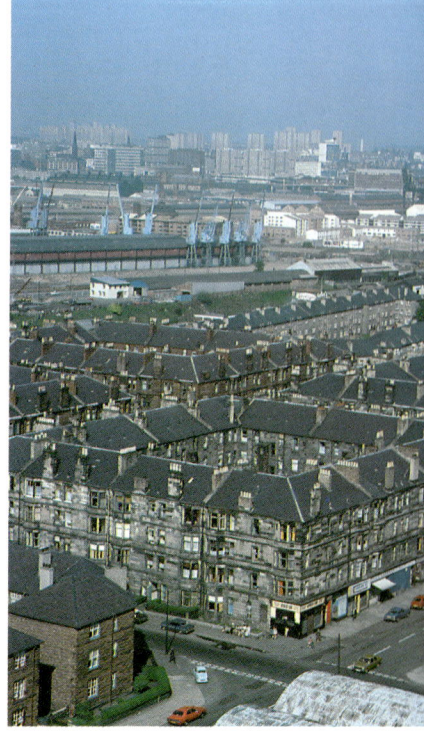

*Old and new ways of housing the population of Glasgow, in Scotland: terraced housing (foreground) and modern high-rise blocks (background).*

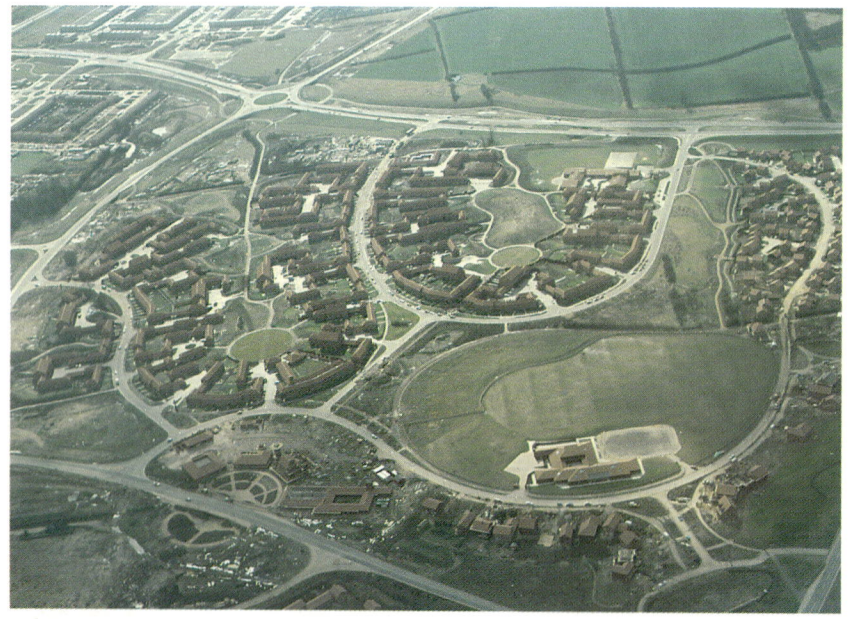

*These new housing estates in Milton Keynes, in the east Midlands, have been built in small groups, with plenty of space available for recreation and relaxation.*

Given the choice, most people would prefer to live in small communities set in pleasant surroundings, with trees and places where children can play. New towns and cities in different parts of the world are being built as clusters of small communities. These have houses in a variety of styles and sizes which are set in woodland or near water. These communities are connected to one another, and to the industrial and business districts, by high-speed roads. As a result, residents of these areas do not have long journeys to work.

In cities, the high price of land in the city centre has resulted in houses and flats being pulled down to make way for tall office blocks, banks and other businesses. Consequently, few people now live in city centres, which are deserted in the evenings and at weekends. To attract people to live in these inner-city areas once more, new blocks of flats like those at the Barbican in the City of London are being built. They are expensive, but conveniently located for those people who need to live near the centre of a city and who enjoy high incomes.

*The luxury flats at the Barbican, in the centre of London.*

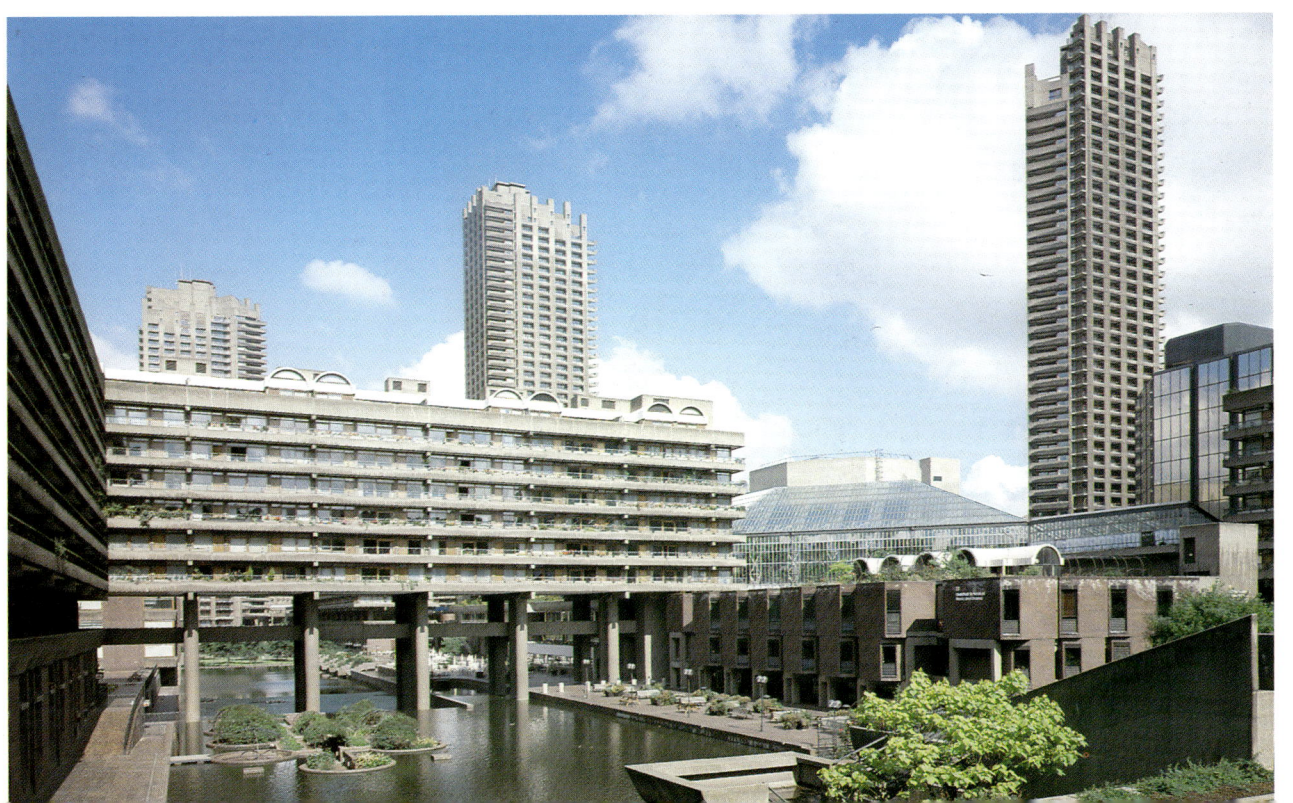

# Places to work

In the past, many towns and cities were formed around mines, factories or shipyards. Houses and factories often shared the same street and this made living conditions dirty, noisy and unpleasant. Industrial cities, such as Manchester and Bradford, grew up in this way and they still bear the scars today.

In more recent times, planners have separated factory sites from housing areas. Industrial estates are built on the edge of cities, or in zones set apart from housing and recreational facilities. Modern machinery is powered by electricity and most factories no longer need to be located near to supplies of raw materials or power. Heavy industries, such as shipbuilding and iron and steel, have contracted. At the same time, there has been a rapid expansion of light industries, especially of 'hi-tech' firms producing silicon chips, micro-circuits and other components used in computers, telecommunications and video equipment.

Hi-tech factories need to be built near a good communications network (e.g. road/rail links) and on cheap land where there is clean air and good power supplies. Country sites are therefore more suitable than cities, and factories are being built outside major urban areas in special 'Science Parks' or technopolises.

*Smoke drifts from industrial chimney stacks over nearby houses in Bradford in Yorkshire, 1947.*

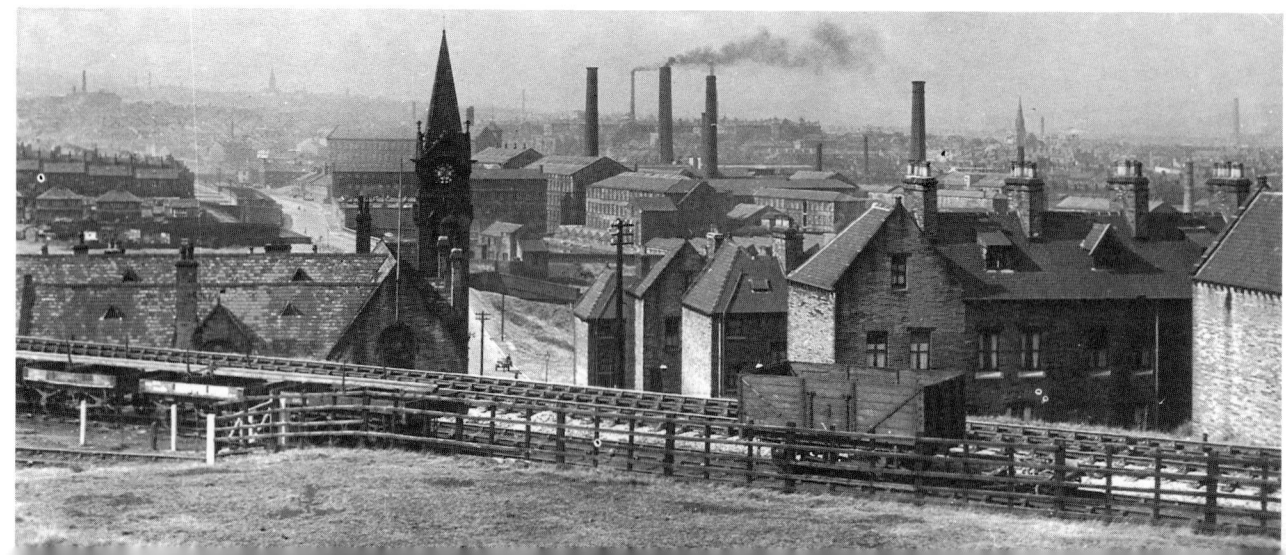

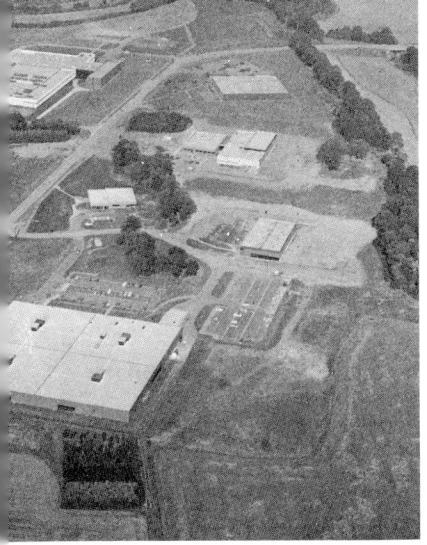

*Kirktown Campus, a science park in Livingston, near Edinburgh in Scotland.*

*This clean modern industrial site in Hendon, north London, causes no pollution problems for nearby housing estates.*

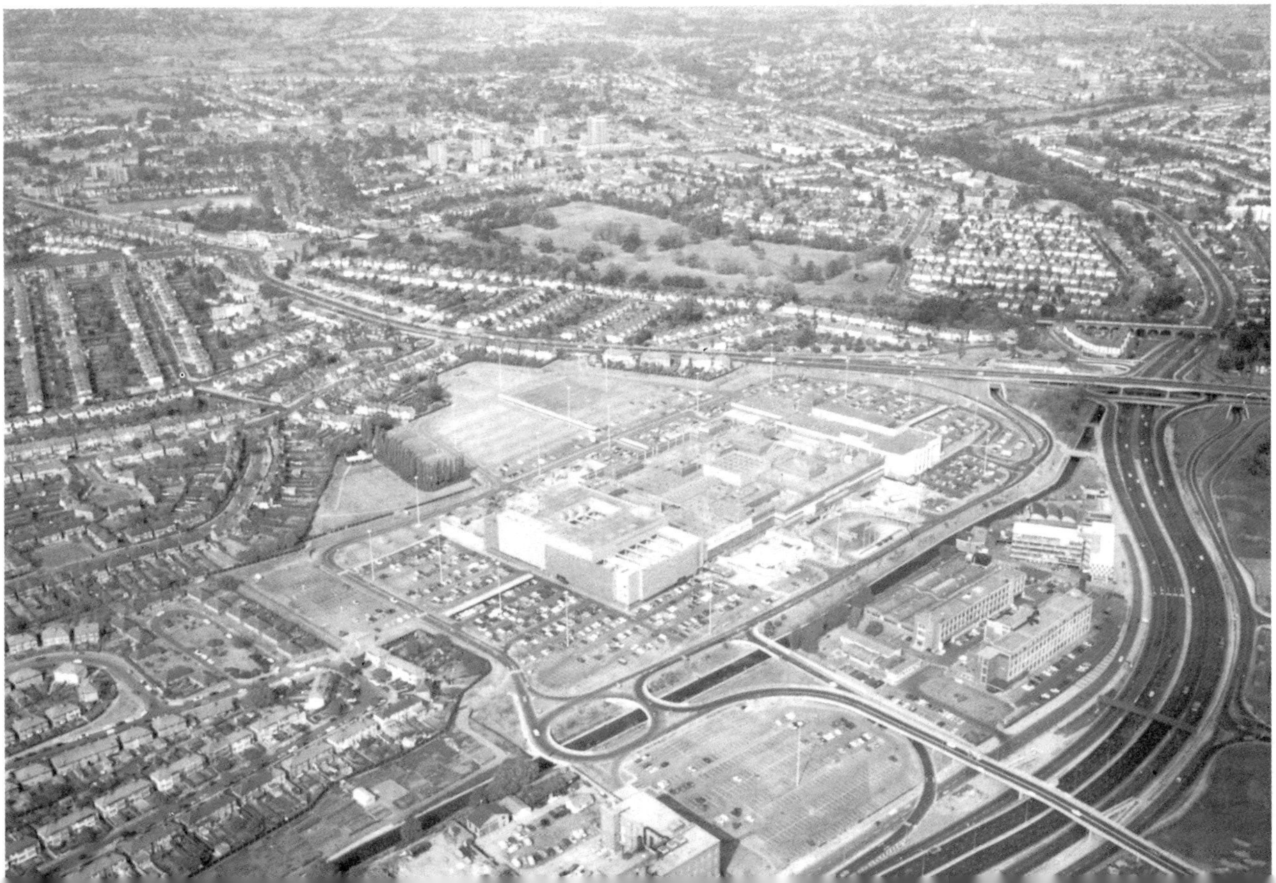

A technopolis is made up of hi-tech firms, universities, research centres and some housing. It is built near a 'mother city' where workers can live, and close to an airport, motorway or railway link. In Japan there are plans for twenty-seven technopolises. They are being built in less-developed regions, such as the southern island of Kyushu and in northern Honshu. They are designed to revive the regions and relieve overcrowding in the older industrial cities of Tokyo, Osaka and Nagoya.

Hi-tech firms are also choosing countryside sites in Britain and the United States, particularly those areas which are near towns and cities where workers can live in pleasant surroundings. The route of the M4, between London and Bristol, and 'Silicon Glen', between Edinburgh and Glasgow, are expanding hi-tech regions. In the United States, the area on the south side of San Francisco Bay is called Silicon Valley, because of the high concentration of electronics firms in the region.

# Shopping

In the last forty years, there has been an enormous increase in the number of people who own cars and, as a result, shopping habits have changed. City centres have become congested with traffic and consequently large stores in central business districts have lost some of their customers. Some councils are trying to attract people back to the city centres by improving public transport services, pulling down old buildings and opening new shopping malls.

In Newcastle, part of the run-down central area has been demolished and a large indoor mall, called Eldon Square, has been created. The mall has two levels and is visited by about 100,000 people each day. There is a bus station at ground level and an underground 'Metro' station nearby which links Eldon Square by rail with the built-up areas along both banks of the River Tyne.

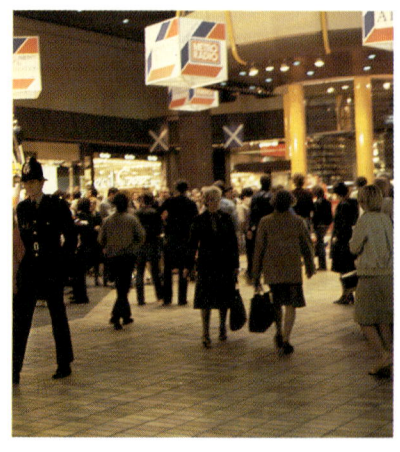

*The interior of the shopping mall at Eldon Square, in Newcastle, north-east England.*

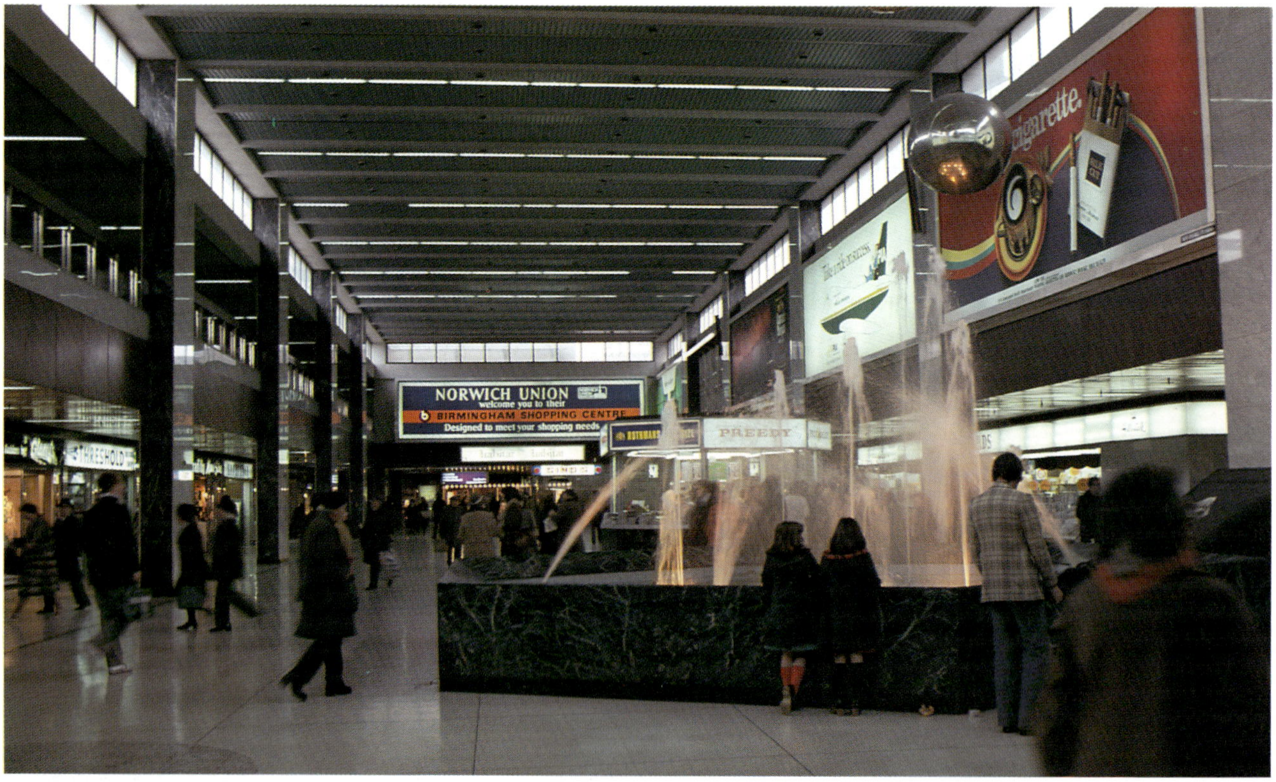

*The Bull Ring shopping centre in Birmingham, a typical covered mall complex.*

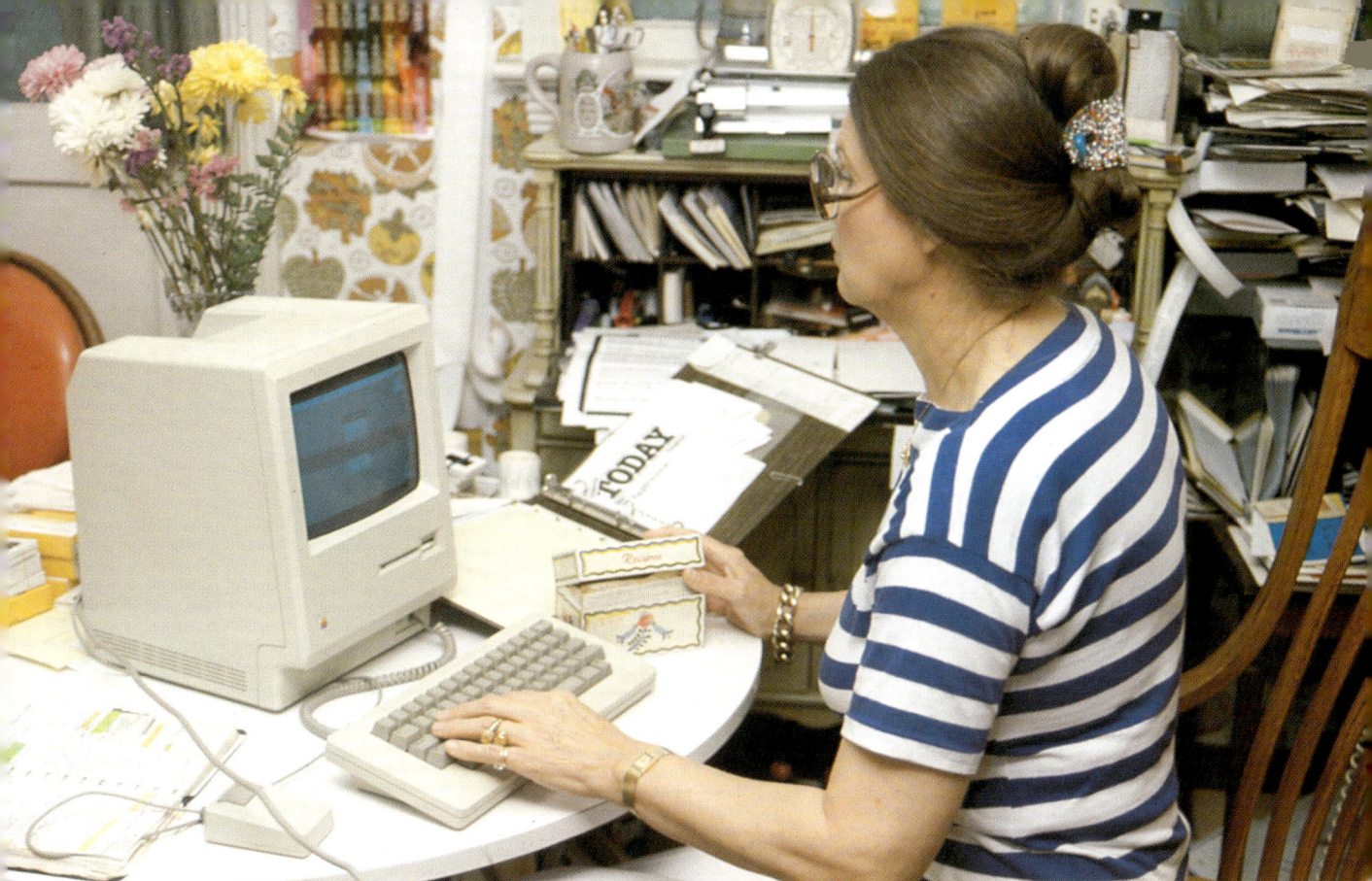

*Shopping from home by personal computer will save both time and effort.*

To meet the needs of people who like to shop by car, large shopping malls have also been developed on the outskirts of built-up areas. These 'green field' sites are placed close to main roads and have plenty of parking space. In the future, larger and more luxurious malls are likely to be found outside cities. Already there are malls whose temperature is carefully controlled and which contain ice-skating rinks, gardens, lakes and waterfalls. People visit these malls for entertainment as well as to shop.

Shopping in the future may also be done from the home, especially for everyday goods such as food and clothing. In an experiment being conducted in Nottingham, some homes have been linked to the city's stores by means of personal computers. Shopping lists entered on these computers are received by the stores and the ordered goods are delivered the next day. Payment from the customer's bank account is also made by computer.

# Leisure

The changing ways in which we spend our leisure time are bringing about new developments in our cities and the surrounding countryside. We are gradually spending less time at work and therefore we have more time for holidays and other leisure activities. People are increasingly using their free time to take part in leisure activities, especially outdoor and indoor games. As a result, many towns and cities are building large sports centres, equipped with facilities for all sorts of sports and leisure pursuits. In the future, these centres will become larger and may well include such things as artificial lakes, ski slopes and ice-skating rinks.

The popularity of museums, art galleries, theatres and concert halls, has led to new cultural centres being opened. In Paris, for example, the Pompidou Centre, with its art museum, library and other attractions, has proved very popular.

*The fascinating design of the Pompidou Centre in Paris (below) has aroused fierce debate. The most noticeable of its unusual features are the escalators, which are placed on the outside of the building.*

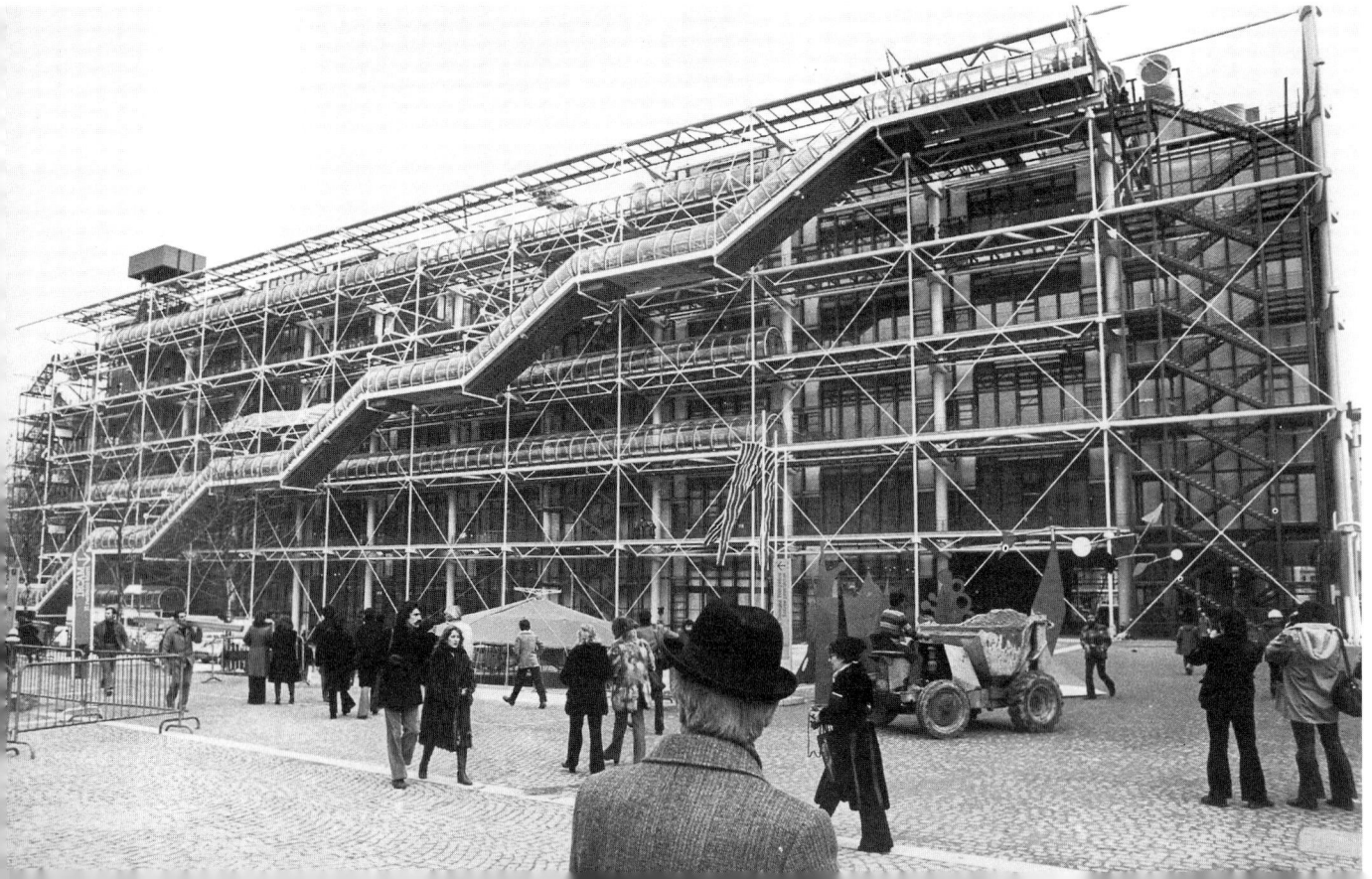

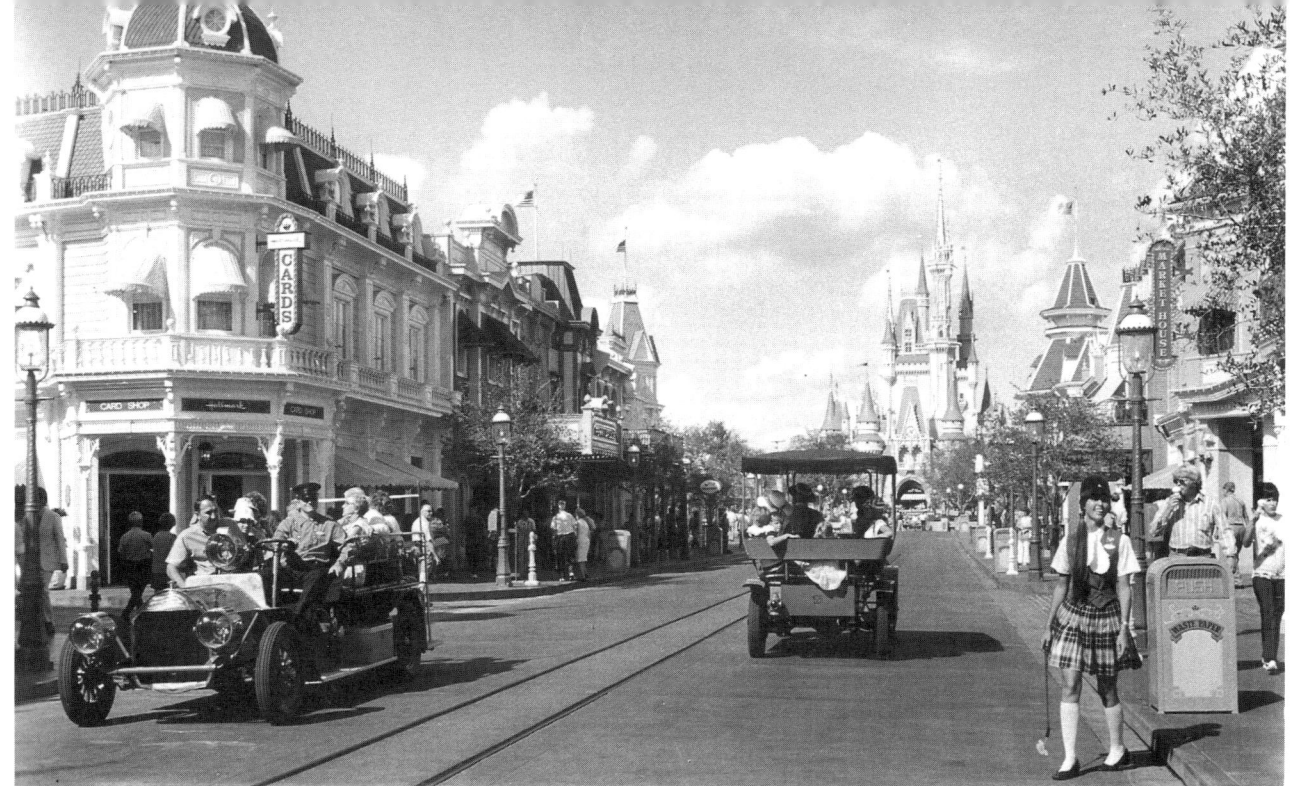

*The imaginative exhibits of Disneyworld in Florida, which attract hundreds of thousands of visitors each year.*

As their living standards rise, people generally spend more time and money on leisure activities. They are also able to travel longer distances to enjoy them. To meet this demand, 'theme parks' are being built in countryside areas which can be easily reached by car. The first theme park was built thirty years ago by Walt Disney on the outskirts of Los Angeles. It was called Disneyland and proved so popular that a similar park, Disneyworld, was built on the other side of the United States near Orlando in Florida.

In Britain there are six small theme parks and more are planned for the future. At Corby in Northamptonshire, a theme park to be called Wonderworld is planned, based on the theme of Great Britain. It will be entirely under cover, with a glass building housing ten pavilions. Each pavilion will have a different theme such as 'Film Making' or 'Energy'. Sporting facilities are planned for an indoor stadium and an outdoor sports area. Seven hotels, a concert hall and a golf course have also been included in the design.

# *Chapter Five*
# Experiments in living

## Energy from the sun

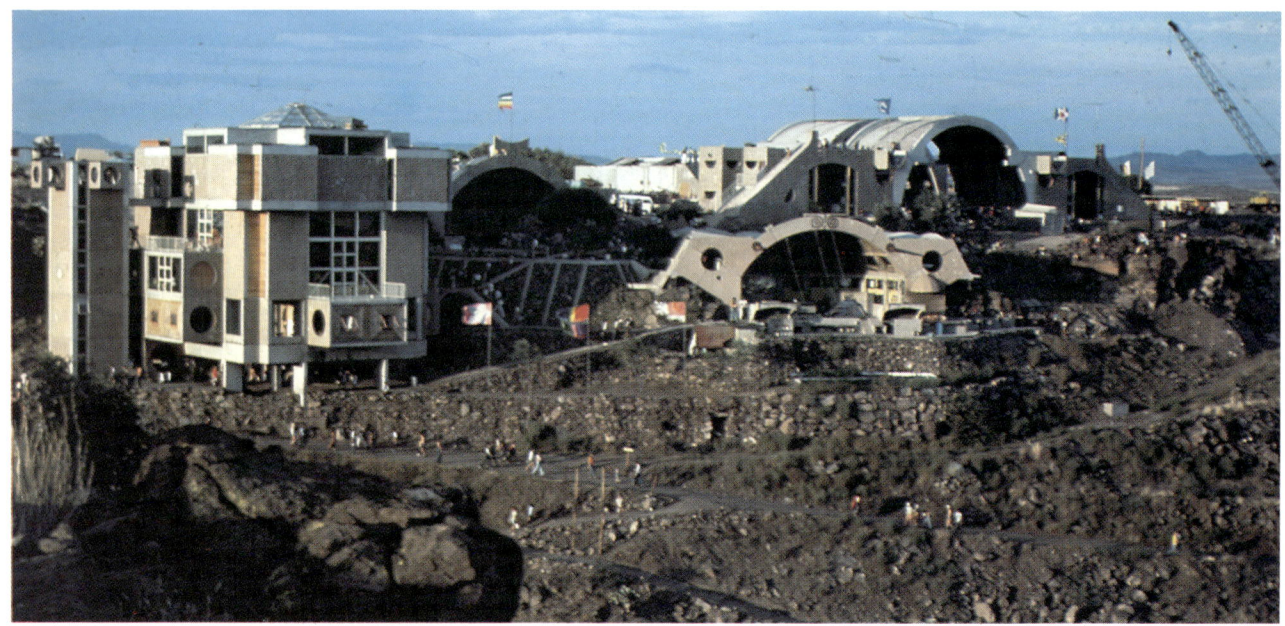

How would you like to live in a part of the world which is warm all through the year? Would you miss anything?

Many people in the USA have left the colder, northern parts of the country and moved to the south and south-west, to what they call the 'sun belt'. As the sun-belt towns and cities grow rapidly, people have begun to realize that the sun has more to offer than warm winter days. For example, the long hours of sunshine have made the sun belt a good place in which to develop a large tourist industry.

In the Arizona desert, about 113 kilometres (70 miles) north-west of Phoenix, a new town is being

*Construction work being carried out on the new town of Arcosanti near Phoenix, Arizona.*

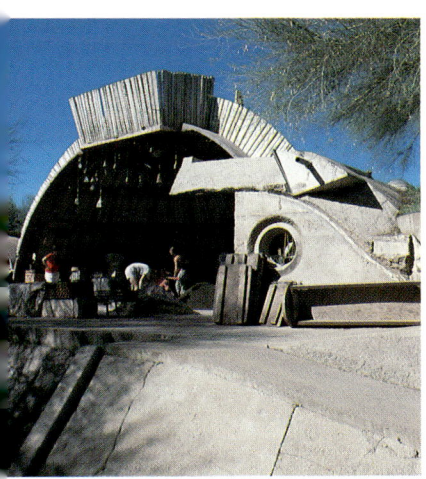

*One of the domes at Arcosanti that will provide an energy efficient home and work place.*

built which will provide an entirely new way of housing and supporting the town-dwellers of the future. The new town has been named Arcosanti. As you can see from the photographs, it has not yet been finished, but the building is going on steadily. Soon it is hoped that it will house 35,000 people, who will enjoy a very modern way of life in the middle of the Arizona desert. The life blood of this new city will be energy trapped from the sun.

The main buildings in the town are huge domes in which people will work and live. The domes are built into rock faces. These will enable the domes to stay cooler in the hot summer and warmer in winter. The heat for air conditioning, energy for cooking and lighting and power for workshops will all come from solar energy. It is planned to place huge polythene envelopes around the domes. These will provide an artificial environment in which food crops and plants can be grown. Moisture and temperature inside the envelopes will be controlled to provide ideal growing conditions.

Even in colder countries, like Britain, we are now learning how to use the energy of the sun to heat hot-water systems in homes and offices. In towns and cities in the future, we are likely to see greater efforts to use solar panels as a way of producing energy more efficiently and keeping bills down.

*Some homes in Britain are having solar panels installed to provide energy.*

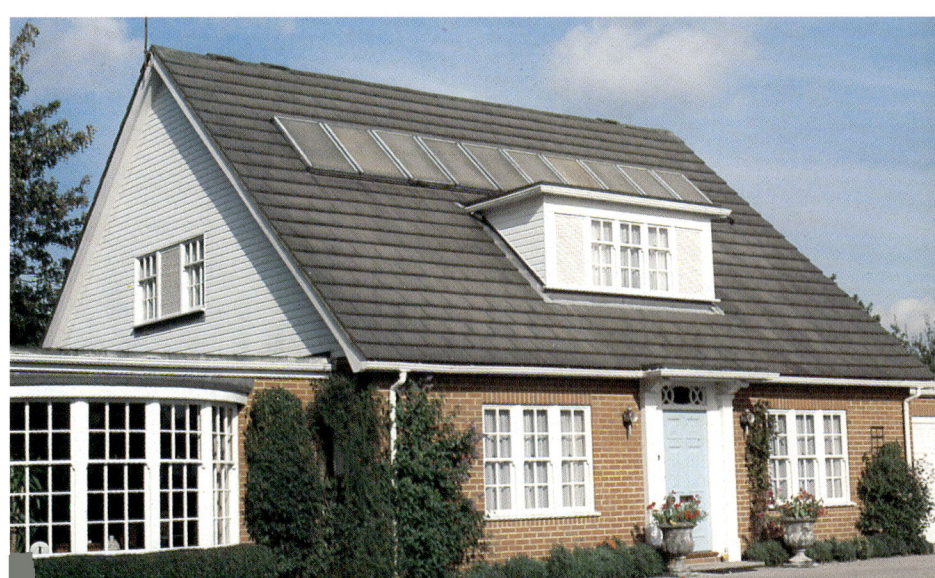

# Harnessing the sea

In Kuwait, and those countries which lie around the Red Sea and the Arabian Gulf, the desert climate makes supplies of fresh water very scarce. Traditionally, most people in the region were herders or traders, until huge reserves of oil were discovered. The wealth earned by the oil industry has brought about very rapid changes in these countries. New cities, factories and houses have been built. Workers from other countries have been attracted to Kuwait by the high wages offered in the oil industry and in other jobs. However, the modern factories and increased population have created a demand for larger quantities of fresh water than the natural supplies could meet.

The photograph shows a desalination plant, a place where salt water is processed to make drinking water. Sea water is heated until about half of it has evaporated. The water vapour that is produced passes to a cooler container, where it condenses into fresh water. Because so much fuel is needed to heat large quantities of sea water, this is a very expensive process. However, Kuwait and other oil-producing countries are so wealthy that they can afford to build desalination plants to obtain water for drinking, irrigating crops and for the factories. The new water supply has also enabled Kuwait to modernize some of its traditional industries, such as its fish- and shrimp-canning works.

As some countries turn to new processes of water production to meet the needs of their cities, other countries are working on new ideas for obtaining energy when oil supplies eventually run out or become too expensive. In Britain, there has been a great deal of research into the use of the energy of tides to make electricity. It has been suggested that the Severn estuary, the Wash and the Mersey

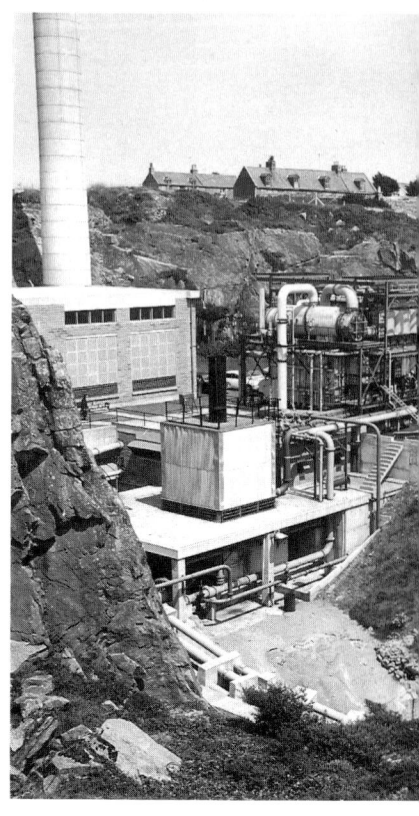

*The desalination plant at Jersey. Each day it processes over 1.5 million gallons of water.*

estuary are ideal sites for tidal barrages. As the tidal waters move in towards the land they can be captured behind the barrage. At low tide, the stored water is allowed to rush down to the low-tide level. As it does so, it turns dynamos which generate electricity. Once the barrage is built, the electricity is cheap to produce. Why do you think the people of Liverpool like this idea? Can you think of any disadvantages of tidal barrages?

*Two types of tidal barrage which could be used to tap energy to make electricity.*

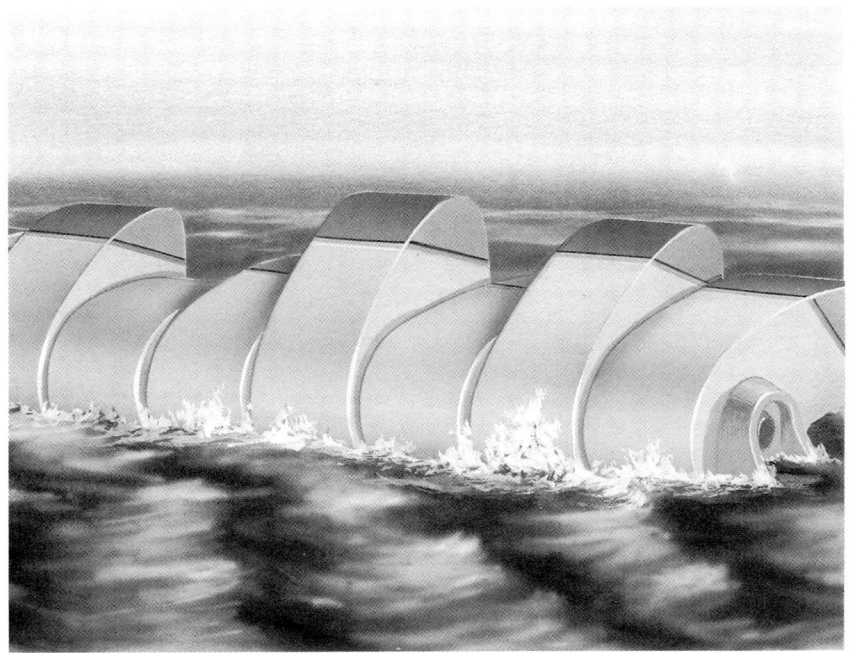

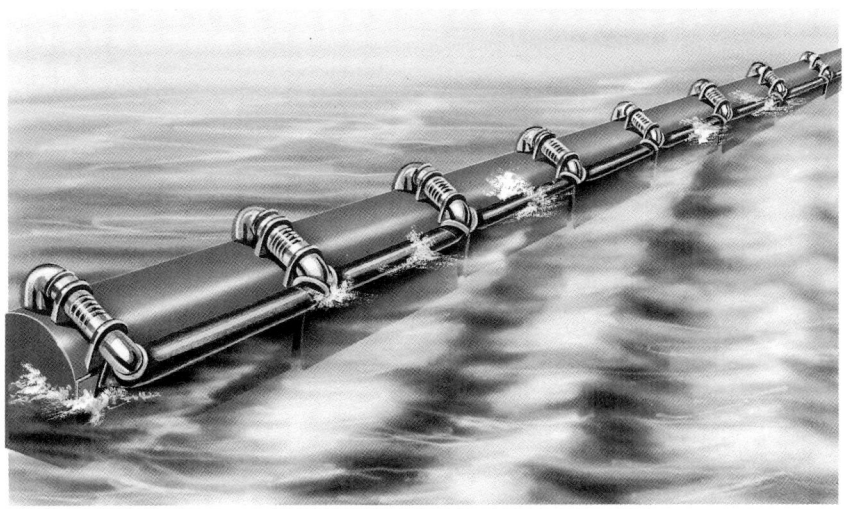

# Cities for a single group

When people retire, they no longer earn any wages. They have to live on their pensions and on the money they saved while they were working. Some elderly people live for many years after they have retired and so they have to be very careful about how they spend their money.

One thing over which they have no control is the amount of taxes and rates they have to pay. In Britain, people who own their own homes have to pay rates to their local councils, whether they have retired or not. If the pensions and the savings of retired people are high enough, they also have to pay income tax.

In the USA, people have to pay local taxes instead of rates. Some of the local taxes are used to pay for schools in their cities. Some old people argue that if they do not have young children they should not have to pay for schools. So, in a few places they have tried to do something about this problem.

*The comfortable homes of the residents of Sun City, USA.*

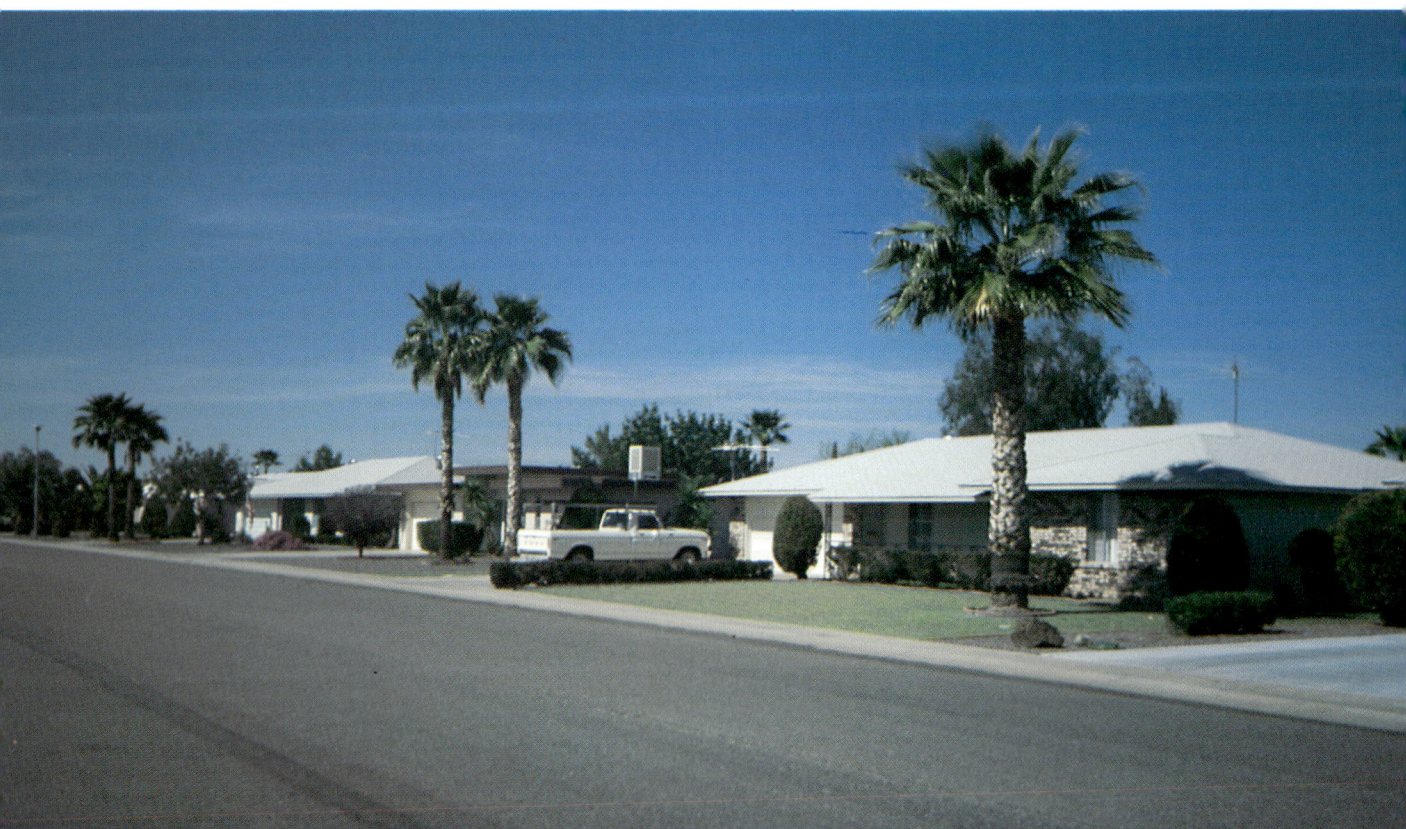

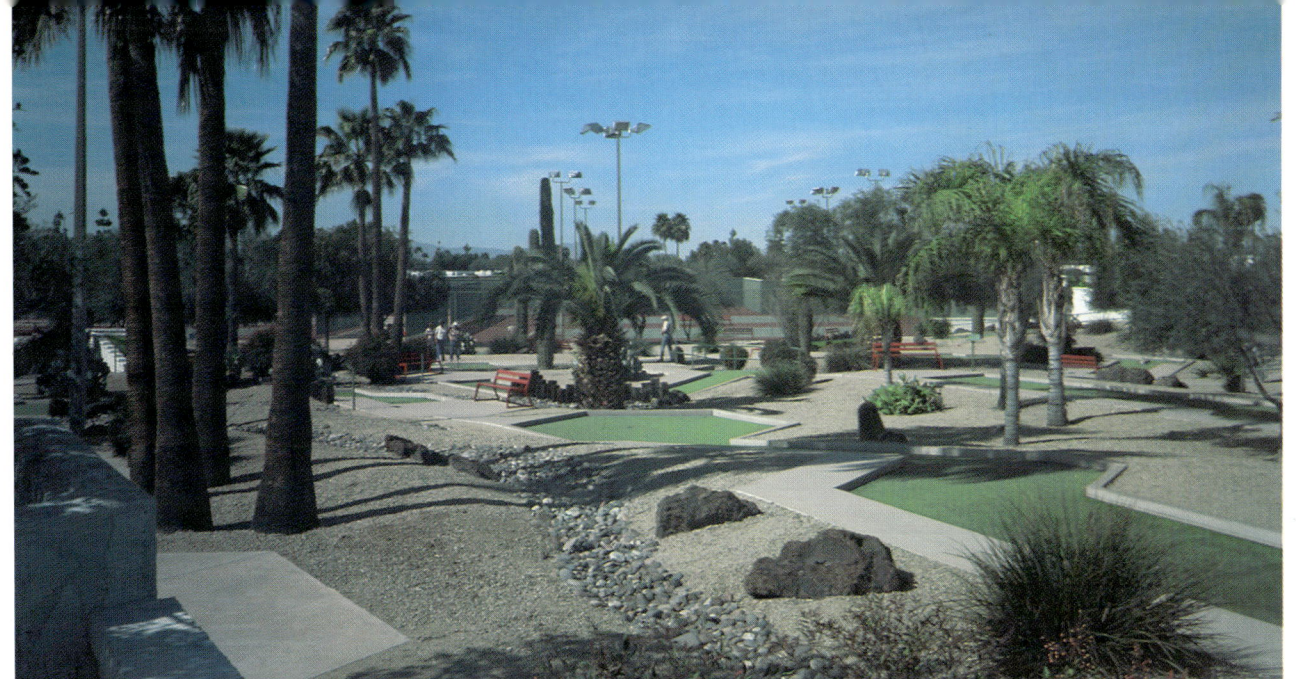

*The leisure facilities in Sun City are excellent, allowing its citizens every opportunity to enjoy their retirement.*

The photographs show Sun City in the USA. It is in the sun belt and has been built for a population of 30,000 people. It is a city built for the elderly, with comfortable homes, gardens, parks and attractive shopping centres. There are sports and leisure centres and concert halls, but there are no schools. In fact, families with young children are not wanted in Sun City. Grandchildren do not stay with their grandparents long enough for them to need to go to school. Since they have kept young children out of their town, the elderly people of Sun City do not have to pay taxes to support schools. It is a city for a single group – the elderly save their own money by keeping out the young.

Many people say that the Sun City folk are selfish. Others say it is a very unnatural place, because there are no young people living there. What do you think? Could you design a city for young people only? What taxes or rates would you save?

If some people grow more selfish, or if some groups become very powerful, they may decide to build cities in the future in which they themselves are safe and comfortable. The rest of the people might then be left to fend for themselves.

# Separate living

Today, all our towns and cities contain people of different origins. Some have moved to the city from other parts of the country. Others belong to different religious groups and follow different customs of dress and behaviour. People of different nationalities and colours live in the same city.

One hundred years ago, when millions of immigrants were flooding into the USA, the country was called 'the melting pot'. The Americans then took pride in the fact that people from all over the world migrated to their country and became English-speaking Americans. However, even at that time, people from different countries formed groups in different parts of the USA. Many Irish families settled in Boston, many Jewish and Italian families were found in parts of New York. This is true of the British in London today – Southall is known for its Indian families, Kilburn for the Irish, and Golders Green has many Jewish families.

However, in some parts of the world, people have been deliberately kept apart in the cities in which they live. The best example in Europe is Berlin. A wall has been built across the city to stop people who live in the east, in the communist German Democratic Republic, from moving west to the Federal Republic (West Germany) or vice versa.

In South Africa, the policy of apartheid is practised. Apartheid separates people solely according to their race or colour. The Black population is not allowed to live in White areas of the cities and, until recently, Blacks were forced to travel in separate sections of buses and trains. Even the beaches of the seaside resorts are allocated to single racial groups. This brutal and unpleasant system has allowed the White people of South Africa to have a very high standard of living and to control the

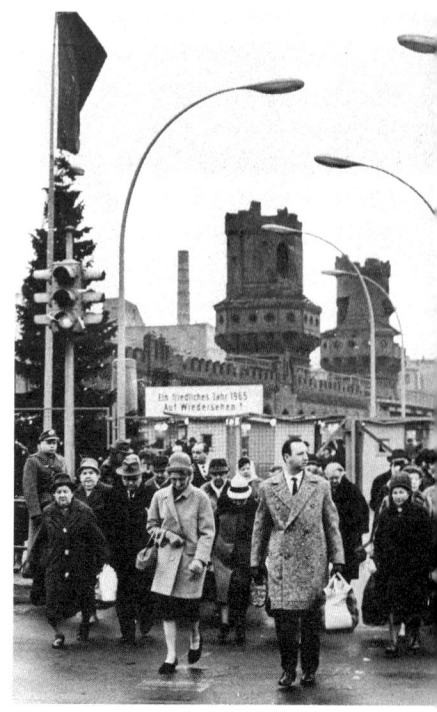

*Residents of West Berlin take one of the rare opportunities when the wall is opened to visit relatives in the east of the city.*

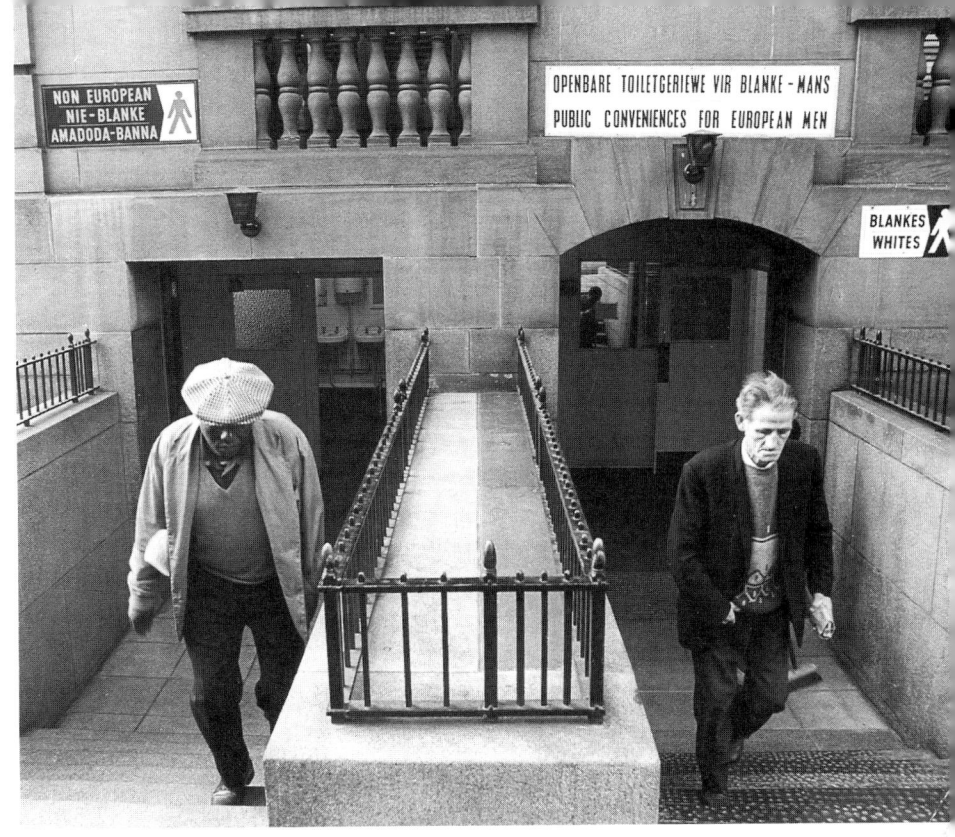

*Separate toilets for Blacks and Whites in Johannesburg, South Africa. Apartheid affects every area of life in the country, denying the Blacks the most basic rights.*

*The face of apartheid: this shanty town, Crossroads, was home to about 20,000 Blacks who were crammed together in conditions of extreme poverty.*

country even though they are greatly outnumbered by the Black population.

Both these examples of separate living force certain groups to live in particular ways. Why do most of the people of the world believe it better for the different groups in our towns and cities to mix? The future may see big changes in the cities of South Africa. Do you think that change may be less likely in Berlin?

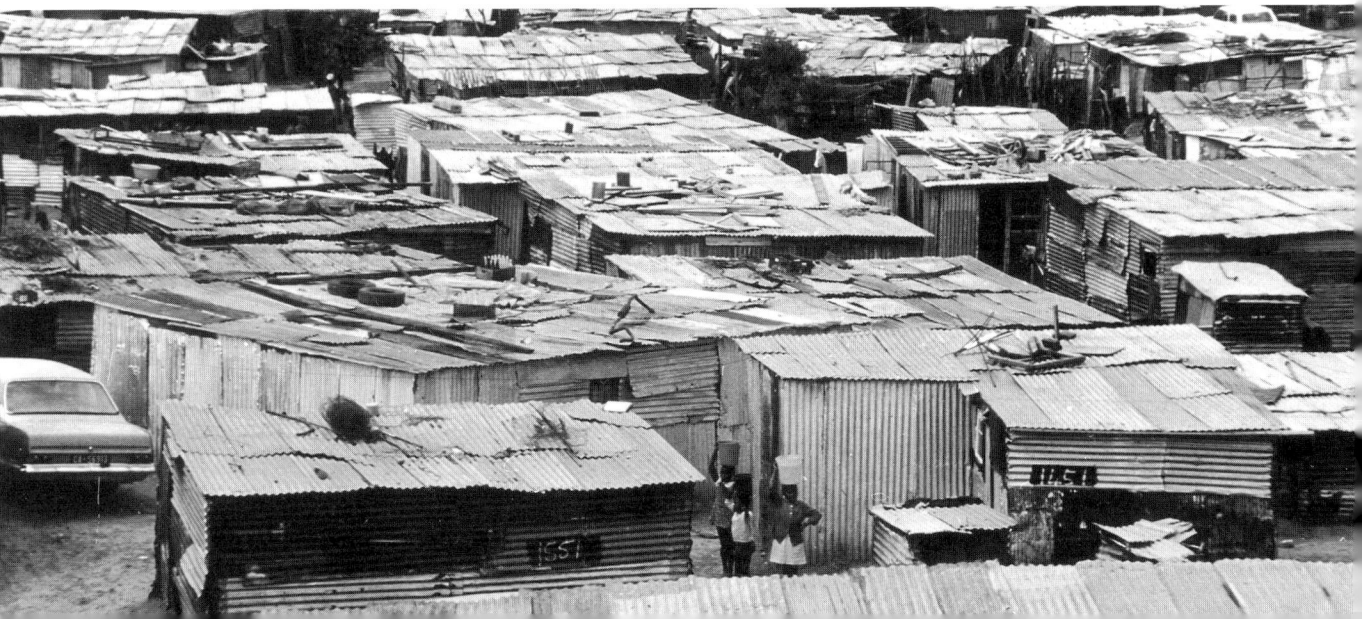

## Chapter Six
## Things to do

### The future in your town

What will cities look like in the twenty-first century? If we could return to a town or city we know in fifty or one hundred years time, we should still recognize some of the buildings and landmarks because they will have been preserved as places of interest or as historic buildings. Edinburgh will still have its Royal Mile, its castle and Princes Street Gardens, while landmarks in London will include the Tower, St. Paul's Cathedral and Piccadilly Circus. The greatest changes are likely to be in the shops and the appearance of buildings and houses, as well as travel and leisure facilities.

What will your town or part of the city look like in the future? Think about which parts of your town

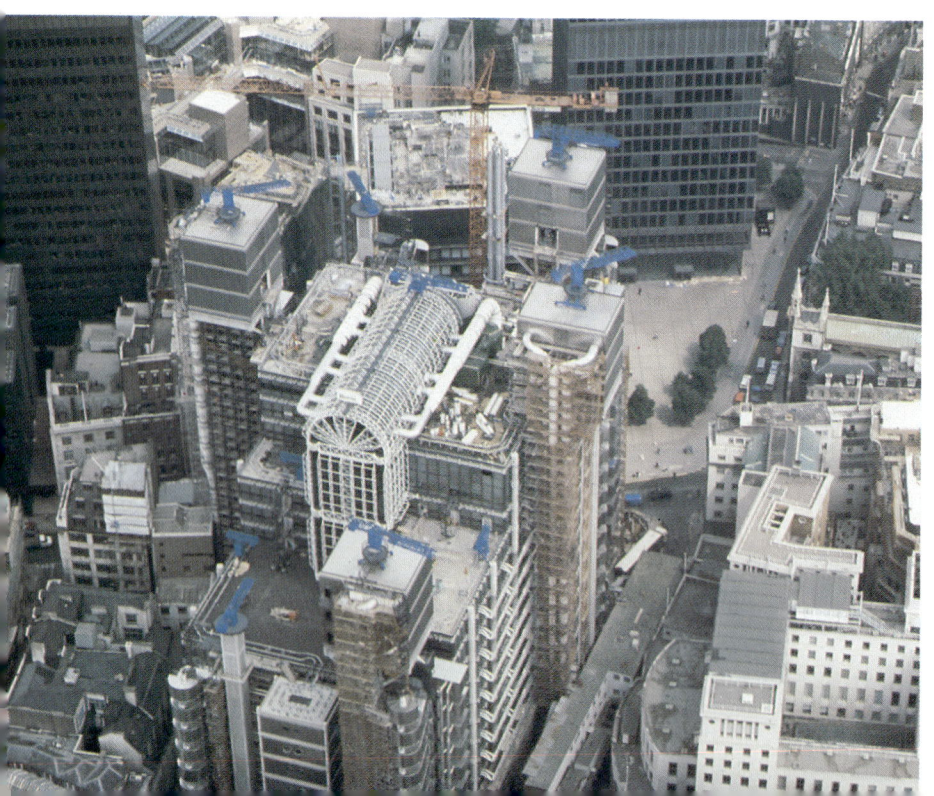

*The shape of things to come? The unusual design of the new Lloyds building in London.*

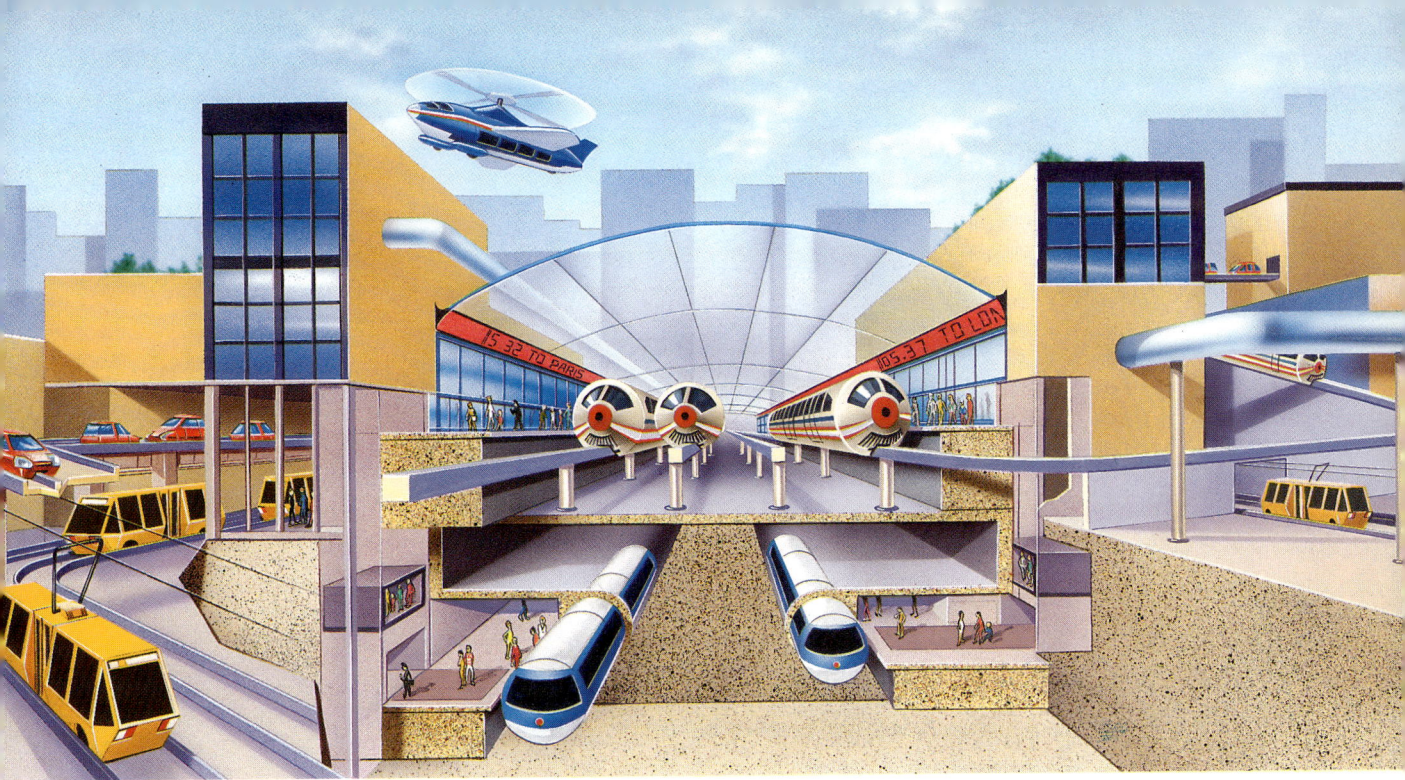

*Some of the transport systems that may be found in the city of the future.*

should be preserved and which pulled down or altered. For example, you might decide that the town hall will be kept, but that the roads around it will be replaced with gardens, trees and lakes. Draw sketches of different parts of your town as you imagine they will look.

Private cars and other vehicles which congest our city roads at present may be replaced by a rapid transit system, with automatic vehicles running on special tracks between the suburbs and city centre. Here is an artist's impression of these vehicles arriving at a terminus. Make sketches of a rapid transit system passing through the centre of your city or along a main road near your home. Make models of the cars, trains and helicopters.

Write, or record on tape, a diary of one day in your life in the year 2050. Do you think you would go to school or instead have lessons from a screen linked by computer to a learning centre? Think about how you would do your shopping, how you would spend your spare time and the kind of things you would eat.

# Homes and leisure in the future

### Future homes

Imagine you are a passenger in a time-ship which takes you forward into the middle of the twenty-first century. What kinds of buildings will people be living in in the year 2050? Will they be prefabricated homes fitted together like pieces of Lego, or will they be dome-shaped with plastic and glass panels? What other shapes might be used? How will they be heated? Make a sketch or model of what a home of the future will look like.

Today's TV sets will be antiques by the year 2050, but people are still likely to want to be entertained at home. Perhaps you can think of new ways to watch concerts, games and other events in the home and of some unusual features that will mark the home of the future.

**Below:** *An experimental solar-panelled home in Albuquerque, New Mexico.*

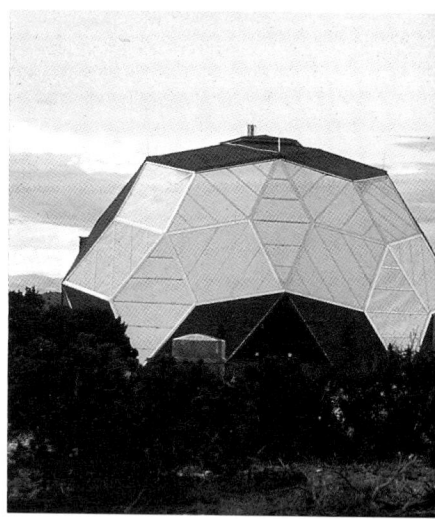

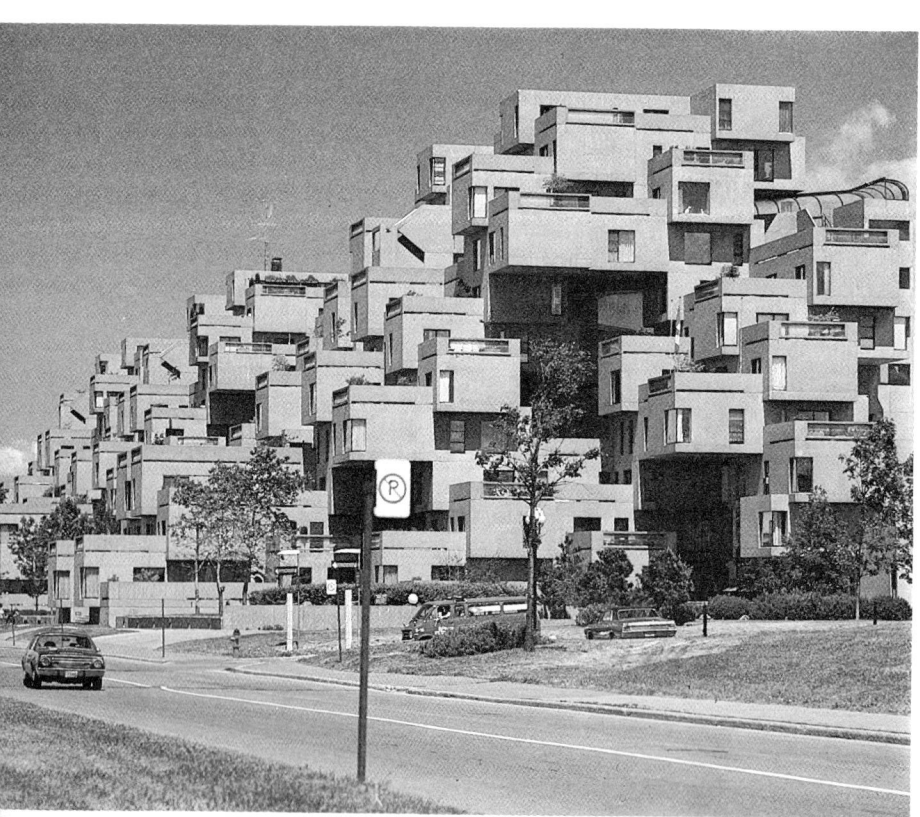

**Left:** *These homes in Montreal, Canada, have been fitted together in blocks to produce the unusual overall shape of the building.*

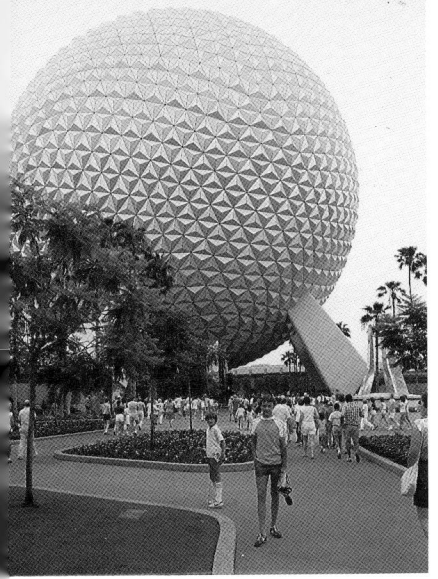

*Spaceship Earth, one of the features of the Epcot Centre in Florida.*

*The Gate of the Golden Sun, Peking, one of the world's great landmarks reproduced at the Epcot Centre's Futureworld.*

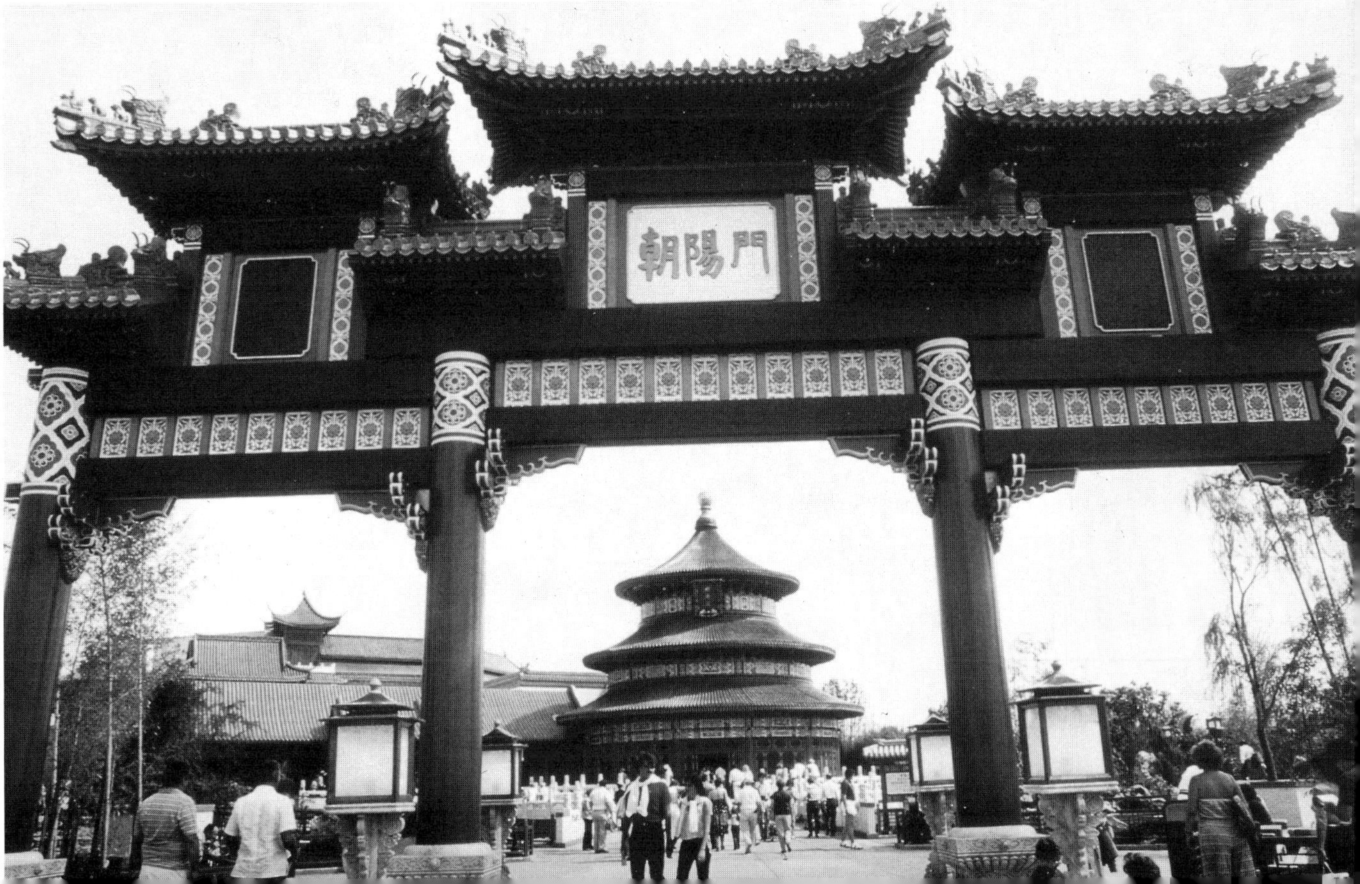

## A theme park

In Florida, the Walt Disney Organization has built a new theme park near Disneyworld, which is called the Epcot Centre. One part of the park is the World Showcase. Here nine countries have built exhibitions, shops and other attractions to show visitors what their countries are like. The remainder of the Epcot Centre is called Futureworld and visitors travel by monorail from one exhibition building to another.

In Britain, the theme park at Alton Towers in Staffordshire offers visitors exciting rides like the corkscrew roller-coaster.

Imagine you are asked to help design a theme park on a site near your town. Draw a plan of the park and write a guide for visitors describing the attractions they can visit in the park. Tape a commentary which visitors can use when they visit one of the attractions in the park.

# Glossary

**Apartheid** The policy of racial separation which has been practised in the Republic of South Africa since 1948.

**Commuter** A person who travels a considerable distance daily to work. Commuters travel from the country and suburbs to work in the city.

**Conurbation** A large urban area formed by the growing together of a number of towns.

**Desalination** The removal of salt from seawater so that it can be used as drinking water, for irrigation and in factories and homes.

**Developing World** The poorer underdeveloped countries which make up most of Africa, Asia, Central and South America.

**Facilities** Items provided in the house such as hot and cold water, a bathroom, cloakroom and central heating.

**Heliport** An airport designed and used by helicopters.

**Hi-tech industries** Firms making silicon chips, micro-circuits and specialized parts used in computers and other electronic equipment.

**Inner city** An area near the centre of a city which is densely populated and contains old, poor-quality housing. It is characterized by poverty and the loss of jobs and people.

**Megalopolis** A cluster of towns and cities which are linked to one another to form a large urban region.

**Redevelopment** The modernization of old parts of the city by the removal of old housing and factories, and replacement by new roads and modern housing and offices.

**Shopping mall** A planned shopping centre with a number of stores under one roof which share the same car park.

46

| | |
|---|---|
| *Solar energy* | Energy obtained from the sun. |
| *Suburbs* | Outer parts of a city which consist mainly of houses. |
| *Technopolis* | A development of hi-tech firms with research centres and other facilities close to a 'mother' city. |
| *Theme park* | A recreational centre containing a variety of activities based on a central idea. The activities are set in a large open space or park, often with lakes, hotels and other amenities. |
| *Traffic congestion* | The clogging of city streets by the large number of vehicles which use them. |
| *Water vapour* | Water which has been turned into a gas. |

# Books to Read

*Wayland Atlas of the World* (Wayland, 1985)
*The Red Sea and Persian Gulf*, ed. Pat Hargreaves (Wayland, 1982)
*How Towns Grow and Change*, Bolwell and Lines (Wayland, 1985)
*City Life* series (Macdonald)
*Living in the Future*, Mark Lambert (Wayland, 1985)
*Living in Famous Cities* series (Wayland)

## Picture Acknowledgements

Hutchison 6, 7 (bottom), 9 (top), 15 (bottom), 16 (both), 19, 25, 26 (top); Photri 7 (top), 11, 31, 45 (top); Topham 8, 14, 15 (top), 17, 18 (top), 23 (bottom), 28, 30 (bottom), 33, 44 (bottom, right); Aerofilms 10 (bottom), 12, 24 (top), 29 (bottom); Shell 10 (top); Laurie Bolwell 34, 35; Cliff Lines 13, 38, 39; Bruce Coleman 18 (bottom), 26 (bottom), 27; Milton Keynes Development Corporation 20, 21; Livingston Development Corporation 29 (top); Eldon Associates 30 (top); Lloyds of London 42; Camerapress 32, 36, 40, 41 (both), 45; Picturepoint 44 (bottom, left); Artwork by Malcolm Walker 10, 22, 24; Maltings Partnership 37, 43.

# Index